Small Animal Parasites: Biology and Control

Guest Editors

DAVID S. LINDSAY, PhD
ANNE M. ZAJAC, DVM, PhD

VETERINARY CLINICS OF NORTH AMERICA: SMALL ANIMAL PRACTICE

www.vetsmall.theclinics.com

November 2009 • Volume 39 • Number 6

SAUNDERS an imprint of ELSEVIER, Inc.

W.B. SAUNDERS COMPANY
A Division of Elsevier Inc.

1600 John F. Kennedy Blvd. • Suite 1800 • Philadelphia, PA 19103-2899

http://www.vetsmall.theclinics.com

VETERINARY CLINICS OF NORTH AMERICA: SMALL ANIMAL PRACTICE Volume 39, Number 6
November 2009 ISSN 0195-5616, ISBN-13: 978-1-4377-1287-2, ISBN-10: 1-4377-1287-8

Editor: John Vassallo; j.vassallo@elsevier.com
Developmental Editor: Theresa Collier

Veterinary Clinics of North America: Small Animal Practice (ISSN 0195-5616) is published bimonthly (For Post Office use only: volume 39 issue 6 of 6) by Elsevier Inc., 360 Park Avenue South, New York, NY 10010-1710. Months of issue are January, March, May, July, September, and November. Application to mail at periodicals postage rates is pending at New York, NY and at additional mailing offices. Subscription prices are $245.00 per year (domestic individuals), $388.00 per year (domestic institutions), $122.00 per year (domestic students/residents), $324.00 per year (Canadian individuals), $477.00 per year (Canadian institutions), $360.00 per year (international individuals), $477.00 per year (international institutions), and $177.00 per year (international and Canadian students/residents). To receive student/resident rate, orders must be accompanied by name of affiliated institution, date of term, and the *signature* of program/residency coordinator on institution letterhead. Orders will be billed at individual rate until proof of status is received. Foreign air speed delivery is included in all *Clinics* subscription prices. All prices are subject to change without notice. **POSTMASTER:** Send address changes to *Veterinary Clinics of North America: Small Animal Practice*, Elsevier Health Sciences Division, Subscription Customer Service, 3251 Riverport Lane, Maryland Heights, MO 63043. Customer Service (orders, claims, online, change of address): Elsevier Periodicals Customer Service, Elsevier Health Sciences Division Subscription Customer Service 3251 Riverport Lane Maryland Heights, MO 63043. Tel: 1-800-654-2452 (U.S. and Canada); 314-447-8871 (outside U.S. and Canada). Fax: 314-447-8029. E-mail: journalscustomerservice-usa@elsevier.com (for print support); journalsonlinesupport-usa@elsevier.com (for online support).

Reprints. For copies of 100 or more of articles in this publication, please contact the Commercial Reprints Department, Elsevier Inc., 360 Park Avenue South, New York, NY 10010-1710. Tel.: 212-633-3812; Fax: 212-462-1935; E-mail: reprints@elsevier.com.

Veterinary Clinics of North America: Small Animal Practice is also published in Japanese by Inter Zoo Publishing Co., Ltd., Aoyama Crystal-Bldg 5F, 3-5-12 Kitaaoyama, Minato-ku, Tokyo 107-0061, Japan.

Veterinary Clinics of North America: Small Animal Practice is covered in *Current Contents/Agriculture, Biology and Environmental Sciences, Science Citation Index, ASCA, MEDLINE/PubMed (Index Medicus), Excerpta Medica, and BIOSIS.*

Printed in the United States of America.

Contributors

GUEST EDITORS

DAVID S. LINDSAY, PhD
Center for Molecular Medicine and Infectious Diseases, Department of Biological
Sciences and Pathobiology, Virginia—Maryland Regional College of Veterinary Medicine,
Virginia Polytechnic Institute and State University, Blacksburg, Virginia

ANNE M. ZAJAC, DVM, PhD
Center for Molecular Medicine and Infectious Diseases, Department of Biological
Sciences and Pathobiology, Virginia—Maryland Regional College of Veterinary Medicine,
Virginia Polytechnic Institute and State University, Blacksburg, Virginia

AUTHORS

ROBERT G. ARTHER, PhD
Manager of Parasitology and Entomology, Bayer HealthCare, Animal Health, Shawnee,
Kansas

MARJORY ARTZER, DVM
Graduate Student of Parasitology, Department of Diagnostic Medicine and Pathobiology,
College of Veterinary Medicine, Kansas State University, Manhattan, Kansas

CLARKE ATKINS, DVM
Diplomate, American College of Veterinary Internal Medicine; Professor of Medicine and
Cardiology, Department of Microbiology and Immunology, College of Veterinary Medicine,
Cornell University, Ithaca, New York

STEPHEN C. BARR, BVSc, MVS, PhD
Diplomate, American College of Veterinary Internal Medicine; Professor, Department
of Clinical Sciences, College of Veterinary Medicine, Cornell University, Ithaca, New York

BYRON L. BLAGBURN, BS, MS, PhD
Department of Pathobiology, College of Veterinary Medicine, Auburn University, Auburn,
Alabama

DWIGHT D. BOWMAN, MS, PhD
Professor of Parasitology, Department of Microbiology and Immunology, College
of Veterinary Medicine, Cornell University, Ithaca, New York

GARY CONBOY, DVM, PhD
Associate Professor, Department of Pathology and Microbiology, Atlantic Veterinary
College-UPEI, Charlottetown, PEI, Canada

MICHAEL W. DRYDEN, DVM, MS, PhD
Department of Diagnostic Medicine/Pathology, College of Veterinary Medicine, Kansas
State University, Manhattan, Kansas

J.P. DUBEY, MVSc, PhD
Senior Scientist, United States Department of Agriculture, Agricultural Research Service, Animal and Natural Resources Institute, Beltsville Agricultural Research Center, Beltsville, Maryland

CHRISTIAN EPE, Dr Med Vet
Diplomate, European Veterinary Parasitology College; Head of Companion Animal Parasiticides Research Group, Novartis Centre de Recherche Santè Animale SA, Switzerland

PATRICIA J. HOLMAN, PhD
Research Associate Professor, Department of Veterinary Pathobiology, College of Veterinary Medicine, Texas A&M University, College Station, Texas

MICHAEL R. LAPPIN, DVM, PhD
Diplomate, American College of Veterinary Internal Medicine; Professor, Department of Clinical Sciences, College of Veterinary Medicine, Colorado State University, Fort Collins, Colorado

DAVID S. LINDSAY, PhD
Professor, Department of Biomedical Sciences and Pathobiology, Virginia-Maryland Regional College of Veterinary Medicine, Blacksburg, Virginia

PATRICIA A. PAYNE, DVM, PhD
Assistant Professor, Department of Diagnostic Medicine and Pathobiology, College of Veterinary Medicine, Kansas State University, Manhattan, Kansas

CHRISTINE A. PETERSEN, DVM, PhD
Assistant Professor, Department of Veterinary Pathology, Iowa State University, Ames, Iowa

KAREN F. SNOWDEN, DVM, PhD
Associate Professor, Department of Veterinary Pathobiology, College of Veterinary Medicine, Texas A&M University, College Station, Texas

Contents

eating infected vectors, causing the release of the organisms into the mouth of the host. Most dogs are diagnosed during the chronic stage of the disease, which is typified by dilated cardiomyopathy and malignant ventricular-based arrhythmias. This article reviews the etiology, epidemiology, pathogenesis, diagnosis, and available therapy for Chagas' disease in dogs.

Christine A. Petersen and Stephen C. Barr

Canine leishmaniasis is a fatal zoonotic visceralizing disease usually associated with tropical areas. The etiologic agent is an obligate intracellular protozoan, *Leishmania infantum*. In 1999, an outbreak of a canine leishmaniasis was reported in a Foxhound kennel in New York, and since that report, several other outbreaks have occurred across the United States in additional Foxhound kennels. Because of the high mortality and transmissibility associated with these outbreaks, it is essential that clinicians be aware of this disease to permit its rapid recognition and institution of control measures. Cases with a travel history may suggest imported disease; these are mainly observed from Southern Europe (eg, south of France, Spain, and Italy). Breeds from these and other endemic areas may be at higher risk of infection with *Leishmania* because of vertical transmission. The purpose of this report is to discuss the clinical signs, epidemiology, diagnosis, control, and treatment of canine leishmaniasis with focus on the aspects of this disease within North America.

Gary Conboy

Cestodes are hermaphroditic flatworms (tapeworms) consisting of a scolex, neck region, and repeating segments. Cestodes lack a mouth, intestine, and body cavity. Life cycles are indirect, with the definitive host acquiring the adult form of the tapeworm by the ingestion of the larval metacestode stage contained in an intermediate host. This article describes the cyclophyllidean and pseudophyllidean groups of infective cestodes. Tapeworm infection is common in dogs and cats in North America. Infection rarely results in clinical disease, but animals infected with tapeworms should be treated. Echinococcosis, though infrequently diagnosed, remains a serious human health threat in North America.

Christian Epe

A variety of nematodes occur in dogs and cats. Several nematode species inhabit the small and large intestines. Important species that live in the small intestine are roundworms of the genus *Toxocara* (*T canis, T cati*) and *Toxascaris* (ie, *T leonina*), and hookworms of the genus *Ancylostoma* (*A caninum, A braziliense, A tubaeforme*) or *Uncinaria* (*U stenocephala*). Parasites of the large intestine are nematodes of the genus *Trichuris* (ie, whipworms, *T vulpis*). After a comprehensive description of their life cycle and biology, which are indispensable for understanding and justifying their control, current recommendations for nematode control are presented and discussed thereafter.

Helminth parasite infection of the canine and feline respiratory tract is uncommon in North America. This article reviews the prevalence, etiology, diagnosis, and treatment of helminth parasite infections in dogs and cats. The diagnosis of parasitic infections caused by helminth parasites of the respiratory tract of cats and dogs is infrequent in most parts of North America. Several fecal examination methods used in the diagnosis of helminthic infections are discussed in this article.

This article is a review of the systematics, taxonomy, biology, prevention, control, and treatment of the canine heartworm, *Dirofilaria immitus*. This filarioid parasite remains one of the most important and dangerous diseases of the dog throughout the United States. The geographic range of the parasite is expanding, and in many parts of the country it has emerged as a threat to canine welfare only in the last 50 or so years. The article also discusses the pathophysiological mechanisms behind the disease induced, the means for diagnosing the disease, and the means of assessing the success of therapy. The treatment of potential complications of heartworm infection, such as post-adulticide thromboembolism, eosinophilic granulomatous pneumonitis, and caval syndrome, is also discussed.

Dogs and cats frequently encounter a diverse variety of mite and lice species, which may result in mild to severe consequences depending on husbandry conditions, the severity of the infestation, and the nature of the localized or systemic defense mechanisms mobilized by the host in response to the parasite. Some of these external parasites are obvious to detect, identify, and control, although others may offer a significant challenge to the practitioner. Traditional acaricide and insecticide formulations, including dips, sprays, powders, and shampoos, have been used to treat and control these infestations. Some of the more recently developed, low-volume, topically applied insecticides and systemically acting macrolide formulations, although not always labeled for specific claims, may offer safe, efficacious, and convenient alternatives. The practitioner may wish to consider these products when implementing treatment and control programs involving these pests.

Flea and tick infestations are common and elimination can be expensive and time consuming. Many advances in control of fleas can be directly linked to improved knowledge of the intricacies of flea host associations, reproduction, and survival in the premises. Understanding tick biology and ecology is far more difficult than with fleas, because North America can have up to 9 different tick species infesting cats and dogs compared to 1 primary flea species. Effective tick control is more difficult to achieve than effective flea control, because of the abundance of potential alternative hosts in the tick life cycle. Many effective host-targeted tick control agents exist, several of which also possess activity against adult or immature fleas and other parasites.

THE CLINICS ARE NOW AVAILABLE ONLINE!

Access your subscription at:
www.theclinics.com

Preface

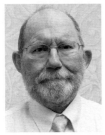 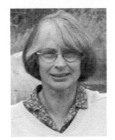

David S. Lindsay, PhD   Anne M. Zajac, DVM, PhD
Guest Editors

We readily accepted the task of editing this book when approached by the editorial staff at Elsevier. We were grateful for the opportunity to work with our colleagues from the American Association of Veterinary Parasitologists and other experts from veterinary colleges and industry. We have asked our authors to compose useful reviews of the important parasites of dogs and cats. They have complied and produced reviews that emphasize the biology, diagnosis, and treatment of parasites found in small animals. New material in these areas is presented to keep the clinician current, while other basic material is provided as a current review. Parasites of emerging importance, such as *Tritrichomonas fetus*, *Trypanosoma cruzi,* and *Leishmania infantum*, are discussed with recent advances in our knowledge presented. Common and familiar parasites (fleas, heartworms, *Giardia* spp) of dogs and cats are discussed in detail with new ideas or options for treatment and control presented. We thank Elsevier for encouraging the use of color pictures in the reviews. These color photographs will enhance the use of the information presented in the text. We believe that this issue of *Veterinary Clinics of North America: Small Animal Practice* will be helpful to the practicing veterinarian and will serve as a source of information upon which to base practical prevention and treatment programs.

David S. Lindsay, PhD
Center for Molecular Medicine and Infectious Diseases
Department of Biological Sciences and Pathobiology
Virginia—Maryland Regional College of Veterinary Medicine
Virginia Polytechnic Institute and State University
Blacksburg, VA 24061, USA

Vet Clin Small Anim 39 (2009) xi–xii
doi:10.1016/j.cvsm.2009.08.003   **vetsmall.theclinics.com**

Anne M. Zajac, DVM, PhD
Department of Biological Sciences and Pathobiology
Virginia—Maryland Regional College of Veterinary Medicine
Virginia Polytechnic Institute and State University
Blacksburg, VA 24061, USA

E-mail addresses:
lindsayd@vt.edu (D.S. Lindsay)
azajac@vt.edu (A.M. Zajac)

The Biology and Control of *Giardia* spp and *Tritrichomonas foetus*

Patricia A. Payne, DVM, PhD*, Marjory Artzer, DVM

KEYWORDS

- *Giardia* • *Tritrichomonas foetus* • Dog • Cat • Diarrhea

This article may seem an odd combination of protozoal parasites to some readers; however, these two protozoal parasites are similar in their origins and both are causative agents of diarrhea in dogs and cats.[1,2] *Giardia* spp and *Tritrichomonas foetus* are both flagellated Protisits and because of their close association with host mucus membranes, they are considered to be muscoflagellates. Both live, feed, and disrupt the intestinal tract of dogs and cats. *Giardia* spp causes diarrhea in both dogs and cats and although *Tritrichomonas foetus* has rarely been found in the diarrheic feces of dogs, it is now considered to be the cause of an emerging infectious diarrheal disease of cats.[1] The in-depth 2007 review article in *Science* highlights several similarities of these two parasites at the molecular level, including metabolic and genetic traits, and suggests that they are of sister lineages.[4] These two protozoal parasites are different, yet interestingly similar in their biology and control (**Fig. 1**).

Diarrhea is a common clinical entity in small animal veterinary practice, and has many possible causes including stress, disturbances in water balance, nutritional and immune status, dietary indiscretion, neoplasia, inflammatory disease, and bacterial, parasitic, or viral pathogens or coinfections with any combination of these.[5,6] Any disruption of the normal intestinal flora and function can lead to an abnormal altered pH within the milieu, resulting in the overpopulation of opportunist pathogens. Stress has an effect on normal function and the immunologic integrity of the gut.[7] Giardiasis and intestinal tritrichomonasis are more common in animals housed in stressful situations, pet stores, puppy mills, shelters, and catteries.[8–10] The host-parasite relationships that cause diarrhea are complex and may be affected by many factors.[11,12]

Special concern for clients who are immunocompromised must be given in regard to proper diagnosis and sanitation measures when their pet has diarrhea.[13] Many

Department of Diagnostic Medicine and Pathobiology, College of Veterinary Medicine, Kansas State University, 333 Coles Hall, Manhattan, KS 66506-5600, USA
* Corresponding author.
E-mail address: payne@vet.k-state.edu (P.A. Payne).

Vet Clin Small Anim 39 (2009) 993–1007
doi:10.1016/j.cvsm.2009.06.007
0195-5616/09/$ – see front matter © 2009 Elsevier Inc. All rights reserved.

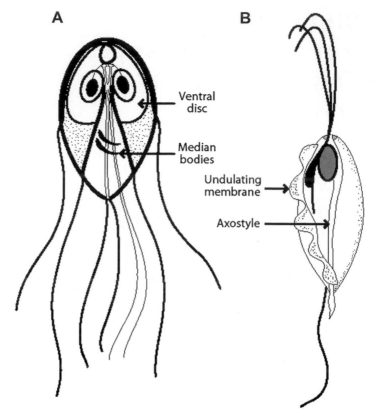

Fig. 1. Trophozoites of *Giardia* spp (*A*) and *Tritrichomonas foetus* (*B*).

species of *Giardia* occur worldwide in many hosts and some do have the potential to be zoonotic; *T foetus* occurs in cattle, pigs, dogs, and cats, and has not been considered to be zoonotic.[1] However, humans may be infected with the venereal trichomand species, *Trichomonas vaginalis*. Practical diagnoses of the underlying parasitologic cause of diarrheal infections in all animals are based on host, site specificity, direct observation, and molecular techniques. Efforts to determine a specific diagnosis are highly recommended. The zoonotic potential of diarrhea of dogs and cats, regardless of causative agent, is possible, and sanitation measures and treatment of all animals in the household when indicated cannot be overemphasized to clients.

GIARDIASIS

Giardiasis is caused by infections with *Giardia* spp parasites and occurs in many animal species including humans, cattle, sheep, goats, dogs, cat, rodents, birds, and amphibians. This cosmopolitan parasite causes a malabsorption syndrome in many of the humans and animals that it parasitizes.[14] The species of this genus is specific in some animals and intertwined in others. Many species and genotypes have been described, and it is recognized that some differ in host range but many are restricted to one host. The prevalence of each of the 7 genetic assemblies varies considerably from country to country.[15]

GENUS *GIARDIA* KUNSTLER 1882

Giardia spp are in the Order Diplomonadida, whose key characteristics include cuplike depressions on the nuclear surface in front of one basal body, three basal body-associated microtubular fibers, and no Golgi, mitrochondria, hydrogenosomes, or axostyle. *Giardia* spp are in the suborder Diplomonadina, family Hexamitidae. These organisms have two karyomastigonts (nuclei and associated flagella) that are arranged in binary symmetry.[2]

There are at least 41 species of *Giardia* that have been described, which live in vertebrates and are distributed in three morphologic groups corresponding to the species *Giardia intestinalis* from man and other animals.[2] However, there are several differing opinions concerning the nomenclature of members of this genus.[1,15] Over the years, the species infecting humans has had several names, several from the scientists who first described the organism or the location within the host, including *Giardia lamblia*, *Giardia duodenalis*, *Giardia intestinalis*, and most recently *Giardia entarica*.

Antonie van Leeuwenhoek first described and sketched the trophozoites and cyst forms in 1681. The Czech physician, Vilem Lambl, has been credited with the actual discovery of *Giardia* spp parasites in 1850 when he observed the organisms in the stools of children with diarrhea. He named these organisms *Cermomonas intestinalis*. Raphael Anatole Émile Blanchard renamed the organism *Lamblia intestinalis* in 1888.[16] Charles Wardell Stiles changed the name to *G lamblia* in 1915 in honor of Professor A. Giard of Paris and Dr F. Lambl of Prague.[17] Some of the species that have remained consistently associated with one host are *Giardia muris* in mice, *Giardia agilis* in amphibians, and *Giardia psittaci* in birds.[1]

The *Giardia* species that is found in humans is considered as a species complex with members discussed in the terms of assemblages that are based on genotypes, determined by various molecular techniques.[1,15,18] The polymerase chain reaction (PCR) techniques that have been used to define the members of the assemblages include glutamate dehydrogenase (GDH), elongation factor 1-α (ef1-α), triphosphate isomerase (TPI), and rDNA.[6,19,20] The 7 genetic assemblages are lettered and most, but not all are species specific.[9,15,20] Assemblages A and B are found in both humans and animals; assemblages C to G are usually host specific with assemblages C and D in canines, assemblage E in hoof stock such as cattle, sheep, goats, pigs, and water buffaloes, and assemblages F in cats and G in rats. It is generally agreed that the genetics of parasites in this genus are still not clearly defined, and because there is now a slight possibility of meiosis and genetic exchange, the nomenclature of this genus, the population genetics, and host specificity are still under intense investigation.[4,15,21]

MORPHOLOGY AND LIFE CYCLE

There are two life stages, the feeding trophozoite and the environmentally stable cyst. *Giardia* spp trophozoites feed in the jejunum and ileum of the small intestine whereas other intestinal flagellates are found in the cecum and colon.[1] The cysts are environmentally stable and dormant yet "spring loaded for action" to excyst on ingestion.[22]

After ingestion of infective cysts, the acidic conditions in the stomach stimulate the relatively quick excystation process that involves changes in the mRNA expression and cell ultrastructure. When the excysting parasites reach the alkaline environment of the small intestine they are exposed to digestive enzymes and bile salts, which enables the completion of the excystation process. The resulting trophozoites (after excystation the four nucleated stage divides in to two trophozoites that each have two nuclei) that emerge from each cyst adhere to enterocytes by means of the ventral disk, start feeding, and establish an infection.[23] The trophozoites, 12 to17 by 7 to 10 μm in size, contain two slender axonemes located inside of the trophozoites, and basal bodies. The four pairs of flagella are located between the two endosome (prominent nucleolus)-filled nuclei in the middle of the cell.[2] *Giardia* spp trophozoites are teardrop-shaped, and have been described as split pears with a flattened ventral surface occupied by the ventral adhesive disk tapering posteriorly to a tail.

The adhesive disk is uniquely adapted for attachment to the mucous epithelial cells lining the intestine. The parasite alternates between attachment and free-swimming phases. The complexities of division and formation of new functional adhesive disks is not fully understood. This information is critical to the understanding of the pathogenesis and treatment protocols for giardiasis because the number of feeding parasites dictates the severity of disease.[22,24–26]

Encystment is an adaptation for survival outside of the host, "packing its bags" so to speak, as it folds in on itself and forms a protective coat around the flagella and internal structures, ready to complete its journey through the host and pass out into the environment. The transformation of the trophozoite to the cyst occurs when the surrounding internal environment changes and the organism is stressed.[27–29] This stress may be due to water reabsorption, or chemical and enzyme clues as the organism passes down through the intestinal tract.[30] Details of this fascinating process can be found in the newly publish article by Midlej and Benchimol.[29] The signals for encystment have yet been fully identified; however, a reduction in the concentration of free cholesterol may be the first molecular signal.[23,28] During the encystment process, encystment proteins are released from vesicles and are the basis of *Giardia* spp fecal antigen tests. The infective cysts (9–13 × 7–9 μm) are passed into the environment in the feces,[1,9] and the cyst is considered to be the diagnostic stage of the parasite.

Cyst excretion from the host is intermittent.[31] The excreted cysts contain a mitotically arrested trophozoite that can remain infectious for months in cool, wet environments.[14,20,27] Knowledge of the biochemical composition and functional properties of the complex outer membranous system have been described in detail, and just how tough these cysts are in the environment are starting to be understood. Cyst environmental survival is a major factor for the high prevalence of giardiasis worldwide.[28,32,33]

Trophozoites are rarely passed directly into the environment. This situation may occur if the intestinal motility is extremely fast and the resulting diarrhea is very liquid. These trophozoites will soon perish outside of the host and will not be infective to other animals or humans.[1]

EPIDEMIOLOGY

The reported incidence and prevalence of giardiasis in humans and animals has been documented worldwide, but varies considerably among populations and geographic locations. Few studies have compared *Giardia* spp isolates from humans and animals living in the same locality or household. *Giardia* spp are transmitted to humans and animals via the fecal oral route. *Giardia* spp cysts are shed in the feces intermittently and are immediately infective. Cysts survive in moist environments and are resistant to most disinfectants, are able to survive water treatment disinfection, and can pass through physical barriers such as filters.[34,35]

Waterborne outbreaks in human populations have been devastating in both rural and urban communities.[6,12] The largest waterborne acute giardiasis outbreak described to date occurred in Norway in the fall of 2004, with more than 1500 people affected. Continuous *Giardia* spp infections, due to poor sanitation, occur in developing countries;[28] however, people living in urban environments are not without risk where *Giardia* is the most common parasite of humans. Hand washing and other common sanitation practices in daycare facilities and food service operations are important to prevent person-to-person spread of the infective cysts to susceptible hosts in these situations.

The incidence of giardiasis in animals is greatest in populations of dogs and cats in confined breeding facilities and animal shelters with poor sanitation and crowded conditions.[12] Animals in unsanitary confined quarters are easily reinfected by grooming infective cysts from their own hair coat or from others. Inanimate objects, such as food bowls and cages in catteries and kennels, may serve as reservoirs of infective cysts.

Risk factors for people include age, location, lifestyle, and immune status; for animals risk factors include being young and housed in a stressful, unsanitary situation.

PATHOGENIC PROCESS

Most dogs and cats are able to ingest infective *Giardia* spp cysts with no adverse effects. Others develop varying degrees of illness and clinical signs. The numbers of cysts ingested plays a role in the resulting pathogenesis. In humans, 10 to 100 cysts are required to establish an infection. It makes sense that the severity of the pathogenesis is related to the dose of infective cysts. If an otherwise healthy individual person or animal ingests a large number of cysts from a contaminated source, the immune system could be overwhelmed and disease would follow.

The host-parasite interaction and resulting pathogenesis at the intestinal villi has been studied intensively in both humans and animals.[9,24,36–38] Initial stress on the animal has been shown to jump-start this pathologic process with *Giardia* spp as well as other organisms and causative agents of diarrhea.[5] T-lymphocyte–mediated pathogenesis is common to this and a variety of other enteropathies. A series of cascading events occurs, starting with the loss of the microvillus brush border after parasite attachment. These events result in disaccharidase insufficiencies and malabsorption of electrolytes, nutrients, and water.[39] The entrocytic injury is mediated by activated host T lymphocytes resulting from the parasite disrupting the epithelial tight junctions, increasing intestinal permeability and destruction of enterocytes.[40,41] It has also been shown that goblet cells in *Giardia* infected dogs become hyperplasic and generate gates, allowing tissue invasion by the trophozoites.[42] Hyper excretion of chloride ions has also been reported.[43] Different strains of *Giardia* parasites have been shown to vary in their ability to cause enterocyte apoptosis.[36] The total effects of parasite attachment and disruption of the intestinal integrity may eventually lead to the development of severe chronic intestinal disorders including inflammatory bowel disease, Crohn disease, and food allergies. Further research using *Giardia* spp as the test model may actually result in new therapeutic targets for these devastating chronic diseases in people and animals.[40]

CLINICAL SIGNS

Infections with *Giardia* are common, but most animals and people remain asymptomatic. The severity of clinical signs varies with age, stress level, immune and nutritional status, as well as species of animal host and strain of parasite.[9,44] The resultant small bowel diarrhea is usually self limiting. However, the clinical signs range from slight abdominal discomfort to severe abdominal pain and cramping, explosive watery, foul-smelling diarrhea, with malabsorption and possible physical growth arrest.[42]

Acute giardiasis develops after an incubation period of 1 to 14 days (average, 7 days) in people and usually lasts 1 to 3 weeks.[17] The prepatent period in dogs is usually 1 to 2 weeks and can last for 24 hours to months.[1,9]

DIAGNOSIS

Giardiasis is often a diagnostic dilemma. *Giardia* spp are one of the most commonly misdiagnosed, underdiagnosed, and overdiagnosed parasites in veterinary practices today. The gold standard technique is fecal flotation with centrifugation in zinc sulfate, stained with Lugol iodine. Other in-clinic techniques include the saline direct fecal smear and the SNAP *Giardia* antigen test (IDEXX Laboratories). Reference laboratories provide additional diagnostic techniques including immunofluorescent assays (IFA) (eg, the MeriFluor *Cryptosporidium/Giardia*) and PCR. The Companion Animal Parasite Council[45] recommends "testing symptomatic (intermittently or consistently diarrheic) dogs and cats with a combination of direct smear, fecal flotation with centrifugation, and a sensitive, specific fecal ELISA optimized for use in companion animals. Repeat testing performed over several (usually alternating) days may be necessary to identify infection."

There are many reasons why fecal flotation is challenging for private practitioners, including poor or no equipment including centrifuges, microscopes, micrometers, availability of proper flotation solutions, and inability to correctly identify the small delicate cysts. Cysts are shed intermittently, and repeated fecal analyses may be needed before cysts are recovered in a sample. Many pseudoparasites, such as yeasts, plant remnants, and debris, have been mistaken for these tiny organisms.[46]

In many clinics the only diagnostic technique used is the direct fecal smear; however, trophozoites are fragile and are often found only in very fresh, diarrheic feces, and can be confused with other flagellates or anything that moves. Trophozoites are rarely seen in direct fecal smears unless the sample is taken directly from the rectum and the feces are diarrheic. Mobile trophozoites have a tumbling or falling-leaf motion. Cysts are difficult to identify in wet mounts, and the sample size is usually inadequate for diagnosis.

The SNAP *Giardia* Test for dogs and cats (IDEXX Laboratories)[47] is available to veterinarians, is easy to use, and reliably identifies *Giardia* spp cyst wall protein shed in dog or cat feces. The enzyme-linked immunosorbent assay (ELISA)-based technology of the SNAP *Giardia* antigen test uses antibodies specific to *Giardia* cyst wall proteins released into the feces during the encystation process. The lateral flow technology allows a blue color to be visualized when antibody binds *Giardia* cyst wall antigen.

There have been several population surveys and comparison studies completed, with interesting results.[3,8,12,13,48–50] Some incongruent results have come from the evaluation of various testing techniques (direct smear, fecal flotation, ELISA), where none of the three methods consistently agreed with the others nor did any one method prove to be superior in a particular group of animals. None of the current methods for diagnosing *Giardia* as the cause of diarrhea in dogs and cats is 100% reliable. Flotation and antigen testing can be used in combination, and if more than one fecal sample is analyzed, a solid accurate diagnosis can be made.

TREATMENT AND CONTROL

There is a strong argument for not treating asymptomatic people and animals for giardiasis.[51] *Giardia* cysts are ubiquitous in the environment, and most people and animals will be exposed to cysts but most will not become ill. On the other hand, treatment of

Giardia in dogs and cats, ill or asymptomatic, has been strongly recommended because of the possible zoonotic risk.[9,52]

In the animal with diarrhea, medical treatment should definitely be initiated. Fenbendazole (50 mg/kg once daily for 3 or 5 days) or the combination product Drontal Plus (febantel-pyrantel-praziquantel, 37.8 mg/kg, 7.56 mg/kg, 7.56 mg/kg, respectively) (febantel is metabolized to fenbendazole) is the most current treatment recommendation for giardiasis in dogs and cats.[1,9,53,54] Fenbendazole, a benzimidazole anthelmintic, binds to the a-tubulin cytoskeleton of trophozoites . Energy metabolism is thus inhibited by lack of glucose uptake.[55]

Veterinarians have routinely treated giardiasis in dogs and cats with metronidazole (22 mg/kg orally twice daily for 5 days). This compound is an effective therapy for diarrhea in dogs and cats regardless of cause, and may definitely be used in combination with fenbendazole to relieve clinical signs and eliminate parasites. Metronidazole is in the nitromidazole class of agents. Once the drug enters the parasite it becomes activated by the reduction of the nitro group and binds covalently to DNA molecules, resulting in irreversible helical damage and death of the organism. This drug should not be used in higher doses in small animals due to the adverse side effects. Tinidazole (Tindamax or Fasigyn) is a second-generation nitroimidazole that is closely related to metronizole.[55] It has recently been approved in the United States for the treatment of giardiasis in people. The mechanism of action is not clearly understood. Ronidazole (Ridzol) is also in the same class of drugs as tinidazole, has been used for treatment of Blackhead in turkeys, and was recently tried for treatment of *T foetus* in cats.[56] There are several other compounds including furazolidone, quinacrine, albendazole, and oxfendazole that have been used for treatment of giardiasis but are not recommended at this time.[9,27,57–59]

Unfortunately, there are many cases of giardiasis in humans and animals that do not respond to initial treatment efforts.[9,60] It is the authors' opinion that reinfection is the most common cause of treatment failure. A thorough review of the treatment protocol including treatment of all contact animals, bathing after treatment, and sanitation of the environment should be performed before resistance to the medications is considered. Increasing dosages of medications, especially metronizole, may result in irreversible side effects.

Because immune status of the host is a primary factor in treatment success, giardiasis in debilitated young animals is definitely much harder to eliminate than in a mature, healthy, well-nourished animal. When animals are in stressful situations such as confinement in animal shelters, pet shops, kennels, or catteries, the added stress will compound the pathologic process and complicate treatment attempts, and adversely affect success.

A *Giardia* vaccine for dogs and cats is available commercially (GiardiaVax, Fort Dodge Animal Health, Overland Park, Kansas) but has not proven to prevent infection in dogs or cats.[61,62] The *Giardia* vaccine is entered in the "not recommended category" in The 2006 American Animal Hospital Association canine vaccine guidelines.[63]

Sanitation measures should include thorough cleaning of all surfaces with detergent and hot, soapy water. Chemical disinfectants have been recommended and evaluated, but there is no substitute for cleanliness. There has been recent interest in the use of ultraviolet light to eliminate *Giardia* cysts from water sources in kennel situations.[64,65]

PUBLIC HEALTH

In his presentation to an Academy in 1915, Charles Atwood Kofoid raised the question of the zoonotic potential of *Giardia* spp and the possible contamination of human food by the cyst-infected feces of vermin such as mice rats and cats. He started the discussion on the multiple biologic problems of host specificity and transformation by the environment that has not yet been resolved.[66]

Is *Giardia* spp zoonotic? This key question is often asked by practicing veterinarians but has not been answered with data. There is no fast and or easy way to determine which assemblage the parasite found in a dog or cat stool belongs to, or if in fact the *Giardia* spp cysts seen actually poses a zoonotic threat to the owner of the animal, the veterinarian and his staff, or the researcher and the caretakers. There is an increasing number of water-related *Giardia* spp epidemics in human populations worldwide, and the significance of nonhuman hosts in these occurrences is still an unresolved issue.[9,12,15,20,35,65] Overlapping of transmission cycles of humans and animals may result in zoonotic transfer. Once the taxonomy issues are resolved, veterinarians may have a better understanding of the risks of and links between the interaction between animal and humans that enables the zoonotic transfer of infection. Currently there is little epidemiologic evidence that strongly supports the importance of zoonotic transmission.[9,20,67,68]

The question that logically follows the previous one concerns treatment options. If *Giardia* spp cysts are found on fecal flotation or the *Giardia* spp cyst antigen is positive, should the animals and all of their housemates be treated? What if only one test is positive? What if the tests are positive and the stool is normal? Should these animals be treated with medications and the animals quarantined? Until all of these questions can be answered definitely, all animals with diarrhea that test positive for *Giardia* spp parasites on fecal flotation or the antigen test should be treated as well as all of their housemates, and bathed on the last day of treatment. If the animal does not have diarrhea, testing for *Giardia* spp antigen is not advised on a routine basis. These decisions can have major consequences if the puppy is one of many in a pet shop, in a group situation in an animal shelter, or in a cohort purpose bred for research.

TRITRICHOMONIASIS

Beginning in 1996, reports of large numbers of trichomonads in feline feces have been reported in the literature.[10,69,70] Thanks to a few determined researchers and their laboratory teams, it is now known that some of these organisms are actually *T foetus*, the same organism that is known to cause early abortions and infertility in naturally bred cattle. Tritrichomoniasis is prevalent among cats in shelters and purebred show cats, and is significantly associated with the history of diarrhea within the cattery.[71] *T foetus* is now the cause of an emerging infectious diarrheal disease of cats worldwide (United States, Britain, Norway, Australia, and Italy).

GENUS *TRICHOMONAS* KOFOID 1920

Parabasalids are anaerobic flagellates without mitochondria. Most of these organisms live as parasites in the alimentary or urogenital tract of vertebrates and invertebrates.[2] Parabasalia are characteristically pear-shaped with one nucleus, and have a rodlike axostyle. Trichomonads do not have a cyst stage. Organisms in the genus *Tritrichomonas* are small flagellates (8–22 μm) with three free anterior flagella and a recurrent one, forming a well-developed undulating membrane. The recurrent flagellum is free posteriorly. There are 20 described species that live in the intestinal tract of nonhuman primates, rodents, swine, birds, reptiles, and amphibians.[2] *Tritrichomonas suis* lives in the nasal cavity, stomach, and intestines of pigs, and is now considered to be identical to *T foetus*.[72] *T foetus* has been recognized for many years as an important venereal transmitted pathogen of bovines that causes infertility and early abortion in naturally bred cattle.[1] More recently, *T foetus* has been recognized as an intestinal pathogen in cats, causing chronic large bowel diarrhea,[71] and has also been found in the feline uterus[72] and, rarely, in the intestinal tract of dogs.[1] *Trichomonas vaginalis* commonly occurs as a venereal disease in people. Men are asymptomatic carriers and women suffer from vaginitis.[1] Because it is difficult to determine the specific genera of trichomonads based on morphology alone, molecular techniques have been developed to identify trichomonads. Diagnosis is usually based on host site specificity and the number of anterior flagella.[1]

MORPHOLOGY AND LIFE CYCLE

T foetus is a flagellated protozoan parasite that measures 6 to 11 by 3 to 4 mm. The organisms reproduce by binary fission within the intestine of the host.[10] It is presumed that cats are infected by direct contact because there is no cyst stage.[73] A recent report found *T foetus* in the uterus of a cat with pyometra. This animal did live in a house with other cats that were diagnosed with enteric tritrichomonads but the route of transmission is unknown.[72]

It is now known that isolates of *T foetus* from cattle are infectious for cats, and that isolates of *T foetus* from cats are infectious for cows. Isolates of *T foetus* from cats do not seem to be as pathogenic for cattle as are cattle isolates.[74,75]

EPIDEMOLOGY

The origin and prevalence of *T foetus* in the feline colon is unknown. It has been reported in this species in the United States as well as other countries including Britain, Switzerland, Norway, and Australia.[76,77] Three epidemiologic studies have been completed and reported in the United States and Britain over the last several years, which agree that the disease is usually found in densely housed young cats whereby fecal-oral transmission may readily occur.[69,72]

The epidemiologic study that was conducted by Gookin and colleagues[78] in 2004 also included data concerning *Giardia* spp infection. It was concluded that there was a high prevalence of *T foetus* infection in purebred domestic show cats. The clearest and most preventable risk factor for infection was a high density (low number of square feet of facility area per cat) of cats housed within a facility.

The British survey was conducted in 2007 with fecal samples from 111 United Kingdom cats with diarrhea. The assessment of *T foetus* infection was determined by PCR. Sixteen (14.4%) samples were found to be positive. In agreement with studies from the United States, infected cats were predominantly of pedigree breed and under 1 year old. The investigators noted that Siamese and Bengal cats specifically were overrepresented in this population.[79]

A more recent study was conducted in pet cats in the United States. There were 173 feline fecal samples analyzed, with 17 (10%) both culture- and PCR-positive. No correlation was found between breed and sex. All positive samples were diarrheic.[80]

From the results of these studies, one cannot help but wonder what effect stress has on the predisposition for disease with this organism.

PATHOGENIC PROCESS

There is little information regarding the pathologic process in naturally infected animals. However, a detailed report of the pathology of experimentally infected cats was presented in 2004.[10] Forty-three sections of colon were evaluated from seven cats with chronic diarrhea and *T foetus* infection. Following experimentally induced infection, *T foetus* organisms colonize the feline ileum, cecum, and colon, resulting in diarrhea. The presence of organisms was associated with multiple changes within the lining of the intestine including infiltration of lymphocytes and neutrophils, loss of goblet cells, and other changes in the mucosa surface. Trichomonads were most commonly found in close proximity to the surface of the mucosa and less frequently compressed within the lumen of the colonic crypts. The investigators concluded that the number of factors mediating pathogenicity of the organism is limited. Identified mechanisms included the possibilities of alterations in the normal intestinal flora, adherence to the epithelium, and elaboration of cytokines and enzymes. These possibilities were extrapolated from the vast array of studies on the pathology of venereal *T foetus* in cattle.

CLINICAL SIGNS

Cats infected with *T foetus* present in good body condition and appetite, with chronic large bowel diarrhea, associated with blood, mucus, flatulence, tenesmus, and anal irritation.[71,78,80] Owners report that the cats pass cow-pie like stools that are malodorous.[81] Cases are usually diagnosed with trichomoniasis after it becomes apparent that the diarrhea is nonresponsive to routine therapies.

Trichomonads are usually commensal organisms causing no clinical signs in their host. Some cats with *T foetus* infection are asymptomatic.

DIAGNOSIS

The diagnosis is made by direct observation of the flagellates in fresh or cultured feces. Flotation solutions will destroy trophozoites.[73] The trophozoites are difficult to distinguish from those of *Giardia* spp and other nonpathogenic intestinal trichomonads such as *Pentatrichomonas hominis.* Trophozoites of *T foetus* and *Giardia* spp are about the same size but they move differently. *Giardia* spp organisms have been said to have motility that resembles the fall of a leaf, whereas trichomonads move erratically.[82] *T foetus* cannot be reliably distinguished from the nonpathogenic *P hominis.*[82,83] Cultivation of feline feces in the commercially available transport and test system (InPouch TF-Feline, Biomed Diagnostics Inc, San Jose, California) has been recommended and is now considered to be the gold standard diagnostic test for *T foetus* in felines.[84] As with other causes of diarrhea, bacterial, viral, other parasites, and nutritional problems need to be ruled out before a diagnosis of tritrichomoniasis can be made.

TREATMENT AND CONTROL

There is no approved treatment for *T foetus* in cats. Treatment of infected animals is difficult, and although many medications have been suggested and used alone or in combination, success is limited. The medications that have been evaluated include paromomycin, metronidazole, sulfamethoxine, fenbendazole, furazolidine, enrofloxacin, gentamycin, and cephalexin. Diarrhea did improve during the treatment of the animals but none of the antimicrobials were effective in resolution of clinical signs.[71] More recently, tinidazole was also found to be relatively ineffective.[85] However, ronidazole was shown to be effective (30 mg/kg once a day for 10 days) in cats that were experimentally infected.[56,81] Ronidazole is not readily available but may be obtained through compounding pharmacies in the United States. This drug must be used with caution because it will cause neurologic side effects. Other routine measures to relieve diarrheal symptoms such as dietary changes have also failed to help resolve symptoms.

Once again, sanitation of the environment and the animals in a cattery is critical, with animals shedding trichomonads into the environment and constant grooming activities of themselves and their kittens after defecation. These organisms do not survive for any length of time outside the host, but cats are fastidious and will definitely reingest these parasites readily.

PUBLIC HEALTH

The possibility of cat to human transmission has been alluded to, but has not been suspected or proved.[81]

SUMMARY

There is a vast amount of information available for *Giardia* spp in pets and humans, but the investigations of *T foetus* in cats is still new and information relatively sparse. The most obvious reason for this disparity is that *Giardia* is a historic and well-known human pathogen and *T foetus* is not. The one obvious common denominator in the incidence of these two parasites in pets is being housed in densely populated areas such as breeding kennels and catteries, and therefore most likely to be under stress.

These two protozoal parasites are different, yet interestingly similar in their biology and control. The host-parasite relationships of these two parasites are complex and may be affected by many factors. The zoonotic potential of diarrhea of dogs and cats, regardless of causative agent, is possible, and sanitation measures and treatment of all animals in the household cannot be overemphasized to clients.

ACKNOWLEDGMENT

The authors thank Mal Rooks Hoover, Graphic Designer Specialist, for her illustration of the trophozoites.

REFERENCES

1. Bowman D. Protozoans. Georgis' parasitology for veterinarians, 8th edition. St. Louis: Saunders; 2009. p. 84–114.
2. Brugerolle G, Lee JJ. Order diplomonadida. In: Lee JJ, Leedale GF, Bradbury P, editors. An illustrated guide to the protozoa. 2nd edition. Lawrence (KS): Allen Press; 2000. p. 1132–208.
3. Gookin JL, Birkenheuer AJ, St. John V, et al. Molecular characterization of trichomonads from feces of dogs with diarrhea. J Parasitol 2005;91(4):939–43.
4. Morrison HG, McArthur AG, Gillin FD, et al. Genomic minimalism in the early diverging intestinal parasite *Giardia lamblia*. Science 2007;317(5846):1921–6.
5. Buret AG. How stress induces intestinal hypersensitivity. Am J Pathol 2006; 168(1):3–5.
6. Thompson RC. The zoonotic significance and molecular epidemiology of *Giardia* and giardiasis. Vet Parasitol 2004;126(1–2):15–35.
7. Lappin MR. Enteric protozoal diseases. Vet Clin North Am Small Anim Pract 2005; 35(1):81–8, vi.
8. Scaramozzino P, Di Cave D, Berrilli F, et al. A study of the prevalence and genotypes of *Giardia duodenalis* infecting kennelled dogs. Vet J 2008.

9. Thompson RC, Palmer CS, O'Handley R. The public health and clinical significance of *Giardia* and *Cryptosporidium* in domestic animals. Vet J 2008;177(1): 18–25.

10. Yaeger MJ, Gookin JL. Histologic features associated with *Tritrichomonas foetus*-induced colitis in domestic cats. Vet Pathol 2005;42(6):797–804.

11. Buret AG. Mechanisms of epithelial dysfunction in giardiasis. Gut 2007;56(3): 316–7.

12. Meireles P, Montiani-Ferreira F, Thomaz-Soccol V. Survey of giardiasis in household and shelter dogs from metropolitan areas of Curitiba, Parana state, Southern Brazil. Vet Parasitol 2008;152(3–4):242–8.

13. Hill SL, Cheney JM, Taton-Allen GF, et al. Prevalence of enteric zoonotic organisms in cats. J Am Vet Med Assoc 2000;216(5):687–92.

14. Adam RD. Biology of *Giardia lamblia*. Clin Microbiol Rev 2001;14(3):447–75.

15. Caccio SM, Ryan U. Molecular epidemiology of giardiasis. Mol Biochem Parasitol 2008;160(2):75–80.

16. Faubert G. Immune response to *Giardia duodenalis*. Clin Microbiol Rev 2000; 13(1):35–54, table.

17. Giardiasis. CDCPDX 1. Available at: http://www.dpd.cdc.gov/dpdx/HTML/Giardiasis.htm. Accessed December 15, 2008.

18. Eligio-Garcia L, Cortes-Campos A, Jimenez-Cardoso E. Classification of *Giardia intestinalis* isolates by multiple polymerase chain reaction (multiplex). Parasitol Res 2008;103(4):797–800.

19. Vasilopulos RJ, Rickard LG, Mackin AJ, et al. Genotypic analysis of *Giardia duodenalis* in domestic cats. J Vet Intern Med 2007;21(2):352–5.

20. Xiao L, Fayer R. Molecular characterisation of species and genotypes of *Cryptosporidium* and *Giardia* and assessment of zoonotic transmission. Int J Parasitol 2008;38(11):1239–55.

21. Cooper MA, Adam RD, Worobey M, et al. Population genetics provides evidence for recombination in *Giardia*. Curr Biol 2007;17(22):1984–8.

22. Lauwaet T, Davids BJ, Reiner DS, et al. Encystation of *Giardia lamblia*: a model for other parasites. Curr Opin Microbiol 2007;10(6):554–9.

23. Gallego E, Alvarado M, Wasserman M. Identification and expression of the protein ubiquitination system in *Giardia intestinalis*. Parasitol Res 2007;101(1):1–7.

24. Davids BJ, Palm JE, Housley MP, et al. Polymeric immunoglobulin receptor in intestinal immune defense against the lumen-dwelling protozoan parasite *Giardia*. J Immunol 2006;177(9):6281–90.

25. Hansen WR, Fletcher DA. Tonic shock induces detachment of *Giardia lamblia*. PLoS Negl Trop Dis 2008;2(2):e169.

26. Tumova P, Kulda J, Nohynkova E. Cell division of *Giardia intestinalis*: assembly and disassembly of the adhesive disc, and the cytokinesis. Cell Motil Cytoskeleton 2007;64(4):288–98.

27. DuBois KN, Abodeely M, Sakanari J, et al. Identification of the major cysteine protease of Giardia and its role in encystation. J Biol Chem 2008;283(26): 18024–31.

28. Hausen MA, Freitas JC Jr, Monteiro-Leal LH. The effects of metronidazole and furazolidone during *Giardia* differentiation into cysts. Exp Parasitol 2006;113(3): 135–41.

29. Midlej V, Benchimol M. *Giardia lamblia* behavior during encystment: how morphological changes in shape occur. Parasitol Int 2008;58:72–80.

30. Lujan HD, Mowatt MR, Nash TE. The molecular mechanisms of Giardia encystation. Parasitol Today 1998;14(11):446–50.

31. Thompson J, Yang R, Power M, et al. Identification of zoonotic *Giardia* genotypes in marsupials in Australia. Exp Parasitol 2008;120(1):88–93.
32. Chavez-Munguia B, Cedillo-Rivera R, Martinez-Palomo A. The ultrastructure of the cyst wall of *Giardia lamblia*. J Eukaryot Microbiol 2004;51(2):220–6.
33. Chavez-Munguia B, Omana-Molina M, Gonzalez-Lazaro M, et al. Ultrastructure of cyst differentiation in parasitic protozoa. Parasitol Res 2007;100(6):1169–75.
34. Caccio SM, Thompson RC, McLauchlin J, et al. Unravelling *Cryptosporidium* and *Giardia* epidemiology. Trends Parasitol 2005;21(9):430–7.
35. Smith HV, Caccio SM, Cook N, et al. *Cryptosporidium* and *Giardia* as foodborne zoonoses. Vet Parasitol 2007;149(1–2):29–40.
36. Chin AC, Teoh DA, Scott KG, et al. Strain-dependent induction of enterocyte apoptosis by *Giardia lamblia* disrupts epithelial barrier function in a caspase-3-dependent manner. Infect Immun 2002;70(7):3673–80.
37. Lee P, Abdul-Wahid A, Faubert GM, et al. Comparison of the local immune response against *Giardia lamblia* cyst wall protein 2 induced by recombinant *Lactococcus lactis* and *Streptococcus gordonii*. Microbes Infect 2009;11(1):20–8.
38. Ringqvist E, Palm JE, Skarin H, et al. Release of metabolic enzymes by *Giardia* in response to interaction with intestinal epithelial cells. Mol Biochem Parasitol 2008;159(2):85–91.
39. Buret AG. Immunopathology of giardiasis: the role of lymphocytes in intestinal epithelial injury and malfunction. Mem Inst Oswaldo Cruz 2005;100(Suppl 1):185–90.
40. Buret AG. Pathophysiology of enteric infections with *Giardia duodenalius*. Parasite 2008;15(3):261–5.
41. Palmer CS, Traub RJ, Robertson ID, et al. Determining the zoonotic significance of *Giardia* and *Cryptosporidium* in Australian dogs and cats. Vet Parasitol 2008;154(1–2):142–7.
42. Ponce-Macotela M, Gonzalez-Maciel A, Reynoso-Robles R, et al. Goblet cells: are they an unspecific barrier against *Giardia intestinalis* or a gate? Parasitol Res 2008;102(3):509–13.
43. Troeger H, Epple HJ, Schneider T, et al. Effect of chronic *Giardia lamblia* infection on epithelial transport and barrier function in human duodenum. Gut 2007;56(3):328–35.
44. Sahagun J, Clavel A, Goni P, et al. Correlation between the presence of symptoms and the *Giardia duodenalis* genotype. Eur J Clin Microbiol Infect Dis 2008;27(1):81–3.
45. CAPC guidelines, Protozoa: giardiasis guidelines. Available at: http://www.capcvet.org/recommendations/giardia.html.
46. Dryden MW, Payne PA, Smith V. Accurate diagnosis of *Giardia* spp and proper fecal examination procedures. Vet Ther 2006;7(1):4–14.
47. IDEXX. SNAPP *Giardia* Test for dogs and cats. Available at: http://www.idexx.com/animalhealth/testkits/giardia_feline/index.jsp.
48. Artzer M, Payne PA, Dryden MW, et al. Post treatment evaluation of *Giardia* spp. Proceedings AAVP 53rd Annual Meeting 2008;38:7–19 [abstract].
49. Carlin EP, Bowman DD, Scarlett JM, et al. Prevalence of *Giardia* in symptomatic dogs and cats throughout the United States as determined by the IDEXX SNAP *Giardia* test. Vet Ther 2006;7(3):199–206.
50. Geurden T, Berkvens D, Casaert S, et al. A Bayesian evaluation of three diagnostic assays for the detection of *Giardia duodenalis* in symptomatic and asymptomatic dogs. Vet Parasitol 2008;157:14–20.

51. Saffar MJ, Qaffari J, Khalilian AR, et al. Rapid reinfection by *Giardia lamblia* after treatment in a hyperendemic area: the case against treatment. East Mediterr Health J 2005;11(1–2):73–8.

52. Montoya A, Dado D, Mateo M, et al. Efficacy of Drontal(R) Flavour Plus (50 mg praziquantel, 144 mg pyrantel embonate, 150 mg febantel per tablet) against *Giardia* sp in naturally infected dogs. Parasitol Res 2008;103(5):1141–4.

53. Merck veterinary manual, treatment: giardiasis. Available at: http://www.merckvetmanual.com/mvm/index.jsp?cfile=htm/bc/21300.htm.

54. Payne PA, Ridley RK, Dryden MW, et al. Efficacy of a combination febantel-praziquantel-pyrantel product, with or without vaccination with a commercial *Giardia* vaccine, for treatment of dogs with naturally occurring giardiasis. J Am Vet Med Assoc 2002;220(3):330–3.

55. Gardner TB, Hill DR. Treatment of giardiasis. Clin Microbiol Rev 2001;14(1):114–28.

56. Gookin JL, Copple CN, Papich MG, et al. Efficacy of ronidazole for treatment of feline *Tritrichomonas foetus* infection. J Vet Intern Med 2006;20(3):536–43.

57. Barr SC, Bowman DD, Frongillo MF, et al. Efficacy of a drug combination of praziquantel, pyrantel pamoate, and febantel against giardiasis in dogs. Am J Vet Res 1998;59(9):1134–6.

58. Barr SC, Bowman DD, Heller RL. Efficacy of fenbendazole against giardiasis in dogs. Am J Vet Res 1994;55(7):988–90.

59. Barr SC, Bowman DD, Heller RL, et al. Efficacy of albendazole against giardiasis in dogs. Am J Vet Res 1993;54(6):926–8.

60. Escobedo AA, Cimerman S. Giardiasis: a pharmacotherapy review. Expert Opin Pharmacother 2007;8(12):1885–902.

61. Anderson KA, Brooks AS, Morrison AL, et al. Impact of *Giardia* vaccination on asymptomatic *Giardia* infections in dogs at a research facility. Can Vet J 2004;45(11):924–30.

62. Stein JE, Radecki SV, Lappin MR. Efficacy of *Giardia* vaccination in the treatment of giardiasis in cats. J Am Vet Med Assoc 2003;222(11):1548–51.

63. Paul MA, Carmichael LE, Childers H, et al. 2006 AAHA canine vaccine guidelines. J Am Anim Hosp Assoc 2006;42(2):80–9.

64. Li D, Craik SA, Smith DW, et al. Survival of *Giardia lamblia* trophozoites after exposure to UV light. FEMS Microbiol Lett 2008;278(1):56–61.

65. Linden KG, Shin GA, Faubert G, et al. UV disinfection of *Giardia lamblia* cysts in water. Environ Sci Technol 2002;36(11):2519–22.

66. Kofoid CA, Christinsen EB. On the life-history of *Giardia*. www. 2008. Ref Type: Electronic Citation.

67. De Santis-Kerr AC, Raghavan M, Glickman NW, et al. Prevalence and risk factors for *Giardia* and coccidia species of pet cats in 2003–2004. J Feline Med Surg 2006;8(5):292–301.

68. Sulaiman IM, Fayer R, Bern C, et al. Triosephosphate isomerase gene characterization and potential zoonotic transmission of *Giardia duodenalis*. Emerg Infect Dis 2003;9(11):1444–52.

69. Gookin JL, Breitschwerdt EB, Levy MG, et al. Diarrhea associated with trichomonosis in cats. J Am Vet Med Assoc 1999;215(10):1450–4.

70. Romatowski J. *Pentatrichomonas hominis* infection in four kittens. J Am Vet Med Assoc 2000;216(8):1270–2.

71. Foster DM, Gookin JL, Poore MF, et al. Outcome of cats with diarrhea and *Tritrichomonas foetus* infection. J Am Vet Med Assoc 2004;225(6):888–92.

72. Dahlgren SS, Gjerde B, Pettersen HY. First record of natural *Tritrichomonas foetus* infection of the feline uterus. J Small Anim Pract 2007;48(11):654–7.
73. Zajac AM, Conboy GA. Fecal examination for the diagnosis of parasitism. Veterinary clinical parasitology. 7th edition. Ames (IA): Blackwell; 2006. p. 3–148.
74. Stockdale H, Rodning S, Givens M, et al. Experimental infection of cattle with a feline isolate of *Tritrichomonas foetus*. J Parasitol 2007;93(6):1429–34.
75. Stockdale HD, Dillon AR, Newton JC, et al. Experimental infection of cats (*Felis catus*) with *Tritrichomonas foetus* isolated from cattle. Vet Parasitol 2008; 154(1–2):156–61.
76. Bissett SA, Gowan RA, O'Brien CR, et al. Feline diarrhoea associated with *Tritrichomonas* cf. *foetus* and *Giardia* co-infection in an Australian cattery. Aust Vet J 2008;86(11):440–3.
77. Frey CF, Schild M, Hemphill A, et al. Intestinal *Tritrichomonas foetus* infection in cats in Switzerland detected by in vitro cultivation and PCR. Parasitol Res 2008;104:783–8.
78. Gookin JL, Stebbins ME, Hunt E, et al. Prevalence of and risk factors for feline *Tritrichomonas foetus* and *Giardia* infection. J Clin Microbiol 2004;42(6):2707–10.
79. Gunn-Moore DA, McCann TM, Reed N, et al. Prevalence of *Tritrichomonas foetus* infection in cats with diarrhoea in the UK. J Feline Med Surg 2007;9(3):214–8.
80. Stockdale HD, Givens MD, Dykstra CC, et al. *Tritrichomonas foetus* infections in surveyed pet cats. Vet Parasitol 2008;160:13–7.
81. Gookin JL, Dybas D. An owners guide to diagnosis and treatment of cats infected with *Tritrichomonas foetus*. Available at: http://www.cvm.ncsu.edu/docs/documents/ownersguide_tfoetus_revised042808.pdf. Accessed April 28, 2008.
82. Gookin JL, Levy MG. Discrimination of *Tritrichomonas foetus* and *Giardia* by light microscopy. www. 2008. Ref Type: Electronic Citation.
83. Gookin JL, Foster DM, Poore MF, et al. Use of a commercially available culture system for diagnosis of *Tritrichomonas foetus* infection in cats. J Am Vet Med Assoc 2003;222(10):1376–9.
84. Biomed. Available at: http://www.biomeddiagnostics.com/pilot.asp?pg=Tfoetus-feline.
85. Gookin JL, Stauffer SH, Coccaro MR, et al. Efficacy of tinidazole for treatment of cats experimentally infected with *Tritrichomonas foetus*. Am J Vet Res 2007; 68(10):1085–8.

Toxoplasmosis and Other Intestinal Coccidial Infections in Cats and Dogs

J.P. Dubey, MVSc, PhD[a],*, David S. Lindsay, PhD[b],
Michael R. Lappin, DVM, PhD[c]

KEYWORDS

- Coccidiosis • Diagnosis • Treatment • Isospora
- Toxoplasma • Neospora

Toxoplasma gondii and related coccidians are intracellular protozoan parasites. Coccidia are obligate intracellular parasites normally found in the intestinal tract. Virtually all warm-blooded animals, including humans, are commonly infected with coccidia.[1] Until, the discovery of the life cycle of *T. gondii* in 1970, coccidia were considered host-specific parasites with infection generally confined to intestines. In addltlon, coccidia of dogs and cats were classified in the genus *Isospora*, and were thought to be of little or no biologic or clinical significance.[2] Since then, a lot has been learnt about public health and biological significance of canine and feline coccidia, and they are now classified into several distinct genera: *Toxoplasma*, *Neospora*, *Isospora* (also called *Cystoisospora*), *Hammondia*, *Besnoitia*, *Sarcocystis*, *Cryptosporidium*, and *Cyclospora*.[2] Only parasites belonging to *Toxoplasma*, *Neospora*, and *Isospora* of cats and dogs are discussed in detail here (**Tables 1** and **2**).

BASIC LIFE CYCLE

All coccidians have an asexual and a sexual cycle, resulting in the production of an environmentally resistant stage, the oocyst (**Figs. 1–10**). In some genera, such as *Sarcocystis*, the asexual and sexual cycles occur in different hosts, whereas in *Isospora* both cycles may occur in the same host; in *Toxoplasma* both cycles occur in

---

[a] United States Department of Agriculture, Agricultural Research Service, Animal and Natural Resources Institute, Beltsville Agricultural Research Center, Building 1001, Beltsville, MD, 20705-2350, USA
[b] Department of Biomedical Sciences and Pathobiology, Virginia-Maryland Regional College of Veterinary Medicine, Virginia Tech, 1410 Prices Fork Road, Blacksburg, VA 24061-0342, USA
[c] Department of Clinical Sciences, College of Veterinary Medicine, Colorado State University, Fort Collins, CO 80523, USA
* Corresponding author.
E-mail address: jitender.dubey@ars.usda.gov (J.P. Dubey).

Vet Clin Small Anim 39 (2009) 1009–1034
doi:10.1016/j.cvsm.2009.08.001
0195-5616/09/$ – see front matter

Table 1
Summary of biology of coccidia of cats

Species and References	Oocyst Size[a]	Stage Excreted	Main Life Cycle	Development Site[b]	Extraintestinal Cycle in Cat	Tissue Cysts	Pathogenicity[c]
Isospora felis[3–5]	40 × 30	Unsporulated	One-host	Villar epithelium	No	One-zoite[e]	Mild
Isospora rivolta[4–6]	22 × 20	Unsporulated	One-host	Villar epithelium	No	One-zoite	Mild
Toxoplasma gondii[7,8]	12 × 10	Unsporulated	Two-host	Villar epithelium	Yes	Many[f]	Mild
Hammondia hammondi[7,9]	12 × 11	Unsporulated	Two-host	Villar epithelium	No	Many[g]	None
Besnoitia							
Wallacei[10]	17 × 12	Unsporulated	Two-host	Lamina propria	No	Many[h]	None
Darlingi[11]	12 × 11	Unsporulated	Two-host	Lamina propria	No	Many +	None
Oryctofelisi[12]	12 × 11	Unsporulated	Two-host	Lamina propria	Yes	Many[h]	None
Sarcocystis spp[13]	11 × 9[d]	Sporulated	Two-host	Lamina propria	No	Many[i]	None

a Average size of unsporulated oocyst in micrometers.
b Schizonts in the small intestine of the cat.
c Pathogenicity for the cat.
d Sporocyst.
e These cysts contain 1 sporozoite and have been found only in experimentally infected animals fed oocysts.
f Tissue cysts are microscopic, and contain many bradyzoites in almost all tissues of the cat.
g Tissue cysts are not found in the cat; they are found mainly in muscles of rodents fed H. hammondi oocysts.
h Besnoitia cysts are found only in the intermediate hosts and can be macroscopic.
i Sarcocystis cysts (sarcocysts) are often macroscopic and occur only in the intermediate.

Table 2
Summary of biology of coccidia of dogs

Species and References	Oocyst Size[a]	Stage Excreted	Main Life Cycle	Development Site[b]	Extraintestinal Cycle in Dog	Tissue Cysts	Pathogenicity[c]
Isospora canis[14,15]	38 × 30	Unsporulated	One-host	Villar epithelium	No	One-zoite[e]	Mild
Isospora ohioensis[16]	24 × 20	Unsporulated	One-host	Villar epithelium	No	One-zoite	Mild
Isospora neorivolta[17]	i	Unsporulated	One-host	Villar epithelium and lamina propria	No	Unknown	Unknown
Isospora burrowsi[18,19]	20 × 17	Unsporulated	One-host	Villar epithelium and lamina propria	No	One-zoite	Unknown
Neospora caninum[20,21]	12 × 10	Unsporulated	Two-host	Unknown	Yes	Many[f]	Mild
Hammondia heydorni[21-23]	12 × 11	Unsporulated	Two-host	Villar epithelium	No	Rare[g]	None
Sarcocystis spp[13]	11 × 9[d]	Sporulated	Two-host	Lamina propria	No	Many[h]	None

[a] Average size of unsporulated oocyst in micrometers.
[b] Schizonts in the small intestine of the dog.
[c] Pathogenicity for the dog.
[d] Sporocysts.
[e] These cysts contain 1 sporozoite and have been found only in experimentally infected animals fed oocysts.
[f] Tissue cysts are microscopic, contain many bradyzoites, and are found in the central nervous system and muscles.
[g] Tissue cysts are not confirmed.
[h] Sarcocystis cysts are often macroscopic and occur only in the intermediate hosts.
[i] Oocysts are considered to be the same size as I. ohioensis but were not described.

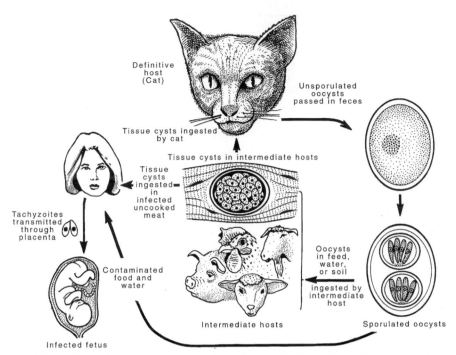

Fig. 1. Life cycle of *Toxoplasma gondii*. (*From* Dubey JP. Toxoplasmosis – a waterborne zoonosis. Vet Parasitol 2004;126:57–72; with permission.)

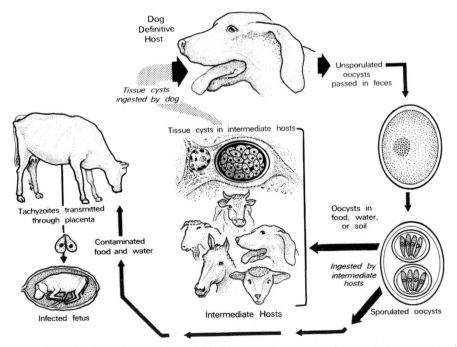

Fig. 2. Life cycle of *Neospora caninum*. (*From* Dubey JP. Recent advances in Neospora and neosporosis. Vet Parasitol 1999;84:350; with permission.)

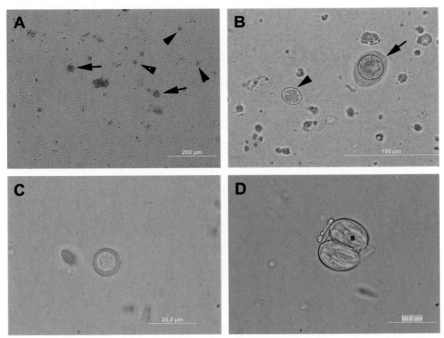

Fig. 3. Coccidial oocysts from dog feces. (*A*) Oocysts of *Isospora canis* (*arrows*) and *I. ohioensis* type (*arrowheads*). Unstained. (*B*) Higher-power view of oocysts of *I. canis* (*arrow*) and *I. ohioensis* type (*arrowhead*). Unstained. (*C*) Unsporulated oocyst of *Neospora/Hammondia* type. Unstained. (*D*) Sporulated oocyst of *Neospora/Hammondia* type. Note the 2 sporocysts each with 4 sporozoites (S). Unstained.

one host (the cat), and only the asexual cycle occurs in nonfeline hosts. The host that excretes the oocyst is called the definitive host, and those hosts wherein only the asexual cycle occurs are called intermediate hosts.

A representative coccidian life cycle is best described as follows. Oocysts are passed unsporulated in feces (**Fig. 3**A–C; **Fig. 4**; **Fig. 10**C). After exposure to warm (20°C) environmental temperatures and moisture, oocysts sporulate, forming 2 sporocysts. Within each sporocyst are 4 sporozoites (**Fig. 3**D; **Fig. 10**D). The sporozoites are banana-shaped and are the infective stage. The sporozoites can survive environmental exposure inside the oocysts for many months. After the ingestion of sporulated oocysts by cats or dogs, sporozoites excyst in the intestinal lumen, and the sporozoites initiate the formation of schizonts or meronts. During schizogony or merogony, the sporozoite nucleus divides into 2, 3, or more nuclei, depending on the parasite and the stage of the cycle. After nuclear division, each nucleus is surrounded by cytoplasm, forming a merozoite (**Fig. 5**B, D; **Fig. 6**A; **Fig. 7**B–D; **Fig. 9**B). The number of merozoites within a schizont varies from 2 (see **Fig. 7**B) to several hundred, depending on the stage of the cycle and the species of coccidia. Merozoites are released from the schizont when the infected host cell ruptures. The number of schizogonic cycles varies with the parasitic species. First-generation merozoites repeat the asexual cycle and form second-generation schizonts, or transform into male (micro) and female (macro) gamonts. The microgamont divides into many tiny microgametes (**Fig. 5**C; **Fig. 7**F; **Fig. 9**D). A microgamete fertilizes a macrogamete (**Fig. 7**E; **Fig. 9**C), and an oocyst wall is formed around the zygote (see **Fig. 5**D). The life cycle is completed when unsporulated oocysts are excreted in feces.

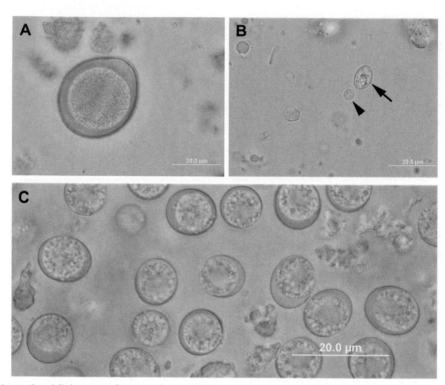

Fig. 4. Coccidial oocysts from cat feces. (*A*) Unsporulated oocysts of *Isospora felis*. Unstained. (*B*) Sporocyst of *Sarcocystis* sp (*arrow*) and an oocyst of *Cryptosporidium* sp (*arrowhead*). Unstained. (*C*) Numerous unsporulated oocysts of *Toxoplasma gondii*. Unstained.

ISOSPORA SPP

Members of the genus *Isospora*, the most commonly recognized coccidians infecting dogs or cats, are species specific for the definitive host. At least 4 species, *I. canis*, *I. ohioensis*, *I. burrowsi*, and *I. neorivolta*, infect dogs, and 2 species, *I. felis* and *I. rivolta*, infect cats.

The life cycle of *Isospora* infecting dogs and cats is similar to the basic coccidian intestinal cycle, except an asexual cycle can also occur in the definitive or intermediate host. On ingestion by definitive or suitable paratenic (intermediate) hosts, oocysts excyst in the presence of bile, and free sporozoites invade the intestine. Some sporozoites penetrate the intestinal wall and enter mesenteric lymph nodes or other extraintestinal tissues, where they form enlarging monozoic cysts (see **Fig. 8**). If no replication occurs, the term paratenic host, rather than intermediate host, is used. Monozoic cysts of *Isospora* may remain in extraintestinal tissues of paratenic hosts for the life of the host. Ingestion of monozoic cysts in paratenic hosts leads to intestinal infection in the definitive dog and cat host. The life cycle after the ingestion of paratenic host is the same as after the ingestion of sporulated oocysts from feces. The significance of the paratenic host in the life cycle of dogs and cats is unknown because the direct fecal-oral cycle is very efficient.

Clinical Findings

Enzootic infections are frequently found in catteries or kennels where animals are congregated.[24–27] Clinical signs are most apparent in neonates. Diarrhea with weight

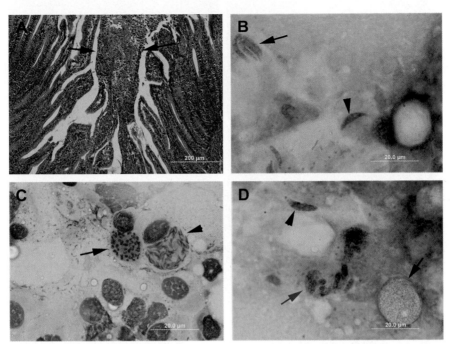

Fig. 5. Lesions and developmental stages of *Isospora ohioensis* in dogs. (*A*) The arrows bracket a necrotic area of small intestine. Hematoxylin and eosin stain. (*B*) Schizont in which merozoites are still attached (*arrow*) and a fee merozoite (*arrowhead*). Giemsa stain. (*C*) Immature (*arrow*) and mature (*arrowhead*) microgamonts. Giemsa stain. (*D*) Schizont (*orange arrow*), free merozoite (*arrowhead*), and an oocyst (*black arrow*). Giemsa stain.

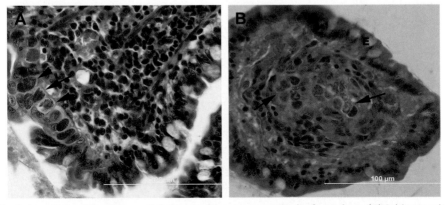

Fig. 6. Location of developmental stages of *Isospora neorivolta* from dogs. (*A*) Schizont with merozoites (*arrow*) and microgamonts (*arrowheads*) in epithelial cells of a villous. Hematoxylin and eosin stain. (*B*) Cross section of a villous demonstrating developmental stages (*arrows*) in the lamina propria. The epithelial (E) portion of the villous is readily observed. Hematoxylin and eosin stain.

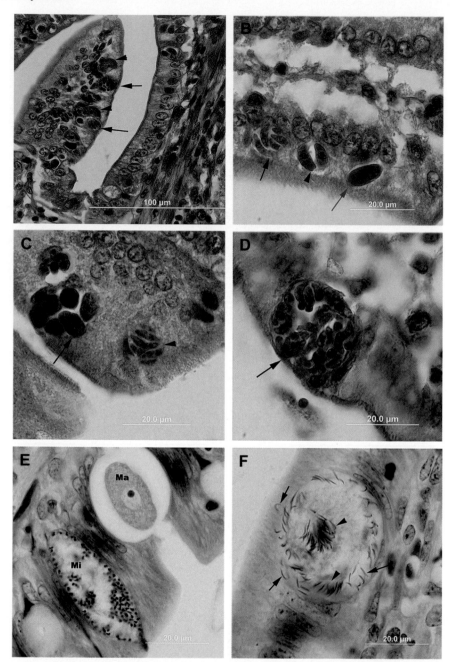

Fig. 7. Asexual and sexual stages of *Isospora felis* from cats. (*A*) Asexual stages (*arrows*) and macrogamonts (*arrows*) and in a villous. Hematoxylin and eosin stain. (*B*) Asexual stages demonstrating an immature schizont (*orange arrow*), a schizont with merozoites (*black arrow*), and 2 large merozoites (*arrowhead*). Hematoxylin and eosin stain. (*C*) Asexual stages demonstrating a group of immature schizont (*arrow*) and a schizont with merozoites (*arrowhead*). Hematoxylin and eosin stain. (*D*) Schizont containing many merozoites (*arrow*). Hematoxylin and eosin stain. (*E*) Microgamont (Mi) with numerous nuclei and a macrogamont (Ma) in feline enterocytes. Iron-hematoxylin stain. (*F*) Microgamont containing many microgametes. Some microgametes (*arrows*) are at the periphery and appear fully developed, whereas others are still in groups (*arrowheads*). Iron-hematoxylin stain.

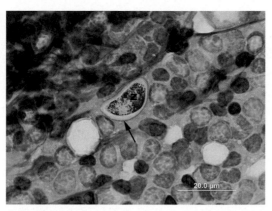

Fig. 8. Unizoic cyst of *Isospora felis* in a lymph node. Note the cyst wall (*arrow*) and the periodic acid Schiff reaction positive zoite (Z). Periodic acid Schiff reaction.

loss and dehydration and, rarely, hemorrhage is the primary sign attributed to coccidiosis in dogs and cats. Anorexia, vomiting, mental depression, and ultimately death may be seen in severely affected animals.

Intestinal coccidiosis may be manifest clinically when dogs or cats are shipped or weaned, or experience a change in ownership. Diarrhea might result from the extraintestinal stages of *Isospora* returning to the intestines. Pathogenesis of intestinal coccidiosis of cats and dogs is not well understood because clinical disease has not been reliably produced in experimentally infected animals, and clinical signs are not correlated with the number of oocysts found in feces. Little is known of the virulence of the different strains of these parasites.[15]

Diagnosis

Intestinal coccidial infection in dogs and cats is diagnosed by identification of the oocysts with any of the fecal flotation methods commonly used to diagnose parasitic infections. In dogs, only *I. canis* can be identified with certainty by oocyst size and shape (see **Fig. 3**A, B). The oocysts of the other 3 species of *Isospora*, namely *I ohioensis*, *I. burrowsi*, and *I neorivota*, may overlap in size, and their distinction is not clinically important. The 2 species of *Isospora* occurring in cats can be readily distinguished by oocyst size. Although oocysts of these *Isospora* are passed unsporulated in freshly excreted feces, they sporulate partially by the time fecal examination is made. Partially sporulated oocysts contain 2 sporocysts without sporozoites. *Isospora* species may sporulate within 8 hours of excretion, and these *Isospora* are highly infectious. In cats, *I. felis* oocysts are twice the size of *I. rivolta*. In extreme cases epithelial casts may be found in feces, and schizonts, merozoites, and partially formed oocysts can be found in smears made in normal saline (not water).

Treatment

The primary goal of treatment of *Isospora* spp infections is to resolve diarrhea in puppies and kittens.[24] Whereas controlled data are generally not available for most protocols listed in **Table 3**, there is anecdotal evidence that administration of drugs can lessen morbidity and mortality, and lessen oocyst shedding. Supportive care such as fluid therapy for correction of dehydration should be administered as indicated.

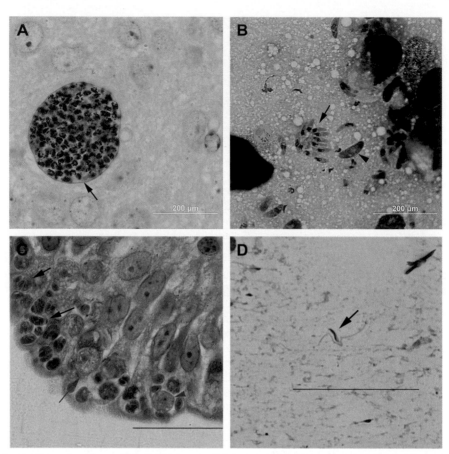

Fig. 9. Life cycle stages of *Toxoplasma gondii* from cats. (*A*) Tissue cyst in the brain. Note the periodic acid Schiff reaction positive bradyzoites and the thin tissue cyst wall (*arrow*). Periodic acid Schiff reaction. (*B*) Intestinal stages in an intestinal smear. Note the schizonts containing small merozoite (*arrow*) and the larger merozoite (*arrowhead*). Giemsa stain. (*C*) Histologic section of small intestine containing enteroepithelial stages. Asexual stages (*black arrows*), a developing macrogamont (*orange arrowhead*), and oocyst (*orange arrow*). Hematoxylin and eosin stain. (*D*) A single microgamete (*arrow*) in an intestinal smear. Note the 2 flagella. Giemsa stain.

The majority of the drugs listed in **Table 3** have only a coccidiostatic effect on the organisms and so infection may not be cleared. In addition to the potential for gastrointestinal irritation, some sulfa drugs have other significant side effects including induction of keratoconjunctivitis sicca, cholestasis, hepatocellular necrosis, and thrombocytopenia.[28,29] The activity of ponazuril, diclazuril, and toltrazuril against apicomplexans has been studied recently.[30–35] These drugs are currently preferred for the treatment of *Isospora* spp infection by many clinicians. Ponazuril is available in the United States as a treatment for *Sarcocystis neurona* infection in horses (Marquis Paste, Bayer Animal Health). This product can be purchased by veterinarians and diluted for use in puppies or kittens. Most compounding pharmacies alternatively will provide appropriate concentrations of ponazuril for use in small animals by prescription.

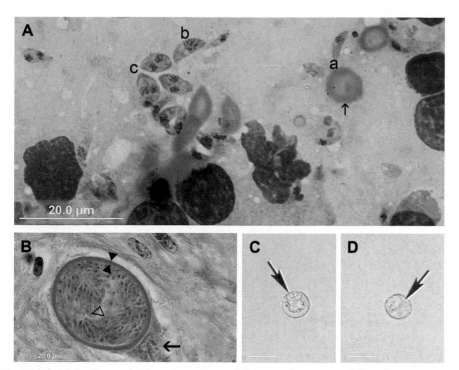

Fig. 10. Life cycle stages of *Neospora caninum*. (*A*) Impression smear of liver from an exper-imentally infected mouse depicting numerous tachyzoites. Notice that tachyzoites vary in dimension, depending on the stage of division: (a) a slender tachyzoite, (b) tachyzoite before division, (c) 3 dividing tachyzoites compared with the size of a red blood cell (*arrow*). Giemsa stain. (*B*) Histologic section of a tissue cyst inside a neuron in spinal cord of a congen-itally infected calf. Note the thick cyst wall (*opposing arrowheads*) enclosing slender brady-zoites (*open triangle*). The host cell nucleus (*arrow*) is cut at an angle. Hematoxylin and eosin stain. (*C*) Unsporulated oocyst (*arrow*) with a central undivided mass in feces of a dog. Unstained (bar = 10 μm). (*D*) Sporulated oocyst (*arrow*) with 2 internal sporocysts. Unstained (bar = 10 μm). (*Data from* Dubey JP, Schares G, Ortega-Mora LM. Epidemiology and control of neosporosis and *Neospora caninum*. Clin Microbiol Rev 2007;20:323–67; with permission.)

Depending on the protocol used, infection may or may not be eliminated in all puppies or kittens. In addition, repeated infection with *Isospora* spp can occur. Thus, it is unclear whether there is value in repeating diagnostic testing after success-ful treatment of clinical disease. Treatment of all other "in-contact" dogs or cats may lessen the likelihood of repeat infection, but also increases expense to the owner and increases the risk for drug-associated side effects. *Isospora* spp are very resistant to routine disinfectants used in small animal practice. If there is a problem with recurrent coccidiosis in a kennel or cattery, potential transport hosts should be controlled, and the treatment of all animals combined with careful environmental cleaning as well as steam cleaning of surfaces may be indicated. In shelters with recurrent problems with coccidiosis, it is recommended that ponazuril be used prophylactically by admin-istering a dose to all puppies or kittens at 2 to 3 weeks of age (http://www.sheltermedicine.com/portal/is_parasite_control.shtml).

Diarrhea associated with *Isospora* spp infections is generally self-limited or rapidly responsive to drug therapy. Thus, puppies and kittens with persistent diarrhea and

Table 3
Drug protocols commonly used to treat *Isospora* spp infections in dogs and cats

Drug	Protocols	Species
Amprolium	– 300–400 mg (total) for 5 d – 110–200 mg (total) daily for 7–12 d – 60–100 mg/kg (total) daily for 7 d – 1.5 tablespoon (23 ml)/gallon (3.8 L) (sole water source) not to exceed 10 d	D
Amprolium/Sulfadimethoxine	150 mg/kg of amprolium and 25 mg/kg of sulfadimethoxine for 14 d	D
Diclazuril[a]	25 mg/kg daily for 1 d	C
Furazolidone	8–20 mg/kg once or twice daily for 5 d	D, C
Ponazuril[a]	– 20 mg/kg daily for 1–3 d – 30 mg/kg, weekly for 2 treatments – 50 mg/kg, once	D, C
Quinacrine	10 mg/kg daily for 5 d	C
Sulfadimethoxine	50–60 mg/kg daily for 5–20 d	D, C
Sulfadimethoxine/Ormetoprim	55 mg/kg of sulfadimethoxine and 11 mg/kg of ormetoprim for 7–23 d	D
Toltrazuril[a]	10–30 mg/kg daily for 1–3 d	D
Trimethoprim/Sulfonamide	–>4 kg animal: 30–60 mg/kg trimethoprim daily for 6 d –<4 kg animal: 15–30 mg/kg trimethoprim daily for 6 d	D, C

Abbreviations: D, dog; C, cat.
[a] These drugs are likely to have a cidal effect against *Isospora* spp and so are most likely to result in elimination of infection. The other drugs are static, so infection may persist after clinical resolution of diarrhea.
Data from the Companion Animal Parasite Council recommendations (www.capcvet.org.)

Isospora spp oocyst shedding should be evaluated thoroughly for other coinfections or diseases that could potentiate *Isospora* spp associated disease.

Prevention

Coccidiosis tends to be a problem in areas of poor sanitation. The fecal shedding of large numbers of environmentally resistant oocysts makes infection likely under such conditions. Animals should be housed so as to prevent contamination of food and water bowls by oocyst-laden soil or infected feces. Feces should be removed daily and incinerated. Oocysts survive freezing temperatures. Runs, cages, food utensils, and other implements should be disinfected by steam cleaning or immersion in boiling water or by 10% ammonia solution. Animals should have limited access to intermediate hosts and should not be fed uncooked meat. Insect control is essential in animal quarters and food storage areas because cockroaches and flies may serve as mechanical vectors of oocysts. Coccidiostatic drugs can be given to infected bitches before or soon after whelping to control the spread of infection to puppies.[24]

TOXOPLASMA GONDII

Toxoplasma gondii is an intestinal coccidian of cats with all nonfeline species as intermediate hosts.[8,36,37] Unlike other coccidian parasites, it has adapted to be transmitted in several ways, including fecal-oral, carnivorism, and transplacental (see **Fig. 1**). Other minor modes of transmission include transfusion of fluids or transplantation of organs.

The coccidian phase of the (enteroepithelial) cycle is found only in the definitive feline host (**Fig. 9**B–D). Most cats are thought to become infected by ingesting intermediate hosts infected with tissue cysts (**Fig. 9**A). Bradyzoites are released in the stomach and intestine from the tissue cysts when the cyst wall is dissolved by digestive enzymes. Bradyzoites penetrate the epithelial cells of small intestine and initiate the formation of schizonts (see **Fig. 9**B, C). After an undetermined number of generations, merozoites released from schizonts form male or female gamonts (see **Fig. 9**C, D). The rest of the cycle proceeds as in other coccidians. The entire enteroepithelial cycle of *T. gondii* can be completed within 3 to 10 days after ingestion of tissue cysts, and occurs in most naive cats. However, after ingestion of sporulated oocysts, the formation of oocysts is delayed until 18 days or more, and only 20% of cats fed oocysts will develop patency. Thus, the fecal-oral cycle of *T. gondii* in cats is not very efficient.[8]

Only cats are known to produce *T. gondii* oocysts. However, some vertebrates and invertebrates can be a transport host for *T. gondii* oocysts. Dogs can eat cat feces infected with *T. gondii* oocysts and these oocysts may pass unexcysted in dog feces. In addition, dogs can roll over in feces of infected cats and people can then become infected by petting these dogs.[38] *T. gondii* oocysts have been identified in feces of naturally infected dogs.[39]

The extraintestinal development of *T. gondii* is the same for all hosts, including dogs, cats, and people, and is not dependent on whether tissue cysts or oocysts are ingested. After the ingestion of oocysts, sporozoites excyst in the lumen of the small intestine and penetrate intestinal cells, including the cells in the lamina propria. Sporozoites divide into 2 by an asexual process known as endodyogeny, and thus become tachyzoites. Tachyzoites are lunate in shape, approximately 6 by 2 μm, and multiply in almost any cell of the body. If the cell ruptures they infect new cells. Otherwise, tachyzoites multiply intracellularly for an undetermined period and eventually encyst. Tissue cysts grow intracellularly and contain numerous bradyzoites (see **Fig. 9**A). Bradyzoites differ biologically from tachyzoites in that they can survive the digestive process in the stomach, whereas tachyzoites are usually killed. Tissue cysts vary in size from 5 to 70 μm and usually conform to the shape of the parasitized cell. Tissue cysts are separated from the host cell by a thin (<0.5 μm) elastic wall (see **Fig. 9**A). Tissue cysts are formed in the central nervous system (CNS), muscles, and visceral organs, and probably persist for the life of the host.

Parasitemia during pregnancy can cause placentitis followed by spread of tachyzoites to the fetus. In people or sheep, congenital transmission occurs usually when the woman or ewe becomes infected during pregnancy. Little is known of transplacental toxoplasmosis in dogs. Many kittens born to queens infected with *T. gondii* during gestation became infected transplacentally or via suckling. Clinical illness is common, varying with the stage of gestation at the time of infection, and some newborn kittens shed oocysts.

The type and severity of clinical illness with *T. gondii* infections are dependent on the degree and localization of tissue injury. Why some infected dogs or cats develop clinical toxoplasmosis while others remain well is not fully understood. Age, sex, host species, strain of *T. gondii*, number of organisms, and stage of the parasite ingested may account for some of the differences. Postnatally acquired toxoplasmosis is generally less serious than prenatally acquired infection. Stress may also aggravate *T. gondii* infection. Concomitant illness or immunosuppression may make a host more susceptible because *T. gondii* proliferates as an opportunistic pathogen. Clinical toxoplasmosis in dogs is often associated with canine distemper or other infections, such as ehrlichiosis, or with glucocorticoid therapy.[37] In some cases, however, predisposing disorders cannot be found. The prevalence of canine toxoplasmosis historically has decreased with the routine use of distemper vaccines. Unlike dogs, clinical toxoplasmosis in cats is considered a primary disease. At present there is no conclusive evidence that concomitant infections with feline leukemia virus, feline immunodeficiency virus (FIV), and *Bartonella* spp infections modify the course of *T. gondii* infection in cats.[8,40]

Clinical Findings

Cats

Clinical toxoplasmosis is most severe in transplacentally infected kittens.[37] Affected kittens may be stillborn or may die before weaning. Kittens may continue to suckle until death. Clinical signs reflect inflammation of the liver, lungs, and CNS. Affected kittens may have an enlarged abdomen because of enlarged liver and ascites. Encephalitic kittens may sleep most of the time or cry continuously.

Anorexia, lethargy, and dyspnea due to pneumonia have been commonly recognized features of postnatal toxoplasmosis. Other clinical signs include persistent or intermittent fever, anorexia, weight loss, icterus due to hepatitis or cholangiohepatitis, vomiting, diarrhea, abdominal effusion, hyperesthesia on muscle palpation, stiffness of gait, shifting leg lameness, dermatitis, loss of vision, and neurologic deficits.[8,36,37,41–61] In 100 cats with histologically confirmed toxoplasmosis, clinical syndromes were diverse but infection of pulmonary (97.7%), CNS (96.4%), hepatic (93.3%), pancreatic (84.4%), cardiac (86.4%), and ocular (81.5%) tissues were most common.[42] Clinical signs may be sudden or may have a slow onset. The disease may be rapidly fatal in some cats with severe respiratory or CNS signs. Anterior or posterior uveitis involving one or both eyes is common. Iritis, iridocyclitis, or chorioretinitis can occur alone or concomitantly. Aqueous flare, keratic precipitate, lens luxation, glaucoma, and retinal detachment are common manifestations of uveitis. Chorioretinitis may occur in both tapetal and nontapetal areas. Ocular toxoplasmosis occurs in some cats without polysystemic clinical signs of disease.

Dogs

Clinical signs may be localized in respiratory, neuromuscular, or gastrointestinal systems, or may be caused by generalized infection.[8,36,37,62–66] The neurologic form of toxoplasmosis may last for several weeks without involvement of other systems, whereas severe disease involving the lungs and liver may kill dogs within a week. Generalized toxoplasmosis is seen mostly in dogs younger than 1 year and is characterized by fever, tonsillitis, dyspnea, diarrhea, and vomiting. Icterus usually results from extensive hepatic necrosis. Myocardial involvement is usually subclinical, although arrhythmias and heart failure may develop as predominant findings in some older dogs.

The most dramatic clinical signs in older dogs have been associated with neural and muscular systems. Neurologic signs depend on the site of lesion in the cerebrum, cerebellum, or spinal cord. Seizures, cranial nerve deficits, tremors, ataxia, and paresis or paralysis may be seen. Dogs with myositis may initially show abnormal gait, muscle wasting, or stiffness. Paraparesis and tetraparesis may rapidly progress to lower motor neuron paralysis. Canine toxoplasmosis is clinically similar to *Neospora caninum* infection, which was previously confused with toxoplasmosis (see neosporosis later). Although these diseases are similar, toxoplasmosis seems to be more prevalent in cats and neosporosis in dogs.

There are only a few reports of ocular lesions associated with toxoplasmosis in dogs. Retinitis, anterior uveitis, iridocyclitis, ciliary epithelium hyperplasia, optic nerve neuritis, and keratoconjuctivitis have been noted. Severe keratoconjuctivitis was recently reported in a dog on prolonged topical corticosteroid therapy.[67]

Diagnosis

Clinical signs, serum chemistry, cytology, radiology, fecal examination, and serology can aid diagnosis.[8,37,42,44,51,52,54,56] Routine hematologic and biochemical parameters may be abnormal in cats and dogs with acute systemic toxoplasmosis. Nonregenerative anemia, neutrophilic leukocytosis, lymphocytosis, monocytosis, and eosinophilia are most commonly observed. Leukopenia of severely affected cats may persist until death, and is usually characterized by an absolute lymphopenia and neutropenia with an inappropriate left shift, eosinopenia, and monocytopenia.

Biochemical abnormalities during the acute phase of illness include hypoproteinemia and hypoalbuminemia. Hyperglobulinemia has been detected in some cats with chronic toxoplasmosis. Marked increases in serum alanine aminotransferase (ALT) and aspartate aminotransferase (AST) have been noted in animals with acute hepatic and muscle necrosis. Dogs generally have increased serum alkaline phosphatase activity with hepatic necrosis, but this occurs less frequently in cats. Serum creatine kinase activity is also increased in cases of muscle necrosis. Serum bilirubin levels have been increased in animals with acute hepatic necrosis, especially cats that develop cholangiohepatitis or hepatic lipidosis. Cats or dogs that develop pancreatitis may show increased serum amylase and lipase activities. Cats often show proteinuria and bilirubinuria. Cats with pancreatitis may have reduced serum total calcium with normal serum albumin concentrations.

Tachyzoites may be detected in various tissues and body fluids by cytology during acute illness. Tachyzoites are rarely found in blood, cerebrospinal fluid (CSF), fine-needle aspirates, and transtracheal or bronchoalveolar washings, but are more common in the peritoneal and thoracic fluids of animals developing thoracic effusions or ascites.

Inflammatory changes are usually noted in body fluids. In suspected feline toxoplasmosis of the nervous system, CSF protein levels were within reference ranges to a maximum of 149 mg/dL, and nucleated cells were a maximum of 28 cells/mL. Lymphocytes predominate, but a mixture of cells may be found.

Thoracic radiographic findings, especially in cats with acute disease, consist of a diffuse interstitial to alveolar pattern with a mottled lobar distribution. Diffuse symmetric homogeneous increased density due to alveolar coalescence has been noted in severely affected animals. Mild pleural effusion can be present. Abdominal radiographic findings may consist of masses in the intestines or mesenteric lymph nodes or homogeneous increased density as a result of effusion. Loss of contrast in the right abdominal quadrant can indicate pancreatitis.

Despite the high prevalence of serum antibodies in cats worldwide, the prevalence of T. gondii oocysts (**Fig. 4**C) in feces is very low. In general, less than 1% of cats shed oocysts on any given day.[68] Because cats usually shed T. gondii oocysts for only 1 to 2 weeks after their first exposure, oocysts are rarely found on routine fecal examination. Moreover, cats usually are not clinically ill and do not have diarrhea during the period of oocyst shedding. Although cats are considered immune to reshedding of oocysts, they may shed a few oocysts after rechallenge with different strains more than 6 years later. Clinical pharmacological doses of corticosteriods do not reactivate shedding of oocysts.

T. gondii oocysts in feline feces are morphometrically indistinguishable from oocysts of *Hammondia hammondi* and *Besnoitia* spp (see **Table 1**), which also occur in cats. Oocysts of these coccidians can be differentiated only by sporulation and subsequent animal inoculation. If 10- to 12-μm sized oocysts are found, they should be considered to be *T. gondii* until proved otherwise. Further inoculations should be attempted only in a diagnostic laboratory with competence in this procedure because of the infectious nature of the organism.

Because of their small size, oocysts of *T. gondii* are best demonstrated by centrifugation using Sheather sugar solution. Five to 10 g of feces are mixed with water to a liquid consistency, and the mixture is strained with gauze. Two parts Sheather sugar solution (500 g sugar, 300 mL water, and 6.5 g melted phenol crystals) are added to one part fecal suspension and centrifuged in a capped centrifuge tube. Care should be taken not to fill the tube to the top, to prevent spills or aerosols. After centrifugation at 1000 *g* for 10 minutes, remove 1 to 2 drops from the meniscus with a dropper, place on a microscope slide, cover with a coverslip, and examine at low-power (×100) magnification. *T. gondii* oocysts are about one-fourth the size of *I. felis* oocysts and one-eighth the size of eggs of *Toxocara cati* (the common roundworm of the cat).

Once infected, animals harbor toxoplasmic tissue cysts for life. IgG in kittens born to chronically infected queens is transferred in colostrum and persists for 8 to 12 weeks after birth. Serologic surveys indicate that *T. gondii* infections are prevalent worldwide. Approximately 30% of cats and dogs in the United States have *T. gondii* antibodies. The prevalence of seropositivity increases with age of the cat or dog because of the chance of exposure rather than susceptibility.

Multiple serologic tests for the detection of antibodies have been used in the diagnosis of toxoplasmosis. The use of these tests in cats has been reviewed.[37] No single serologic assay exists that can definitively confirm toxoplasmosis. The magnitude of titer is not associated with severity of clinical signs. The measurement of serum antibodies in healthy cats cannot predict the oocyst-shedding period. In general, for assessing human health risk, serologic test results from healthy cats can be interpreted as follows. (1) A seronegative cat is not likely currently shedding oocysts but will likely shed oocysts if exposed; this cat poses the greatest public health risk. (2) A seropositive cat is probably not currently shedding oocysts and is less likely to shed oocysts if reexposed or immunosuppressed. It is still recommended that potential exposure to oocysts be minimized.

Because antibodies occur in the serum of both healthy and diseased cats, results of these serologic tests do not independently prove clinical toxoplasmosis. Antibodies of the IgM class are commonly detected in the serum or aqueous humor of clinically ill or FIV-infected cats, but not healthy cats, and they may be a better marker of clinical disease than IgG or IgA. *T. gondii* IgM is occasionally detected in the serum of cats with chronic or reactivated infection, and does not always correlate with recent exposure. A tentative antemortem diagnosis of clinical toxoplasmosis in dogs or cats can be based on the following combination of serology and clinical parameters: (1) serologic evidence of recent or active infection consisting of high IgM titers, or fourfold or greater, increasing or decreasing, IgG or other antibody titers (after treatment or recovery); (2) exclusion of other causes of the clinical syndrome; (3) beneficial clinical response to an anti-*Toxoplasma* drug.

Therapy

Treatment of *T. gondii* infection is indicated to decrease oocyst shedding in acutely infected cats, and to control the signs of clinical toxoplasmosis in dogs and cats.

Multiple drugs have been administered to cats to shorten the oocyst shedding period.[37] As discussed, ingestion of bradyzoites results in an enteroepithelial cycle that generally only lasts days, so duration of drug therapy can be short. The drugs most commonly available are listed in **Table 4**.

It is difficult to induce clinical toxoplasmosis in dogs or cats without concurrent immune suppression, so controlled studies on the effect of treatments are lacking. Based on studies in vitro or in other research species, clindamycin, potentiated sulfas, azithromycin, and ponazuril have activity against *T. gondii* and are relatively safe to use in dogs and cats (see **Table 4**). Clindamycin hydrochloride or a trimethoprim-sulfonamide combination has been used most frequently by one of the authors (M.L.) for the treatment of clinical toxoplasmosis in dogs and cats. Clindamycin has been used successfully for the treatment of a variety of clinical signs including fever, myositis, uveitis, and CNS disease.[52,59,69] The primary problems associated with clindamycin include gastrointestinal irritation in some animals and induction of small bowel diarrhea, possibly from changing the normal anaerobic flora of the gastrointestinal tract. However, coagulation abnormalities or *Clostridium difficile* toxins were not detected in experimentally treated cats.[70,71]

Azithromycin has been used successfully in a limited number of cats, but the optimal protocol is unknown (Lappin MR, unpublished data, 2009). Pyrimethamine combined with sulfa drugs or azithromycin is effective for the treatment of human toxoplasmosis, but commonly results in toxicity in cats.[37]

Ponazuril has been shown to inhibit *T. gondii* in vitro and to be useful for the treatment of toxoplasmosis in rodent models.[30,31] In addition, the drug was administered to a dog with a *T. gondii* associated conjunctival mass that recurred after clindamycin therapy, with no known further recurrence.[67]

Cats with systemic clinical signs of toxoplasmosis, such as fever or muscle pain combined with uveitis, should be treated with anti-*Toxoplasma* drugs in combination with topical, oral, or parenteral corticosteroids to avoid secondary lens luxations and glaucoma. *T. gondii*-seropositive cats with uveitis that are otherwise normal can be treated with topical glucocorticoids alone unless the uveitis is recurrent or persistent. In these situations, administration of a drug with anti-*T. gondii* activity may be beneficial. Some dogs and cats with CNS disease will require supportive care such as anticonvulsants.

Table 4
Drug protocols used to treat *Toxoplasma gondii* infections in dogs (D) and cats (C)

Drug	Protocol	Species
Inhibition of oocyst shedding		
Clindamycin	− 50 mg/kg, PO or IM, every 24 h for 1–12 d − 12.5–25 mg/kg, PO or IM, every 12 h for 1–2 d	C
Toltrazuril	− 5–10 mg/kg, PO, every 24 h for 2 d	C
Systemic infections		
Clindamycin	− 3–13 mg/kg, PO or IM, every 8 h for a minimum of 4 wk − 10–20 mg/kg, PO or IM, every 12 h for a minimum of 4 wk	D
Clindamycin	− 8–17 mg/kg, PO or IM, every 8 h for a minimum of 4 wk − 10–12.5 mg/kg, PO or IM, every 12 h for a minimum of 4 wk	C
Trimethoprim- sulfonamide	15 mg/kg, PO, every 12 h for a minimum of 4 wk	D, C
Azithromycin	10 mg/kg, PO, every 24 h for a minimum of 4 wk	C

PO, by mouth; IM, intramuscularly.

Clinical signs not involving the eyes or the CNS usually resolve within the first 2 to 3 days of clindamycin or trimethoprim-sulfonamide administration; ocular and CNS toxoplasmosis respond more slowly to therapy. If fever or muscle hyperesthesia is not decreasing after 3 days of treatment, other causes should be considered. Recurrence of clinical signs may be more common in cats treated for less than 4 weeks.

There is no evidence to suggest that any drug can totally clear the body of the *T. gondii*, so recurrence of clinical illness can occur in infected dogs or cats. In addition, infected dogs and cats will generally always be seropositive and so there is little clinical use in repeating serum antibody titers after the initial diagnostic workup. Administration of immunosuppressive doses of cyclosporine A (CsA) or glucocorticoids has been associated with activated toxoplasmosis in some cats. Because administration of drugs does not eliminate the organism from canine or feline tissues, whether to test patients and treat positive animals with a drug with anti-*T. gondii* activity before administering CsA or glucocorticoids is of unknown benefit. Cats experimentally infected with *T. gondii* and treated with clindamycin at 20 mg/kg by mouth for 21 days did not repeat *T. gondii* oocyst shedding when immune-suppressed with dexamethasone.[72] In contrast, some cats in the control group repeated oocyst shedding, which suggested a clindamycin effect. In another unpublished research study (Lappin MR, unpublished data, 2009), cats with activation of chronic toxoplasmosis resulting in systemic illness after administration of CsA had extremely high blood levels, reflecting the wide range of bioavailability sometimes detected in cats. These findings led to the recommendation that *T. gondii*-seropositive cats to be administered CsA should have trough levels of CsA determined approximately 2 weeks after initiating CsA. If the levels are high, the dose of CsA should be decreased immediately.

The prognosis is poor for cats and dogs with disseminated toxoplasmosis, particularly in those that are immunocompromised.[53] In some research cats with experimental intravenous *T. gondii* inoculation, administration of clindamycin had a potential paradoxic effect.[72,73]

Prevention

Preventing toxoplasmosis in dogs and cats involves measures intended to reduce the incidence of feline infections and subsequent shedding of oocysts into the environment. Kittens raised outdoors usually become infected shortly after they are weaned and begin to hunt. Cats should preferably be fed only dry or canned, commercially processed cat food. The prevalence of canine and feline toxoplasmosis has been higher in countries where raw meat products are fed to pets. Freezing or g-ray irradiation can kill tissue cysts without affecting meat quality. Household pets should be restricted from hunting and eating potential intermediate hosts or mechanical vectors, such as cockroaches, earthworms, and rodents. If meat is provided, it should always be thoroughly cooked, even if frozen before feeding. Cats should be prevented from entering buildings where food-producing animals are housed or where feed storage areas are located. At present there is no vaccine to prevent oocyst shedding or clinical disease.

Public Health Considerations

Although oocysts are key in the epidemiology of toxoplasmosis, there is no correlation between toxoplasmosis in adults and cat ownership. Most cats become infected from carnivorousness soon after weaning, and shed oocysts for only short periods (<3 weeks) thereafter. Cats found to be shedding *T. gondii* oocysts should be hospitalized for this period and treated to eliminate shedding, particularly when a pregnant woman is present in the household. To prevent inadvertent environmental contamination, cat owners should practice proper hygienic measures on a routine basis. Because infected cats rarely have diarrhea and they groom themselves regularly, direct fecal exposure from handling infected cats is unlikely. Oocysts were not detected in fur of cats that had shed large numbers of T. gondii oocysts.

Litter boxes should be changed daily, because usually at least 24 hours are necessary for oocysts to reach the infective stage. Oocyst sporulation depends on environmental temperature. Unsporulated oocysts are more susceptible to disinfection and environmental destruction; therefore, control efforts should be directed at this stage. Litter pans should be disinfected with scalding water. Cat feces should be disposed of in the septic system, incinerated, or sealed tightly in a plastic bag before placing in a sanitary landfill. Only organic litters that are biodegradable should be placed in the septic system. High-temperature composting to kill oocysts remains to be proved. Under no circumstances should litter boxes be dumped into the environment.

Oocysts survive best in warm, moist soil, a factor that helps to explain the high prevalence of disease in temperate and tropical climates. Oocysts also withstand exposure to constant freezing temperature, drying, and high environmental temperature for up to 18 months or more, especially if they are covered and out of direct sunlight. A cat's natural instinct to bury or hide its feces provides the protected environment for oocyst survival. Children's sandboxes should be covered to prevent cats from defecating in them. Mechanical vectors, such as sow bugs, earthworms, and houseflies, have been shown to contain oocysts, and cockroaches and snails are additional mechanical vectors. Control of these invertebrates will help reduce the spread of infection. Dogs that commonly roll in cat feces can be examined for their potential to act as mechanical vectors for oocysts.

Sporulated oocysts resist most disinfectants, and only 10% ammonia is effective when it is in contact with contaminated surfaces for 10 minutes. Because of the time required for chemical disinfection and the fumes produced by ammonia, immersing litter pans in boiling or scalding water usually is the easiest means of disinfection. Steam cleaning can decontaminate hard impervious surfaces.

Outbreaks of human infections have been reported when oocyst-contaminated dust particles were inhaled or ingested. Dispersion of oocysts can also occur by earth-moving or cultivating equipment, shoes, animal feet, wind, rain, and fomites. Streams can become contaminated via water runoff. Stray and wild cats have been known to contaminate streams. A report of military recruits infected by drinking oocyst-contaminated stream water in a jungle has been made. Water from streams or ponds should always be boiled before drinking. Heating utensils to 70°C for at least 10 minutes will kill oocysts.

NEOSPORA CANINUM

Neospora caninum is morphologically similar to T. gondii.[20,21,74] The tachyzoites and tissue cysts of N. caninum resemble those of T. gondii under the light microscope (see **Fig. 10**A, B). The domestic dog and the coyote (Canis latrans) are the definitive host.[75–77] As with other coccidia, herbivores likely become infected from ingesting oocysts shed by the definitive host and by subclinical congenital infection from transplacental transmission. Tachyzoites are 5 to 7 by 1 to 5 μm, depending on the stage of division (see **Fig. 10**A). The tachyzoites divide into 2 zoites by endodyogeny. In infected carnivores, tachyzoites are found within macrophages, polymorphonuclear cells, spinal fluid, and neural and other cells of the body. Individual organisms are ovoid, lunate, or globular; they contain 1 or 2 nuclei and are arranged singly, in pairs, or in groups of 4 or more. Cell necrosis occurs after rapid intracellular replication of tachyzoites. Widespread dissemination of tachyzoites to many organs may occur in the acute phases, with subsequent restriction to neural and muscular tissues in more chronically affected dogs.

Tissue cysts (up to 100 μm in diameter) are found mainly in neural cells (brain, spinal cord, peripheral nerves, and retina). Tissue cysts may be round or elongated. The cyst wall is up to 4 μm thick (see **Fig. 10**B) and encloses slender periodic acid Schiff positive bradyzoites.[20,21] Rupture of tissue cysts is associated with a granulomatous inflammatory reaction in the involved tissue. Oocysts are shed unsporulated in dog feces 5 days or later after ingesting tissue cysts, and are 10 to 14 μm in diameter (see **Fig. 10**C). Sporulation occurs outside the body. Sporulated oocysts contain 2 sporocysts, each with 4 sporozoites (see **Fig. 3**D; **Fig. 10**D).

Naturally occurring infections in dogs have been found throughout the world.[78–84] Seroprevalence of clinically healthy dogs is usually much less than 20% but much greater than the prevalence of clinical illness, suggesting subclinical infections. Purebred dogs, especially German shorthaired pointers, Labrador retrievers, boxers, golden retrievers, basset hounds, and greyhounds, have been noticeably prevalent in published case reports.[79] Experimental transmission in dogs can occur after oral (carnivorousness) and parenteral (experimental) administration, but transplacental transmission may be the predominant route in natural infections. Suppositions are that the chronically infected bitch develops parasitemia during gestation, which spreads transplacentally to the fetus. Successive litters from the same subclinically infected dam may be born infected. However, transplacental transmission alone will not be able to propagate *N. caninum* infection in nature. Most, but not all, puppies in a litter have clinical manifestations. Other pups may carry the infection subclinically, with reactivation in later life with immunosuppressive illnesses or administration of modified live virus vaccines or glucocorticoids. In contrast to toxoplasmosis, underlying immunodeficiencies or concurrent illnesses are not consistently detected in canine neosporosis. Postnatal infections may be more frequent than initially recognized.

Dogs

It is likely that many dogs diagnosed with toxoplasmosis before 1988 actually had neosporosis. In general, clinical findings in dogs are similar to those of toxoplasmosis, but neurologic deficits and muscular abnormalities predominate. Clinical signs may also include those of hepatic, pulmonary, and myocardial involvement, but any tissue can become involved. Both pups and older dogs are clinically affected, and the infections can be transmitted congenitally. The most severe and frequent infections have been in young (<6 months) dogs that presented with ascending paralysis of the limbs. In the youngest pups, signs are often noticed beginning at 3 to 9 weeks of age. Features that distinguish neosporosis from other forms of paralysis are gradual muscle atrophy and stiffness, usually as an ascending paralysis; the pelvic limbs are more severely affected than the thoracic limbs. Paralysis progresses to rigid contracture of the muscles of the affected limb. This arthrogryposis is a result of the scar formation in the muscles from lower motor neuron damage and myositis. In some pups, joint deformation and genu recurvatum may develop. Cervical weakness, dysphagia, megaesophagus, and ultimately death occur. In some dogs, the progression may become static. Dogs do not develop severe intracranial manifestations and maintain alert attitudes. Dogs can survive for months with hand feeding and care, but remain paralyzed with associated complications. Older dogs, which are less commonly affected, often have signs of multifocal CNS involvement or polymyositis; less common manifestations result from myocarditis, dermatitis, pneumonia, or multifocal dissemination. Death can occur in dogs of any age.

Experimental studies suggest that *N. caninum* can cause early fetal death, mummification, resorption, and birth of weak pups. Although abortion is a major feature of the disease in cattle, there are no reports of abortion in dogs.

Cats

Natural clinical infections have not been documented, although antibodies to *N. caninum* have been reported in domestic and wild felids.[77]

Diagnosis

Hematologic and biochemical findings have been variable, depending on the organ system of involvement. With muscle disease, creatine kinase and AST activities have been increased. Serum ALT and alkaline phosphatase activities are increased in dogs that develop hepatic inflammation. CSF abnormalities have included mild increases in protein (>20 but <150 mg/dL) and nucleated cell (>10 but <100 cells/dL) concentrations. Differential leukocyte counts included lymphocytes, monocytes and macrophages, neutrophils, and eosinophils in decreasing numbers. CSF results can be within reference limits in some dogs. Electromyographic abnormalities have consisted of spontaneous activity of fibrillation potentials, positive sharp waves, and occasional repetitive discharges. Nerve conduction velocities may be reduced in the most severely affected limbs, especially proximally, but they are often within reference range. Low evoked action potentials may be found with myositis.

Demonstrating serum antibodies to *N. caninum* can help confirm the diagnosis of neosporosis. Serum is reacted with cell-cultured *N. caninum*. Serum indirect fluorescent antibody (FA) titers can vary between laboratories; however, in one reference laboratory, values of 50 or greater are considered positive and values are often greater than 800. CSF can be tested, but titers are of lesser magnitude. Some false-positive titers exist in previously exposed dogs that may be infected, but they remain nonsymptomatic, with values of 800 or greater. Indirect FA IgG titers in most species increase 1 to 2 weeks after infection. Higher indirect FA titer values have been found in clinically versus subclinically affected dogs and in those with the longest duration of illness. However, there is no correlation between the magnitude of titer and clinical signs. There are several enzyme-linked immunosorbent assay methods to detect *N. caninum* antibodies. A direct agglutination test measuring IgG was as sensitive and specific as an indirect FA test, with the advantage of being useful in a variety of host species.

N. caninum may be found in CSF or tissue aspirates and biopsies of some dogs, and may be detected with any material used to stain blood films. Biopsy of affected muscle may yield a definitive diagnosis when organisms are detected. *N. caninum* tachyzoites are similar to *T. gondii* tachyzoites under light microscopy. Tissue cysts of *N. caninum* have thicker walls than those of *T. gondii*. *N. caninum* can be grown in cell culture and in mice. *N. caninum* must be distinguished from *T. gondii* in sections by immunochemical stains. Structural differences can also be detected with transmission electron microscopy. *T. gondii* has a thinner cyst wall, and fewer micronemes and rhoptries. The use of molecular genetics and the polymerase chain reaction to distinguish *Neospora* from other related parasites has been reviewed.

N. caninum oocysts in canine feces are rare. These oocysts are few in number and morphologically resemble oocysts of *T. gondii*, *Hammondia hammondi*, and *H. heydorni*, all of which can be present in feces of dogs.[21–23,75,85,86] Differentiation of these 4 species of coccidia in canine feces is technically difficult and needs the assistance of specialized laboratories.

Therapy

Information on effective therapy for this disease is limited.[37,68] However, drugs used as therapy for toxoplasmosis should be tried early in the course of illness. Clindamycin, sulfadiazine, and pyrimethamine alone or in combination have been administered to treat canine neosporosis.[37] However, clinical improvement is not likely in the presence of muscle contracture or rapidly advancing paralysis. To reduce the chance of illness, all dogs in an affected litter should be treated as soon as the diagnosis is made in one littermate.[81–83] Older (>16 weeks) puppies and adult dogs respond better to treatment. In adult dogs with acute lower motor neuron paralysis from myositis, dysfunction is often more amenable to early treatment because scar contracture is less common. There is no known therapy to prevent a bitch from transmitting infection to her pups.

In dogs, *N. caninum* can be transmitted repeatedly through successive litters and litters of their progeny. This fact should be considered when planning the breeding of *Neospora*-infected bitches. Dogs should not be fed uncooked meat, especially beef. There is no vaccine to combat neosporosis. No drugs are known to prevent transplacental transmission. At present there is no evidence that *N. caninum* infection is zoonotic.

SUMMARY

In conclusion, much needs to be learned concerning the pathogenesis of clinical coccidiosis in dogs. Why coccidiosis occurs after shipping is unknown, and nothing is known of biologic differences among isolates of *Isospora* species of dogs and cats. Transmission of *Isospora felis* in cats in breeding colonies despite very strict hygiene remains an enigma. Prevention of transmission of *T. gondii* oocysts from cat feces to pregnant women, marine mammals, and other endangered animals is a problem. Transmission of *N. caninum* in nature is still not fully known because dogs shed only a few oocysts.

REFERENCES

1. Levine ND. Protozoan parasites of domestic animals and of man. Minneapolis (MN): Minnesota: Burgess; 1973. 1–406.
2. Dubey JP. The evolution of the knowledge of cat and dog coccidia. Parasitology doi:10.1017/S003118200900585X.
3. Shah HL. The life cycle of *Isospora felis* Wenyon, 1923, a coccidium of the cat. J Protozool 1971;18:3–17.
4. Frenkel JK, Dubey JP. Rodents as vectors for feline coccidia, *Isospora felis* and *Isospora rivolta*. J Infect Dis 1972;125:69–72.
5. Dubey JP, Frenkel JK. Extra-intestinal stages of *Isospora felis* and *I. rivolta* (Protozoa: Eimeriidae) in cats. J Protozool 1972;19:89–92.
6. Dubey JP. Life cycle of *Isospora rivolta* (Grassi, 1879) in cats and mice. J Protozool 1979;26:433–43.
7. Dubey JP, Sreekumar C. Redescription of *Hammondia hammondi* and its differentiation from *Toxoplasma gondii*. Int J Parasitol 2003;33:1437–53.
8. Dubey JP. Toxoplasmosis of animals and humans. 2nd edition. Boco Raton (FL): CRC Press; in press.
9. Frenkel JK, Dubey JP. *Hammondia hammondi* gen. nov., sp.nov., from domestic cats, a new coccidian related to *Toxoplasma* and *Sarcocystis*. Z Parasitenkd 1975;46:3–12.
10. Frenkel JK. *Besnoitia wallacei* of cats and rodents: with a reclassification of other cyst-forming isosporoid coccidia. J Parasitol 1977;63:611–28.

11. Dubey JP, Lindsay DS, Rosenthal BM, et al. Establishment of *Besnoitia darlingi* from opossums (*Didelphis virginiana*) in experimental intermediate and definitive hosts, propagation in cell culture, and description of ultrastructural and genetic characteristics. Int J Parasitol 2002;32:1053–64.

12. Dubey JP, Sreekumar C, Lindsay DS, et al. *Besnoitia oryctofelisi* n. sp. (Protozoa: Apicomplexa) from domestic rabbits. Parasitology 2003;126:521–39.

13. Dubey JP, Speer CA, Fayer R. Sarcocystosis of animals and man. Boca Raton (FL): CRC Press; 1989. p.1–215.

14. Lepp DL, Todd KS. Life cycle of *Isospora canis* Neméséri, 1959 in the dog. J Protozool 1974;21:199–206.

15. Mitchell SM, Zajac AM, Charles S, et al. *Cystoisospora canis* Neméséri, 1959 (syn. *Isospora canis*), infections in dogs: clinical signs, pathogenesis, and reproducible clinical disease in beagle dogs fed oocysts. J Parasitol 2007;93: 345–52.

16. Dubey JP. *Isospora ohioensis* sp. n. proposed for *I. rivolta* of the dog. J Parasitol 1975;61:462–5.

17. Dubey JP, Mahrt JL. *Isospora neorivolta* sp. n. from the domestic dog. J Parasitol 1978;64:1067–73.

18. Trayser CV, Todd KS. Life cycle of *Isospora burrowsi* n sp (Protozoa: Eimeriidae) from the dog *Canis familiaris*. Am J Vet Res 1978;39:95–8.

19. Rommel M, Zielasko B. Untersuchungen über den Lebenszyklus von *Isospora burrowsi* (Trayser und Todd, 1978) aus dem Hund [Investigations into the life cycle of *Isospora burrows*; [Trayser and Todd, 1978] of the dog]. Berl Münch Tierärztl Wochenschr 1981;94:87–90 [in German].

20. Dubey JP, Carpenter JL, Speer CA, et al. Newly recognized fatal protozoan disease of dogs. J Am Vet Med Assoc 1988;192:1269–85.

21. Dubey JP, Barr BC, Barta JR, et al. Redescription of *Neospora caninum* and its differentiation from related coccidia. Int J Parasitol 2002;32:929–46.

22. Slapeta JR, Koudela B, Votypka J, et al. Coprodiagnosis of *Hammondia heydorni* in dogs by PCR based amplification of ITS 1 rRNA: differentiation from morphologically indistinguishable oocysts of *Neospora caninum*. Vet J 2002;163:147–54.

23. Sreekumar C, Hill DE, Fournet VM, et al. Detection of *Hammondia heydorni*-like organisms and their differentiation from *Neospora caninum* using random-amplified polymorphic DNA-polymerase chain reaction. J Parasitol 2003;89:1082–5.

24. Dubey JP, Greene CE. Enteric coccidiosis. In: Greene CE, editor. Infectious diseases of the dog and cat. 3rd edition. St Louis (MO): Saunders Elsevier; 2006. p. 775–84.

25. Kirkpatrick CE, Dubey JP. Enteric coccidial infections. *Isospora, Sarcocystis, Cryptosporidium, Besnoitia* and *Hammondia*. Vet Clin North Am Small Anim Pract 1987;17:1405–20.

26. Oduye OO, Bobade PA. Studies on an outbreak of intestinal coccidiosis in the dog. J Small Anim Pract 1979;20:181–4.

27. Olson ME. Coccidiosis caused by *Isospora ohioensis*-like organisms in three dogs. Can Vet J 1985;26:112–4.

28. Trepanier LA. Idiosyncratic toxicity associated with potentiated sulfonamides in the dog. J Vet Pharmacol Ther 2004;27:129–38.

29. Twedt D, Diehl KJ, Lappin MR, et al. Association of hepatic necrosis with trimethoprim sulfonamide administration in 4 dogs. J Vet Intern Med 1997;11:20–3.

30. Mitchell SM, Zajac AM, Davis WL, et al. Efficacy of ponazuril in vitro and in preventing and treating *Toxoplasma gondii* infections in mice. J Parasitol 2004;90: 639–42.

31. Mitchell SM, Zajac AM, Kennedy T, et al. Prevention of recrudescent toxoplasmic encephalitis using ponazuril in an immunodeficient mouse model. J Eukaryot Microbiol 2006;53:S164–5.
32. Lloyd S, Smith J. Activity of toltrazuril and diclazuril against *Isospora* species in kittens and puppies. Vet Rec 2001;148:509–11.
33. Reinemeyer CR, Lindsay DS, Mitchell SM, et al. Development of experimental *Cystoisospora canis* infection models in beagle puppies and efficacy evaluation of 5% ponazuril (toltrazuril sulfone) oral suspension. Parasitol Res 2007;101: S129–36.
34. Daugschies A, Mundt HC, Letkova V. Toltrazuril treatment of cystoisosporosis in dogs under experimental and field conditions. Parasitol Res 2000;86:797–9.
35. Charles SD, Chopade HM, Ciszewski DK, et al. Safety of 5% ponazuril (toltrazuril sulfone) oral suspension and efficacy against naturally acquired *Cystoisospora ohioensis*-like infection in beagle puppies. Parasitol Res 2007;101:S137–44.
36. Dubey JP, Beattie CP. Toxoplasmosis of animals and man. Boca Raton (FL):CRC Press; 1988. p. 1–220.
37. Dubey JP, Lappin MR. Toxoplasmosis and neosporosis. In: Greene CE, editor. Infectious diseases of the dog and cat. 3rd edition. St Louis (MO): Saunders Elsevier; 2006. p. 754–75.
38. Frenkel JK, Lindsay DS, Parker BB. Dogs as potential mechanical vectors of *Toxoplasma gondii*. Am J Trop Med Hyg 1995;53:226.
39. Schares G, Pantchev N, Barutzki D, et al. Oocysts of *Neospora caninum*, *Hammondia heydorni*, *Toxoplasma gondii* and *Hammondia hammondi* in faeces collected from dogs in Germany. Int J Parasitol 2005;35:1525–37.
40. Dubey JP, Lappin MR, Kwok OCH, et al. Seroprevalence of Toxoplasma gondii and concurrent Bartonella spp., feline immunodeficiency virus, and feline leukemia infections in cats from Grenada, West Indies. J Parasitol 2009 [Epub ahead of print].
41. Dubey JP, Carpenter JL. Neonatal toxoplasmosis in littermate cats. J Am Vet Med Assoc 1993;203:1546–9.
42. Dubey JP, Carpenter JL. Histologically confirmed clinical toxoplasmosis in cats— 100 cases (1952–1990). J Am Vet Med Assoc 1993;203:1556–66.
43. Bernsteen L, Gregory CR, Aronson LR, et al. Acute toxoplasmosis following renal transplantation in three cats and a dog. J Am Vet Med Assoc 1999;215:1123–6.
44. Brownlee L, Sellon RK. Diagnosis of naturally occurring toxoplasmosis by bronchoalveolar lavage in a cat. J Am Anim Hosp Assoc 2001;37:251–5.
45. Dubey JP, Zajac A, Osofsky SA, et al. Acute primary toxoplasmic hepatitis in an adult cat shedding *Toxoplasma gondii* oocysts. J Am Vet Med Assoc 1990;197:1616–8.
46. Duncan RB, Lindsay DS, Chickering WR, et al. Acute primary toxoplasmic pancreatitis in a cat. Feline Pract 2000;28:6–8.
47. Foster SF, Charles JA, Canfield PJ, et al. Reactivated toxoplasmosis in a FIV-positive cat. Aust Vet Pract 1998;28:159–63.
48. Heidel JR, Dubey JP, Blythe LL, et al. Myelitis in a cat infected with *Toxoplasma gondii* and feline immunodeficiency virus. J Am Vet Med Assoc 1990;196:316–8.
49. Henriksen P, Dietz HH, Henriksen SA. Fatal toxoplasmosis in five cats. Vet Parasitol 1994;55:15–20.
50. Järplid B, Feldman BF. Large granular lymphoma with toxoplasmosis in a cat. Comp Haematol Int 1993;3:241–3.
51. Little L, Shokek A, Dubey JP, et al. *Toxoplasma gondii*-like organisms in skin aspirates from a cat with disseminated protozoal infection. Vet Clin Pathol 2005;34: 156–60.

52. Lappin MR, Greene CE, Winston S, et al. Clinical feline toxoplasmosis. Serologic diagnosis and therapeutic management of 15 cases. J Vet Intern Med 1989;3: 139–43.
53. Nordquist BC, Aronson LR. Pyogranulomatous cystitis associated with *Toxoplasma gondii* infection in a cat after renal transplantation. J Am Vet Med Assoc 2008;232:1010–2.
54. Park CH, Ikadai H, Yoshida E, et al. Cutaneous toxoplasmosis in a female Japanese cat. Vet Pathol 2007;44:683–7.
55. Peterson JL, Willard MD, Lees GE, et al. Toxoplasmosis in two cats with inflammatory intestinal disease. J Am Vet Med Assoc 1991;199:473–6.
56. Sardinas JC, Chastain CB, Collins BK, et al. *Toxoplasma* pneumonia in a cat with incongruous serological test results. J Small Anim Pract 1994;35:104–7.
57. Thompson J. Toxoplasmosis in dogs and cats in New Zealand. Surveillance 1993; 20:36–8.
58. Singh M, Foster DJ, Child G, et al. Inflammatory cerebrospinal fluid analysis in cats: clinical diagnosis and outcome. J Feline Med Surg 2005;7:77–93.
59. Falzone C, Baroni M, De Lorenzi D, et al. *Toxoplasma gondii* brain granuloma in a cat: diagnosis using cytology from an intraoperative sample and sequential magnetic resonance imaging. J Small Anim Pract 2008;49:95–9.
60. Anfray P, Bonetti C, Fabbrini F, et al. Feline cutaneous toxoplasmosis: a case report. Vet Dermatol 2005;16:131–6.
61. Reppas GP, Dockett AG, Burrell DH. Anorexia and an abdominal mass in a cat. Aust Vet J 1999;77:784–90.
62. Dubey JP, Carpenter JL, Topper MJ, et al. Fatal toxoplasmosis in dogs. J Am Anim Hosp Assoc 1989;25:659–64
63. Dubey JP, Chapman JL, Rosenthal BM, et al. Clinical *Sarcocystis neurona*, *Toxoplasma gondii*, and *Neospora caninum* infections in dogs. Vet Parasitol 2006;137:36–49.
64. Ehrensperger F, Pospischil A. Spontane Mischinfektionen mit Staupevirus und Toxoplasmen beim Hund [Canine concurrent infection with distemper virus and *Toxoplasma* spec]. Dtsch Tierarztl Wochenschr 1989;96:184–6 [in German].
65. Rhyan J, Dubey JP. Toxoplasmosis in an adult dog with hepatic necrosis and associated tissue cysts and tachyzoites. Cancer Pract 1992;17:6–10.
66. van Ham L. Een geval van *Toxoplasma* encefalitis bij de hond [A case of Toxoplasma enoephalitis in the dog]. Vlaams Diergeneesk Tijdsch 1991;60:149–52 [in Dutch].
67. Swinger RL, Schmidt KA, Dubielzig RR. Keratoconjunctivitis associated with *Toxoplasma gondii* in a dog. Vet Ophthalmol 2009;12:56–60.
68. Jones JL, Dubey JP. Waterborne toxoplasmosis - recent developments. Exp Parasitol DOI:10.1016/j.exppara.2009.03.013.
69. Greene CE, Cook JR, Mahaffey EA. Clindamycin for treatment of *Toxoplasma* polymyositis in a dog. J Am Vet Med Assoc 1985;187:631–4.
70. Greene CE, Lappin MR, Marks A. Effect of clindamycin on clinical, hematologic, and biochemical parameters in healthy cats. J Am Anim Hosp Assoc 1993;28: 323–6.
71. Jacobs G, Lappin MR, Marks A, et al. Effect of clindamycin on feline factor-VII activity. Am J Vet Res 1989;50:393–5.
72. Malmasi A, Mosallaneiad B, Mohebali M, et al. Prevention of shedding and re-shedding of *Toxoplasma gondii* oocysts in experimentally infected cats treated with oral clindamycin: a preliminary study. Zoonoses Public Health 2009;56: 102–4.

73. Davidson MG, Lappin MR, Rottman JR, et al. Paradoxical effect of clindamycin in experimental, acute toxoplasmosis in cats. Antimicrob Agents Chemother 1996; 40:1352–9.
74. Dubey JP, Lindsay DS. A review of *Neospora caninum* and neosporosis. Vet Parasitol 1996;67:1–59.
75. McAllister MM, Dubey JP, Lindsay DS, et al. Dogs are definitive hosts of *Neospora caninum*. Int J Parasitol 1998;28:1473–8.
76. Gondim LFP, McAllister MM, Pitt WC, et al. Coyotes (*Canis latrans*) are definitive hosts of *Neospora caninum*. Int J Parasitol 2004;34:159–61.
77. Dubey JP, Schares G, Ortega-Mora LM. Epidemiology and control of neosporosis and *Neospora caninum*. Clin Microbiol Rev 2007;20:323–67.
78. Patitucci AN, Alley MR, Jones BR, et al. Protozoal encephalomyelitis of dogs involving *Neospora caninum* and *Toxoplasma gondii* in New Zealand. N Z Vet J 1997;45:231–5.
79. Lindsay DS, Dubey JP. Canine neosporosis. Vet Parasitol 2000;14:1–11.
80. Dubey JP. Review of *Neospora caninum* and neosporosis in animals. Korean J Parasitol 2003;41:1–16.
81. Dubey JP, Sreekumar C, Knickman E, et al. Biologic, morphologic, and molecular characterization of *Neospora caninum* isolates from littermate dogs. Int J Parasitol 2004;34:1157–67.
82. Dubey JP, Knickman E, Greene CE. Neonatal *Neospora caninum* infections in dogs. Acta Parasitol 2005;50:176–9.
83. Dubey JP, Vianna MCB, Kwok OCH, et al. Neosporosis in beagle dogs: clinical signs, diagnosis, treatment, isolation and genetic characterization of *Neospora caninum*. Vet Parasitol 2007;149:158–66.
84. Reichel MP, Ellis JT, Dubey JP. Neosporosis and hammondiosis in dogs. J Small Anim Pract 2007;48:308–12.
85. Schares G, Vrhovec MV, Pantchev N, et al. Occurrence of *Toxoplasma gondii* and *Hammondia hammondi* oocysts in the faeces of cats from Germany and other European countries. Vet Parasitol 2008;152:34–45.
86. Monteiro RM, Pena HFJ, Gennari SM, et al. Differential diagnosis of oocysts of *Hammondia*-like organisms of dogs and cats by PCR-RFLP analysis of 70-kilodalton heat shock protein (HSP70) gene. Parasitol Res 2008;103:235–8.

Canine Hepatozoonosis and Babesiosis, and Feline Cytauxzoonosis

Patricia J. Holman, PhD, Karen F. Snowden, DVM, PhD*

KEYWORDS

• Parasite • Protozoa • Apicomplexa • Hemoprotozoa
• Tick-borne disease

The apicomplexan protozoans of the genera *Hepatozoon*, *Babesia*, and *Cytauxzoon* are emerging parasite pathogens that are increasingly diagnosed in the pet population. These pathogens are intracellular organisms found in blood that are transmitted by ticks. All of these blood parasites may cause serious, sometimes fatal infections.

AMERICAN CANINE HEPATOZOONOSIS
History and Epidemiology

The genus *Hepatozoon* contains more than 300 species, and canine infections with the parasite *Hepatozoon canis* have been described in dogs on several continents including Europe, the Middle East, Southeast Asia, Africa, and South America since the early 1900s.[1] *Hepatozoon* infections were first detected in dogs in Texas in 1978, and were initially identified as *H canis*.[2] As more clinical cases were characterized, it became evident that the canine parasites in the United States caused more severe, often fatal disease when compared with the clinical presentation of infected dogs in other countries. Based on a variety of clinical, molecular, and immunologic analyses, the etiologic agent causing this disease syndrome in the United States was given the new species name *Hepatozoon americanum* in 1997.[3,4] To date, this species has only been reported in North America. Note that the parasite nomenclature in scientific literature may be confusing in reports published between 1978 and 1997 because the scientific name of *H canis* was used for the North American parasite before naming the new species.

During the last 30 years, hepatozoonosis has been diagnosed in dogs in an expanding range across the southeastern United States, extending from Texas and Oklahoma through the Gulf Coast states, to Georgia and Florida on the east coast.[5,6] The increasing prevalence of canine cases in this geographic region correlates well with the expanding distribution of the Gulf Coast tick vector, *Amblyomma maculatum*.[1]

Department of Veterinary Pathobiology, College of Veterinary Medicine, Mailstop 4467, Texas A&M University, College Station, TX 77843-4467, USA
* Corresponding author.
E-mail address: ksnowden@cvm.tamu.edu (K.F. Snowden).

Vet Clin Small Anim 39 (2009) 1035–1053
doi:10.1016/j.cvsm.2009.08.002
0195-5616/09/$ – see front matter © 2009 Elsevier Inc. All rights reserved.

vetsmall.theclinics.com

In 2 recent surveys, a small number of molecular sequences produced from infected canine blood showed close similarity with sequences from *H canis* as well as *H americanum*, suggesting that both species of parasites may be endemic in the United States.[7,8] Further research is needed to confirm and clarify these findings.

Life Cycle and Transmission

Because sexual reproduction of the parasite occurs in the tick, *A maculatum* is considered the definitive host, with the carnivore host serving as the intermediate host where asexual multiplication takes place. Nymphal ticks become infected with *Hepatozoon* gamonts from the infected canine leukocytes. In about 6 weeks, several hundred infective sporozoites develop in sporocysts inside oocysts in the tick hemocoele as it molts to the adult stage.[6] Larval ticks have also been shown to harbor the *H americanum* organisms, making nymphal stage ticks also capable of transmitting the infection to dogs.[4]

The transmission of this parasite from tick to dog differs from most tick-transmitted infections. Because parasites are not located in the mouthparts of the tick, a dog must ingest the tick to become infected. Sporozoites from oocysts in the tick are released in the dog gastrointestinal tract, enter circulation, and are transported to striated muscle where the parasite develops within phagocytic host cells between the myocytes. Parasites develop into "onion-skin" cysts whose appearance is caused by layers of mucopolysaccharide around the organism (**Fig. 1**A). Parasites multiply asexually by merogony, and merozoites are released into surrounding tissues, triggering a severe localized inflammatory reaction. The lesion is characterized histologically by large numbers of neutrophils as well as macrophages in the granulomas (See **Fig. 1**A), which typically develop within about 1 month of infection.[1] Within about 4 weeks, parasite-infected leukocytes, primarily neutrophils, similarly may be detected in peripheral blood (**Fig. 1**B).[1]

Some *Hepatozoon* spp can be transmitted through predation and ingestion of tissue cysts found in intermediate host tissues; however, this route of transmission has not yet been proven for *H americanum*.[4] Vertical transmission of the *H canis* parasite from bitch to pup has been reported, but this route has not been demonstrated yet for *H americanum*.[9]

Because of the severity of the clinical disease, it has been suggested that the parasite is poorly adapted to the dog, and that it is likely that *H americanum* is a natural parasite of one or more other hosts.[5] The parasite has been identified in naturally

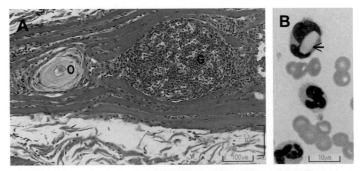

Fig. 1. The tissue and blood stages of *Hepatozoon americanum*. (*A*) A large onion-skin cyst (O) and a neutrophilic granuloma (G) are identified in canine skeletal muscle (hematoxylin-eosin [H&E] stain). (*B*) An intracellular gamont (*arrow*) is in the cytoplasm of a neutrophil in canine peripheral blood (Giemsa stain, original magnification ×1000).

infected coyotes, and has been transmitted between dogs and coyotes through experimentally infected *A maculatum* ticks.[10] *H americanum* or a similar parasite has also been identified in bobcats and ocelots.[11] In a recent study, cotton rats (*Sigmodon hispidus*) and mice (*Mus musculus*) were experimentally infected with *H americanum*, suggesting that rodents could serve as alternative hosts or reservoirs for the parasite.[12] The role of coyotes and other possible wildlife hosts as reservoirs for this infection deserves further investigation.

Diagnosis

Clinical findings
In contrast to the milder disease caused by *H canis*, *H americanum* causes debilitating, usually fatal disease. The most commonly reported clinical signs include stiffness, lameness, reluctance to move, weight loss, and muscle atrophy over time.[1] Hyperesthesia as well as bone and muscle pain reflect the myositis and granulomatous inflammation caused by the parasites in skeletal and cardiac muscle. Fluctuating fevers may be high, and depression can be noted beginning 3 to 5 weeks after infection. Limb edema and periosteal bone proliferation may occur in severe cases. Purulent ocular discharge has also been reported often, sometimes accompanied by decreased tear production. Polyuria and polydipsia associated with secondary glomerulonephritis or renal amyloidosis are reported less frequently.

The severity of clinical signs may wax and wane over time, but untreated dogs usually survive for less that 12 months.[4] However, a persistent infection lasting for 5.5 years has been reported in a single naturally infected dog.[13]

Laboratory findings
The most common hematologic abnormality is a marked leukocytosis and neutrophilia, ranging as high as 200,000 cells/μL.[5] A mild normocytic, normochromic, nonregenerative anemia is also a frequent finding. Platelet counts are usually normal to slightly elevated. If thrombocytopenia is a clinical finding, then concurrent infection with other tick-borne diseases such as ehrlichiosis or babesiosis may be present. Serum chemistry abnormalities are common, including mild elevations in alkaline phosphatase and hypoalbuminemia.[6] Hypoglycemia is also commonly noted, but that finding is an artifact caused by the metabolism of glucose by the high numbers of leukocytes if there is some time lapse between blood collection and performance of the test.[6] Proteinuria is sometimes noted on urinalysis in dogs that develop glomerulonephritis or amyloidosis.

Radiographic findings
Because periosteal bone proliferation is common, lesions that are suggestive of hepatozoonosis can be visualized radiographically. Symmetric lesions range from subtle bone irregularity to smooth lamina thickening, similar to hypertrophic osteopathy.[14] Bony lesions involve long bones most frequently, but periosteal proliferation may also be seen in flat bones such as the pelvis or in vertebrae. In bone scintigraphic studies of experimentally infected dogs, bone lesions occurred within 2 months, with some lesions evident as early as 35 days post infection.[14] The pathogenesis of these bony changes is unclear, but it has been suggested that inflammation stimulated by the parasites causes an increase in the production of specific cytokines that stimulate osteoblastic activity.[14]

Organism identification
The gamont stage of *H americanum* may be observed infrequently in Romanowski-type stained blood films of infected dogs. Blood films should be made promptly

when the blood is collected because parasites may exit cells rapidly.[6] The organisms appear as pale blue to clear oblong structures in the cytoplasm of neutrophils or monocytes (See **Fig. 1**B).[6] Parasitemias are extremely low, so examining buffy coat smears may increase the likelihood of visualizing this stage of the parasite in leukocytes from the peripheral blood. Various special stains have been suggested to enhance parasite detection.[15] Visualization of intracellular parasites provides a definitive diagnosis, but examination of blood films is unreliable, and can be frustrating due to the low number of circulating parasites.

A more rewarding diagnostic approach is skeletal muscle biopsies that demonstrate the parasite and provide a definitive diagnosis. Biopsy samples from the biceps femoris or semitendinosus muscle are frequently collected, although epaxial or other muscles may also be sampled.[6] Histopathologic findings may include the onion-skin cysts, meronts, or granulomas that are frequently neutrophilic (See **Fig. 1**A). A more generalized or multifocal myositis without parasites is also a common finding.

Other diagnostic tests

Although an enzyme-linked immunosorbent assay based antibody detection assay has been described in the scientific literature, immunodiagnostic tests for *H american-um* are not available on a fee-for-service basis.[16] Molecular diagnostic tests using the polymerase chain reaction (PCR) or quantitative PCR to detect *Hepatozoon* spp in canine blood have been reported in the research literature from Europe, South America, and the United States, but no DNA-based tests are currently available in the United States on a fee-for-service basis.[8,17,18]

Treatment

To date, treatment is frustrating because no therapeutic regimen has been successful in curing the parasite infection. Several regimens using combinations of drugs have been suggested for their palliative effects in improving the clinical status of the dog. Short-term use of nonsteroidal anti-inflammatory drugs at standard dosages has been used to provide relief from fever and muscle pain in acute, severe cases.[5] Several weeks of antiparasitic treatments using a combination of trimethoprim-sulfadiazine (Tribrissen), clindamycin (Antirobe, Cleocin), and pyrimethamine (Daraprim) have proven useful in causing remission of clinical disease, although relapses are frequently reported within a few months.[19] Similar results were reported in a small number of dogs treated with the antiprotozoal drug toltrazuril (Baycox), with animals showing a rapid remission of clinical disease, but subsequent relapses.[19]

Dogs respond to a repeated therapeutic regimen during relapses, but the time intervals between relapses typically become shorter in chronic infections. To prevent these relapses, the use of continuous daily treatment with the livestock anticoccidial agent decoquinate (Decoxx) has been encouraging.[5] Dogs that receive twice-daily doses of decoquinate with food have fewer relapses, and those episodes are less severe than in dogs not receiving the treatment.

Control and Prevention

Because the only proven route of transmission for *H americanum* is through *A maculatum*, effective tick vector control on the dog and in the local environment is essential. Note that tick attachment and feeding are not required because dogs become infected through ingestion of the infected tick. Therefore it is important to keep the dog from ingesting ticks while grooming or while scavenging tick-infested prey. The use of some small-volume topical acaricides or amitraz-impregnated collars may be helpful in repelling ticks.

CANINE BABESIOSIS
Introduction

Canine babesiosis is a tick-borne protozoal disease of dogs that may be caused by several distinct members of the apicomplexan family Babesiidae. Pathogenesis and clinical signs of the disease are variable and are influenced by the immune status of the host as well as the species or subspecies of the infecting parasite. *Babesia* spp are capable of producing acute, febrile, and sometimes fatal infections, or the infection may be mild or subclinical. After initial infection, the animal may become a chronic carrier.

Natural infections of *Babesia* spp are transmitted to the dog during feeding by Ixodid vector ticks carrying the protozoan parasite. Dogs may also acquire *Babesia* by blood-to-blood transfer as a result of transfusion of infected blood, skirmish with an infected dog, or mechanical transmission. Vertical transmission from infected dam to offspring may occur.

There are currently 4 known agents of canine babesiosis in the United States. At present, *Babesia gibsoni* is most frequently diagnosed and is distinguished from *Babesia canis vogeli* by its generally smaller size, pleomorphism, and lack of paired piroplasms in the canine red blood cell (**Fig. 2**A). Probably the most familiar of these agents is *B. c. vogeli*, which is distinguished by large paired intraerythrocytic piroplasms (**Fig. 2**B). Two more recently identified species that can cause this disease are: (1) *Babesia conradae*, which has morphologic similarities to *B gibsoni* and to date has only been identified in dogs in California; and (2) the North Carolina *Babesia* sp (**Fig. 2**C), an as yet unnamed piroplasm morphologically similar to *B canis*, identified first in North Carolina and recently diagnosed in a case in Texas.[20–22] It is possible that these newly recognized species are more widespread than is currently realized. If diagnosis is based on morphology, the close similarities between the 2 small piroplasms, *B gibsoni* and *B conradae*, and between the 2 large piroplasms, *B canis* and the North Carolina *Babesia* sp, may lead to misidentification. With the increasing reliance on diagnosis by molecular methods, the distribution of these parasites will be clarified.

Life Cycle and Transmission

The *Babesia* life cycle includes a tick stage and a mammalian host stage. *Babesia* sp-parasitized erythrocytes are taken up by the vector tick while feeding on an infected

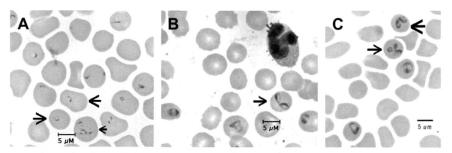

Fig. 2. Blood stage canine *Babesia* spp. (*A*) *Babesia gibsoni* is characterized by ring and small oval piroplasm forms (*arrows*). Other forms including piroplasms with stringy cytoplasm (*small arrow*) occur. (*B*) *Babesia canis* intraerythrocytic paired large piroplasms (*arrow*) distinguish this from the small piroplasm species. (*C*) The North Carolina *Babesia* sp paired piroplasm form (*large arrow*) and a dividing parasite (*small arrow*) are indicated. Single forms of both species are also evident (*B, C*). *Babesia canis* (*B*) and the North Carolina *Babesia* sp (*C*) are morphologically indistinguishable under light microscopy (Giemsa stain, original magnification ×1000).

animal. Within the tick gut, the parasites undergo gamogony. The resulting zygotes develop into kinetes that migrate to different tissues where they undergo multiplication. Kinetes in the salivary glands undergo sporogony, during which development to infective sporozoites requires a molt to the next tick stage. After molting, the tick introduces these infective sporozoites to its next host animal during feeding. This form of transmission is termed transstadial transmission. Transovarial transmission occurs when the kinetes migrate to the tick ovaries and invade the developing eggs. After the eggs are laid, the emerging larval ticks are carrying the parasite. Depending on the *Babesia* species and the vector tick, in some cases the larval stage ticks transmit the *Babesia,* and in others, the tick must molt to the nymphal stage before *Babesia* infection of the mammalian host may occur.[23] Tick species that transmit *Babesia* transovarily are able to carry the protozoan through successive generations, even in the absence of feeding on another infected host. Thus, tick control is extremely important in preventing infection and disease in such situations.

Characterization of Each Species

Babesia gibsoni

Babesia gibsoni, endemic in Asia, the Middle East, and Africa, was regarded as an exotic parasite when first recognized in the United States in 1969 in an imported Malaysian dog.[24] In 1979 the first domestically acquired case was described with the source of infection unclear.[25] A subsequent study of babesiosis in army dogs suggests that the parasite was introduced from Japan.[26] Since that first domestic case, *B gibsoni* has been reported in dogs from more than 29 states.[27,28] Phylogenetic studies have confirmed that *B gibsoni* in the United States, variably referred to as Oklahoma, Okinawa, or Asian strains, is the same as Asian *B gibsoni*.[28,29] It must be noted that a study indicating that the United States isolate is different from the Asian genotype *B gibsoni* [30] was, in fact, making the comparison with *B conradae* (see later discussion), which was later corrected.[31] In the United States, *B gibsoni* Asian genotype is considered less pathogenic than *B conradae*.[32]

B gibsoni is now considered a rapidly emerging pathogen in the United States and is the most commonly diagnosed cause of canine babesiosis.[27,33] Although predominantly reported in the southeastern states, *B gibsoni* is also identified in the 6 westernmost states, and in Indiana, Michigan, West Virginia, Missouri, Oklahoma, and Texas (Patricia Holman, PhD, unpublished findings, 2007).[27,34–39] It is particularly recognized as a growing problem in American Pit Bull and American Staffordshire terrier breeds.[27,36,39] Of note, the Tosa dog (Japanese Mastiff), commonly used in dog fighting in the Aomori Prefecture, Japan, also has a high incidence of *B gibsoni* infection.[40] The Tosa dog breed arose from selective mating of several breeds including the American Pit Bull Terrier.

B gibsoni is transstadially transmitted by *Haemaphysalis* and *Rhipicephalus* ticks outside North America,[41–43] but at this time the vector tick in the United States remains unidentified. Both *Rhipicephalus sanguineus* and *Dermacentor variabilis* are considered possible vectors, but vector competence has not been proven for either tick species. It should be noted that one report[44] suggesting that *R sanguineus* may be the vector of *B gibsoni* was based on studies of *B conradae*, the California small piroplasm of dogs discussed later.[31] To date this tick has not been shown to transmit *B gibsoni* in the United States. It also should be noted that the 2 *Haemaphysalis* species, *H longicornis* and *H bispinosa*, known to vector *B gibsoni* abroad are not indigenous to the United States. Due to the lack of a known tick vector in the United States, the mode of transmission of *B gibsoni* to dogs has been a subject of speculation.[27,37,38] Although the role of the tick in the biology of *Babesia* is well recognized (natural transmission of *Babesia* species requires a tick vector and *Babesia* gameto-genesis occurs in the vector tick), reports of infected dogs in the absence of tick infestation question the role of ticks in transmission of *B gibsoni* in the United States.

Alternative modes of transmission include direct blood transfer via transfusion, mechanically (ie, contaminated hypodermic needle) or fighting, or by vertical transmission from dam to offspring. Vertical transmission of *B gibsoni* has long been suspected due to disease reported in puppies too young to accommodate transmission by ticks, and transplacental transmission was recently experimentally documented.[45] Transfusion acquired cases have been reported, and there is much circumstantial evidence supporting transmission by direct blood transfer during playing or fighting.[36,37,39,46] In fact, *B gibsoni* infection as a result of skirmish is thought to be an important mode of transmission in the United States, where the majority of dogs reported with *B gibsoni* are American Pit Bull or American Staffordshire terriers, 2 breeds with well-recognized interactive aggressive tendencies.

Clinical signs of babesiosis due to *B gibsoni* often include fever, depression, anorexia, splenomegaly, hemolytic anemia, and thrombocytopenia, and may lead to an incorrect diagnosis of idiopathic or immune-mediated hemolytic anemia.[27,33,35,47] Thus, babesia infection should be ruled out before beginning immunosuppressive therapy. Thrombocytopenia is a primary pathologic change in clinical *B gibsoni* infections.[33,36,48] Low hematocrit and hemoglobin values, granulocytosis, and hypoalbuminemia, and elevated alkaline phosphatase, alanine aminotransferase, γ-glutamyltransferase, and bilirubin serum biochemistry values are frequently seen.[35,37] A positive Coombs test is common.[26,47] Puppies are more severely affected than immune competent adult dogs, and subclinical infections in adult dogs are not uncommon.[35,46] However, fatal babesiosis in adults may occur.[37] Survivors may remain carriers of *B gibsoni* for life, and owners should be counseled as to appropriate animal management practices and tick control measures to avoid transmission of the pathogen to other dogs.

Babesia conradae

Babesia conradae is a newly named small piroplasm of dogs.[20] A recent review recaps earlier work on this organism and makes the point that during the time of those studies, the organism was thought to be *B gibsoni*.[31] Thus, this parasite will be listed as *B gibsoni* in most of the references cited herein, but will be referred to as *B conradae* in the text that follows. This name distinction is important because current available serologic and molecular diagnostic tests for the small piroplasm of dogs target *B gibsoni* and are not reliable for detecting infections of *B conradae*. The distinction is especially important in cases of canine babesiosis in California.

To date, infections of *B conradae* have only been identified in Los Angeles County, California.[49] There is serologic evidence that both domestic dogs and coyotes may be infected, but clinical disease has only been documented in the dog. *Rhipicephalus sanguineus* and *D variabilis* ticks have been recovered from dogs that are seropositive for *B conradae*, suggesting a possible role in transmission.[33] Experimental transmission studies revealed that after a *R sanguineus* larval tick fed on a parasitemic dog, sporozoites were found in the nymphal stage salivary glands. These sporozoites indicate biologic development of *B conradae* in *R sanguineus*, and therefore suggest that transstadial transmission may occur via this tick.[31,44] However, the tick failed to transmit *B conradae* to another dog, and the vector tick for *B conradae* remains as yet unproven.

Lethargy, vomiting, pale mucus membranes, and severe hemolytic anemia are the common clinical signs at presentation.[50] Naturally and experimentally infected dogs had splenomegaly and hematological abnormalities including thrombocytopenia and regenerative anemia, hyperbilirubinemia, hypoalbuminemia, and hemoglobinuria.[51] Serum alkaline phosphatase, aspartate aminotransferase, and alanine phosphatase showed mild to moderate elevation. A common gross finding was lymphadenopathy, especially in the hepatic and peripancreatic nodes. *B conradae* immunopathology includes inflammatory cell infiltrates in the liver and glomerulonephritis suggestive of a type II hypersensitivity reaction, contributing to the pathogenesis of the disease.[31,51]

Treatment with imidocarb diproprionate (Imizol) and diminizene aceturate (Berenil, Ganaseg), alone or in combination, results in abatement of clinical signs and may reduce the parasitemia to levels undetectable by microscopic examination of blood films. However, recrudescence is not uncommon.[50,51]

Babesia canis vogeli

Babesia canis was first described by Piana and Galli-Valerio in 1895, and first reported in the United States in 1934.[23,52] This parasite historically has been identified in dogs in the United States by the presence of large paired intraerythrocytic parasites (See **Fig. 2**B).

There are 3 recognized subspecies, including *Babesia canis canis, B c rossi*, and *B c vogeli*, which are differentiated based on vector specificity, geographic occurrence, pathogenicity, differences in cross-immunity, limited serologic cross-reactivity, and molecular characteristics.[53–56]

In addition to subspecies variation in pathogenicity, differences in clinical manifestation also depend on the age of the host and the immunologic response to the parasite.[57] *B c rossi,* considered the most pathogenic, usually culminates in fatal infection even after treatment.[55] Infection by *B c vogeli* generally leads to mild disease in adult dogs, but puppies and debilitated adults are more severely affected.[23,58–60] The pathogenicity of *B c canis* is intermediate between that of *B c vogeli* and *B c rossi*.[55] Of these, only *B c vogeli*, the least pathogenic subspecies, is found in the United States. *B c vogeli* is transmitted by the brown dog tick, *R sanguineus*.[61,62] The tick vectors for *B c canis* and *B c rossi*, *Dermacentor reticulatus*, and *Haemaphysalis leachi,* respectively, are not indigenous to the United States.

B c vogeli is transmitted both transstadially and transovarially by *R sanguineus* ticks.[23] The incubation period of tick-transmitted infection is approximately 10 to 21 days.[62,63] Although reported predominantly in the southeastern United States, a serologic survey of California shelter dogs reported an incidence of 13% in 1994.[49] The disease was recognized as endemic in southeastern greyhound kennels for more than 50 years.[33] With the advent of acaricidal treatments that are safe for use with greyhounds, and with better management practices to reduce risk of tick infestations at racetracks and in kennels, the incidence of babesiosis in this breed likely will decrease.

It was only about a decade ago that 3 subspecies of *B canis* were recognized, each having its own tick vector species, clinical signs and, to some extent, geographic distribution. The recorded descriptions of clinical signs and pathology associated with babesiosis predate this distinction as well as the molecular tools that eventually clarified the relationship among these 3 pathogens. Because disease is more severe in *B c canis* and *B c rossi,* much of the available information is the result of studies or case reports on these 2 subspecies, although this may not always be stated. Babesosis pathology is often presented as an all-encompassing overview that does not distinguish between the more pathogenic species and the less pathogenic *B c vogeli*.

In the United States, *B c vogeli* historically is reported more often in the greyhound than in other breeds, but all breeds are susceptible. Puppies are more severely affected than adult dogs, and present with depression, weakness, anorexia, pallor, anemia (most often regenerative), and thrombocytopenia.[60,64] Splenomegaly is common and the percent parasitemia is variable. Puppies respond well to antibabesial treatment. Infection in adult dogs may lead to mild or chronic illness, and many adult infections are subclinical.[60,62] In the presence of clinical signs, most babesiosis cases are Coombs test positive.

Adult dogs suffer acute babesiosis in reported transfusion acquired cases[59]; this is to be expected because animals receiving transfusions are likely to be debilitated. However, in one report experimental blood transfer caused more severe pathology than did tick-transmitted disease in adult dogs.[62] In contrast, no clinical signs were reported in adult dogs, either asplenic or spleen-intact, that received infected blood from anemic puppies.[60] The recipients did develop a parasitemia and seroconverted. Multiple factors are likely involved in the etiology of the disease.

North Carolina Babesia sp

This large piroplasm was first identified in a 7-year-old dog with lymphoma in North Carolina.[21] To date 2 additional cases have been reported, another in North Carolina and one in Texas.[22,65] It is possible that the distribution is more widespread, but is misdiagnosed as *B canis* due to the morphologic similarity between these 2 species. In fact, the first case in North Carolina was initially thought to be *B canis* infection.[21]

The life cycle of the North Carolina (NC) *Babesia* sp (also referred to as *Babesia* sp (Coco) in the literature) remains yet to be elucidated. The tick vector is unknown. The existence of alternate vertebrate hosts also is unknown at present. Phylogenetics based on ribosomal RNA analyses place this organism most closely related to *Babesia bigemina*, a well-characterized parasite of cattle.[21]

To date NC *Babesia* sp infection has ranged from babesiosis with clinical signs consistent with babesia infection to babesiasis with no clinical signs.[21,22,65] Two of the animals were undergoing treatment for lymphoma and likely were immune-suppressed as a result.[21,22] Both dogs were treated with imidocarb and one eventually tested negative by PCR following treatment. In the third case, there was no indication that the animal was immune-compromised.[65] The pathophysiology of this disease remains to be clarified.

Diagnosis of Babesiosis

Babesia infections may be confirmed microscopically by the observation of intraerythrocytic piroplasms on Romanowski-type stained blood films (See **Fig. 2**). *B gibsoni* and *B canis* historically were differentiated by their morphology in stained blood smears.[50] *B gibsoni* occurs as small (1 × 3.2 μm length) oval or round piroplasms[66] (See **Fig. 2A**). *B gibsoni* is more pleomorphic than *B canis* and may be seen in various forms, such as a delicate ring of bluish cytoplasm surrounding a vacuole with 1 or 2 chromatin dots located at the periphery.[26] Joined paired or tetrad (Maltese cross) forms are not seen, although multiple parasites may occupy a single cell. In contrast, the divided form of *B canis* occurs as larger (2.4 × 5 μm length) paired pear-shaped piroplasms within the erythrocyte [23] (See **Fig. 2B**). Historically the definitive diagnostic form that distinguishes *B canis* from *B gibsoni* infection is joined paired piroplasms.

With the discovery of 2 additional canine *Babesia* species in the United States, identification of the parasite by microscopic examination of stained blood films is no longer reliable for species differentiation. It may be possible to discriminate between the 2 small piroplasms, *B conradae* and *B gibsoni*, if the parasitemia is high because tetrad (also known as Maltese cross) forms are occasionally seen in *B comradae*.[20] Tetrads arise when a single piroplasm produces 4 daughter cells simultaneously, resulting in an X-shaped formation. In cases of low parasitemia, it may not be possible to discriminate between these 2 species. The 2 large piroplasms, B canis and Babesia sp, cannot be distinguished from each other microscopically because of the morphologic similarity between them.

Immunofluorescent antibody tests are available in veterinary medical diagnostic laboratories (fee-for-service). There are tests that report antibody activity to canine Babesia spp, and additional species-specific tests are available for either B gibsoni or B canis.[67] At present, there are no serologic tests available for either B conradae or the NC Babesia sp. Serologic testing is not always useful for diagnosing acute babesiosis because acute cases in puppies or debilitated animals are likely to be seronegative.[60] Subclinical, chronic, and recrudescent cases may be confirmed serologically.

Molecular testing offers the most sensitive and specific method of confirming infection and determining the Babesia species involved. PCR tests for B canis or B gibsoni are available in several fee-for-service diagnostic laboratories. Infections with B conradae or the NC Babesia sp may be identified by research laboratories that specialize in hemoparasitology. A test was recently reported that combines PCR and restriction enzyme polymorphism patterns to distinguish among canine Babesia spp.[68]

Treatment

The only approved drug for canine babesiosis in the United States is imidocarb dipropionate (Imizol). The recommended dosage is 6.6 mg/kg body weight administered either intramuscularly or subcutaneously. Two doses are administered 2 weeks apart. In very young puppies and debilitated older dogs, pretreatment with atropine is recommended. Doxycycline has been shown to have some antibabesial activity (although it does not clear the infection) and is often prescribed along with imidocarb.[69] Imidocarb therapy is effective for B canis infections, alleviating clinical disease and clearing the parasite from the dog.[70,71] B gibsoni infections are more resistant to drug treatment, and dogs treated with imidocarb frequently continue to carry a low parasitemia. Diminizene aceturate (Berenil, Ganaseg) has long been recognized as an effective antibabesial drug, but it is not available in the United States. Diminizene aceturate is very effective for B canis infections, but like imidocarb it does not reliably clear B gibsoni infections.[26] As with imidocarb, diminizene aceturate therapy results in abatement of clinical signs of babesiosis.

Recent research has focused on a therapeutic combination of atovoquone (Mepron) and azithromycin (Zithromax). This combination does have good effect on clinical disease without adverse side effects, but its effectiveness at clearing the parasite is not unequivocal.[72–74] In a recent case in South Africa, a B gibsoni infected dog was treated first with diminizene aceturate, then with 2 doses of imidocarb 3 and 14 days later.[75] At that time, a PCR-based test was positive for B gibsoni. The dog was then treated with a 10-day course of atovoquone and azithromicin, after which the PCR-based test was negative. In several Texas cases, primary treatment with erythromycin (Erythrocin) and atovoquone did not yield negative PCR results, but clinical improvement did occur (Patricia Holman, PhD, unpublished observations, 2008).

Limited information is available on treating infections of the NC Babesia sp. The first case was treated with imidocarb as recommended above, and rapidly improved.[73] Two PCR tests 13 and 64 weeks after diagnosis were negative. The Texas case was treated with 2 doses of imidocarb (7 mg/kg intramuscular) 3 weeks apart, but tested PCR-positive more than 2.5 months after treatment.[22]

Babesiosis due to B conradae responds favorably to treatment with imidocarb or diminizene aceturate, but fatal recrudescence has occurred with both drugs.[50]

Experimentally infected dogs were treated with diminizene aceturate, which reduced the parasitemia to undetectable levels by microscopic examination, but they became parasitemic when splenectomized a year later.[51]

Supportive care may include fluids as needed, blood transfusion when the packed cell volume (PCV) becomes dangerously low, and administration of immunosuppressives to decrease immune-mediated destruction of erythrocytes.

At present, there are no vaccines available that are effective against babesiosis caused by the *Babesia* species found in the United States. Implementation of tick control measures and the prompt removal of any ticks that attach to the animal will help prevent transmission of *Babesia* spp to the dog.

FELINE CYTAUXZOONOSIS
History and Epidemiology

Cytauxzoonosis is a tick-borne disease of cats caused by the protozoan *Cytauxzoon felis* Kier 1979, which was first described as a cause of fatal infection in domestic cats in Missouri.[76–78] Fatalities of *C felis* infected domestic cats were subsequently reported from Arkansas, Georgia, Louisiana, Mississippi, Oklahoma, and Texas.[79–83] The poor prognosis was further supported by an experimental infection study of more than 500 cats in which only a single cat survived.[84] Nevertheless, 20 years after the first report of the fatal disease, a cytauxzoonosis survivor was documented in Oklahoma, followed by additional reports of nonfatal cytauxzoonosis in Oklahoma, Arkansas, Georgia and, more recently, 2 survivors in a study of cats from North and South Carolina and Virginia.[76,85–88] A recent study of healthy free-ranging cats in Florida identified *C felis* in 0.3% using a PCR assay.[89] None of the positive cats was known to have had clinical cytauxzoonosis before testing, suggesting that subclinical *C felis* infection of cats may occur.

To date, feline cytauxzoonosis has been reported in the central states including Indiana, Kansas, Oklahoma, Missouri, and Arkansas, and in the Gulf and Atlantic Coast states south from Texas to as far north as Virginia.[79–82,87,90] The range of the vector tick, *D variabilis*, extends throughout most of the United States, thus it is likely that the disease will be found in additional states with habitat conducive to the bobcat reservoir host.

Life Cycle and Transmission

Cats acquire the protozoan via the bite of a vector tick, which transmits *C felis* sporozoites to the cat. On introduction to the cat, the sporozoites invade endothelial-associated mononuclear phagocytes and multiply, forming a single large schizont within each cell (**Fig. 3A**). Mature schizonts rupture releasing merozoites, which then enter erythrocytes (**Fig. 3B**). The erythrocytic stage piroplasm likely undergoes cycles of multiplication in this stage as dividing forms are observed.[91] Although it was suggested that erythrophagocytosis of infected cells may perpetuate cycles of schizogony,[91] this has not been confirmed. The pathophysiology of the disease results from occlusion of small vessels in the lungs, spleen, and liver with large histiocytic schizont-filled macrophages (See **Fig. 3A**).[88,90]

D variabilis has been shown to be a competent vector of *C felis* by experimental transmission to domestic cats,[92] and there may be other as yet undiscovered tick vectors of this parasite. Cytauxzoonosis in the domestic cat therefore depends on exposure to infected ticks, and cyclic peaks in cases tend to correlate with activity periods of *D variabilis*, a known vector tick, and *Amblyomma americanum*, a possible vector tick.[83,92,93]

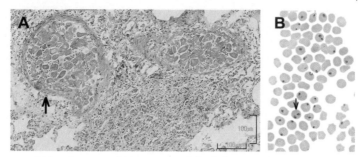

Fig. 3. Tissue and blood stages of *Cytauxzoon felis*. (*A*) Intracellular schizont stages occlude the lumen of a small blood vessel (*large arrow*) in cat lung (H&E stain). (*B*) Numerous intracellular piroplasms localize in erythrocytes in cat peripheral blood (Giemsa stain, original magnification ×1000). Multiple parasites often are seen within an individual erythrocyte (*arrow*).

The North American bobcat (*Lynx rufus*), in which infections are usually asymptomatic, is likely an important reservoir host.[94,95] Recent documentation of *C felis* infections in bobcats in regions of Pennsylvania where cytauxzoonosis has not been found in domestic cats points to the bobcat as the natural and likely reservoir host for this parasite.[96] The finding that domestic cats may carry subclinical infections suggests that they may serve as reservoirs as well.[89]

Clinical Findings

Feline cytauxzoonosis has been reported in cats ranging in age from 2 months to 15 years old.[86,88] The disease is characterized by nonspecific signs of fever, lethargy, anorexia, dehydration, icterus, pallor of the mucous membranes, and dyspnea. Splenomegaly is common. The appearance of intraerythrocytic parasites usually coincides with the development of fever. *C felis* parasitemias ranging from 0.045% to 1.27% are reported for cats that survive cytauxzoonosis, compared with approximately 1% to 20% for those that do not.[83,85,87] Of note, a parasitemia of 50% was observed in a Texas case in which the cat survived (Patricia Holman, PhD, unpublished observation, 2005). Generally at presentation, the PCV is less than 30%, with a decrease to less than 20% as the disease progresses. The most consistent hematologic abnormalities are leukopenia and thrombocytopenia.[83,87] Signs of terminal disease include hypothermia, recumbency, and coma.

Reported clinical chemistry values are variable in fatal cases. In general the clinical chemistry values for total bilirubin, glucose, and alanine transaminase are elevated, whereas albumin and potassium are below reference range.[83,88] Bilirubinuria is common. However, in some cases the clinical chemistry values for blood urea nitrogen, creatinine, alkaline phosphatase, and alanine aminotransferase are within reference ranges.[90]

In many of the documented nonfatal cases, the first clinical signs were lethargy or depression and anorexia, with icterus and dehydration on presentation also reported.[85–87] In many fatal cases, the animals were clearly in advanced state of illness when first presented. The most consistent clinical findings are anorexia, lethargy, depression, and fever that can be elevated to greater than 105°F (40.6°C).[79,81,82,86,90] Other frequent findings include dehydration, anemia, leukopenia, and dyspnea. Vomiting, icterus and enlarged mesenteric lymph nodes, and respiratory harshness were also noted in some cases.

In experimental cytauxzoonosis, the occurrence and degree of the intraerythrocytic stage parasitemia were related to the increase in body temperature, the presence of the schizont stage, and decrease in white blood cells.[91] The pathology associated with C felis infection results primarily from the tissue phase in which schizonts develop in mononuclear phagocytes, leading to venous occlusion in the lung, spleen, liver, and kidney.[91] Postmortem histologic lesions often include protozoal schizonts as large as 60 μm in diameter in the brain, heart, lung, intestine, spleen, lymph node, and kidney.[90,97] Disseminated intravascular coagulation is a common sequela in the pathology of cytauxzoonosis.

Transfer of erythrocytic stage parasites from a bobcat with a subclinical infection to domestic cats resulted in a persistent but nonfatal parasitemia,[92] indicating that this stage of the parasite does not contribute to the pathology of the disease.

Diagnosis

Diagnosis is often made based on the presence of intraerythrocytic piroplasms in Romanowski-type stained blood films (See **Fig. 3**B). Direct diagnosis may be difficult due to low levels of the parasite, variable staining qualities of the parasite, and the difficulty in differentiating C felis from Mycoplasma haemofelis (formerly Haemobartonella) in blood films. Early in infection blood piroplasms may be absent, and repeated evaluation of blood films may be helpful. Additional blood films may still be negative, however, because the clinical disease associated with vascular occlusion caused by the tissue stage of the parasite often precedes the appearance of blood piroplasms. Examination of fine-needle aspirates of spleen, liver, or kidney to detect the schizont stage may be necessary to confirm the diagnosis, and may be beneficial for early diagnosis.[88]

Several veterinary medical research or diagnostic laboratories offer PCR tests for C felis that are highly sensitive and specific.[98] At present, there are no serologic tests widely available for detecting antibodies against the parasite in feline cytauxzoonosis.

Treatment

Whether drug treatment contributes to a favorable outcome in feline cytauxzoonosis is controversial. In nonfatal cases a wide variety of antibiotics have been used, including clindamycin, penicillin G, enrofloxacin (Baytril), and doxycycline (Doxirobe, Vibramycin), singly or in combination with imidocarb diproprionate or diminazene aceturate.[86,87] If imidocarb diproprionate is administered, atropine should be given 30 minutes before the imidocarb to offset possible side effects.[87]

The first reported survivor of the disease was treated with enrofloxacin for 10 days, along with intravenous fluids as necessary, and then with tetracycline for 5 days.[85] A second cat with cytauxzoonosis was treated with diminazene aceturate and survived despite a drop in PCV to 8.5%.[87] Cytauxzoonosis was also successfully treated with imidocarb along with supplemental therapy including heparin (to control the procoagulatory process and prevent the possible development of disseminated intravascular coagulation), isotonic fluids, and a blood transfusion when the PCV dropped to 13.4%.[87] In Texas, a cat with a 50% parasitemia and PCV of 15% was treated with doxycycline, imidocarb (pretreated with atropine), prednisolone, and fluid therapy, and survived the infection (Patricia Holman, PhD, unpublished observation, 2005). Questions remain as to the actual effect of the drugs on the course of infection because many of these treatment regimens have also been followed in fatal cases.

Regardless of the drug therapy used, supportive therapy is a common factor among cytauxzoonosis survivors. Aggressive supportive care should be implemented, including fluid therapy and anticoagulant administration (such as heparin) to prevent disseminated intravascular coagulation. Recovered cats have been reported free of *C felis* by blood film examination.[86,87] However, PCR testing indicates that treated cats may remain carriers of *C felis*.[86] In one case, parasites were detected 2.5 years after clinical illness in the absence of clinical signs (Patricia Holman, PhD, unpublished observation, 2008). Recovered cats should therefore be considered possible reservoirs of infection.

Prevention of cytauxzoonosis includes implementation of tick control measures. Animals that have access to the outdoors should be examined for ticks daily, and any attached ticks removed promptly to prevent transmission of *C felis* to the cat. There is no available vaccine against feline cytauxzoonosis.

It has been suggested that in the nonfatal cases, the cats would have survived the infection without intervention because untreated subclinical *C felis* carrier housemates of symptomatic cats have been reported.[86] On the other hand, subsequent cytauxzoonosis in cohorts in households where deaths due to *C felis* have occurred is also known.[87,90] Of note, in all reported cases of cats with clinical cytauxzoonosis that recovered, at a minimum antimicrobial drugs and supportive therapy were administered.[85-88]

There are no reported experimental controlled studies on the efficacy of imidocarb diproprionate or diminizene aceturate in cytauxzoonosis to date. Experimental use of the antitheilerial drugs parvaquone and buparvaquone (Clexon and Butalex) was detailed in a study of 15 cats.[99] Although *Cytauxzoon* spp are very closely related to *Theileria* species, neither drug was deemed effective when 14 of the 15 cats died. One of 2 control cats infected with the same inoculum unexpectedly survived. These results supported a previous study that concluded that parvaquone likely would not play a practical role in the treatment of feline cytauxzoonosis.[100]

That cats can survive infection with *C felis* may be attributable to several factors (1) there may exist less virulent strains of the parasite[86]; (2) individual variation in immunity and response to the parasite among cats (ie, some cats may not develop severe pathology); (3) schizogony is more limited in survivors, lessening the severity of the disease; or (4) veterinary intervention earlier in the course of disease than in the case of nonsurvivors. The actual number of feline cytauxzoonosis survivors is not known. A recent molecular survey suggests that subclinical infection occurs,[89] which further suggests that the parasite may be more widespread than currently recognized.

SUMMARY

The protozoan parasites causing hepatozoonosis, babesiosis, and cytauxzoonosis have many features in common. These tick-transmitted apicomplexan parasites are becoming more widely recognized as serious canine or feline pathogens. Continuing research efforts and the development of new molecular tools have advanced the basic and applied scientific knowledge about the parasites and their host-pathogen interactions. Recent research efforts have led to the recognition of several new parasite species, and further clarification of the taxonomic identities and biology of these organisms is needed. Additional studies are needed in some cases to clarify the tick vector, to identify reservoir hosts, and to understand transmission patterns and the geospatial distribution of the parasites. With basic scientists working alongside clinicians, improved diagnostic techniques can now be used to detect asymptomatic animals and persistently infected carrier animals, or to determine whether an animal is cured. These techniques and services need to be more widely available to the clinician for use in general patient care. Clinical research efforts are desperately needed to develop better treatment regimens against these parasites.

REFERENCES

1. Panciera RJ, Ewing SA. American canine hepatozoonosis. Anim Health Res Rev 2003;4(1):27–34.
2. Craig TM, Smallwood JE, Knauer KW, et al. *Hepatozoon canis* infection in dogs: clinical, radiographic and hematologic findings. J Am Vet Med Assoc 1978;173: 967–72.
3. Vincent-Johnson NA, Macintire DK, Lindsay DS, et al. A new *Hepatozoon* species from dogs: description of the causative agent of canine hepatozoonosis in North America. J Parasitol 1997;83:1165–72.
4. Baneth G, Mathew JS, Shkap V, et al. Canine hepatozoonosis: two disease syndromes caused by separate *Hepatozoon* spp. Trends Parasitol 2003;19(1): 27–31.
5. Macintire DK, Vincent-Johnson NA, Craig TM. *Hepatozoon americanum* infection. In: Greene CJ, editor. Infectious diseases of the dog and cat. 3rd edition. St Louis MO: WB Saunders; 2006. p. 705–11.
6. Vincent-Johnson NA. American canine hepatozoonosis. Vet Clin North Am Small Anim Pract 2003;33:905–20.
7. Allen K, Li Y, Kaltenboeck B, et al. Diversity of *Hepatozoon* species in naturally infected dogs in the southern United States. Vet Parasitol 2008;154: 220–5.
8. Li Y, Wang C, Allen KE, et al. Diagnosis of canine *Hepatozoon* spp. infection by quantitative PCR. Vet Parasitol 2008;157:50–8.
9. Murata T, Inoue M, Tateyama S, et al. Vertical transmission of *Hepatozoon canis* in dogs. J Vet Med Sci 1993;55:867–8.
10. Garrett JJ, Kocan AA, Panciera MV, et al. Experimental infection of adult and juvenile coyotes with domestic dog and wild coyote isolates of *Hepatozoon americanum* (Apicomplexa: Adeleorina). J Wldl Dis 2005;41(3):588–92.
11. Mercer SH, Jones LP, Rappole JH, et al. *Hepatozoon* sp. in wild carnivores in Texas. J Wildl Dis 1988;24:574–6.
12. Johnson EM, Allen KE, Breshears MA, et al. Experimental transmission of *Hepatozoon americanum* to rodents. Vet Parasitol 2008;151:164–9.
13. Ewing SA, Panciera RJ, Mathew JS. Persistence of *Hepatozoon americanum* (Apicomplexa: Adeleorina) in a naturally infected dog. J Parasitol 2003;89(3): 611–3.
14. Drost WT, Cummings CA, Mathew JS, et al. Determination of time of onset and location of early skeletal lesions in young dogs experimentally infected with *Hepatozoon americanum* using bone scintigraphy. Vet Radiol Ultrasound 2003; 44(1):86–91.
15. Mercer SH, Craig TM. Comparison of various staining procedures in the identification of *Hepatozoon canis* gamonts. Vet Clin Pathol 1988;17:63–5.
16. Mathew JS, Saliki JT, Ewing SA, et al. An indirect enzyme-linked immunosorbent assay for diagnosis of American canine hepatozoonosis. J Vet Diagn Invest 2001;13:17–21.
17. Criado-Fornelio A, Buling A, Cunha-Filho NA, et al. Development and evaluation of a quantitative PCR assay for detection of *Hepatozoon* sp. Vet Parasitol 2007; 150:352–6.

18. Rubini AS, Paduan KDS, Lopes VVA, et al. Molecular and parasitological survey of *Hepatozoon canis* (Apicomplexa: Hepatozoidae) in dogs from rural area of Sao Paulo state, Brazil. Parasitol Res 2008;102:895–9.

19. Macintire DK, Vincent-Johnson NA, Kane CW, et al. Treatment of dogs infected with *Hepatozoon americanum*: 53 cases (19897–1998). J Am Vet Med Assoc 2001;218(1):77–82.

20. Kjemtrup AM, Wainwright K, Miller M, et al. *Babesia conradae*, sp. nov., a small canine *Babesia* identified in California. Vet Parasitol 2006;138(1/2):103–11.

21. Birkenheuer AJ, Neel J, Ruslander D, et al. Detection and molecular characterization of a novel large *Babesia* species in a dog. Vet Parasitol 2004;124: 151–60.

22. Holman PJ, Backlund B, Wilcox A et al. First out of state case of canine babesiosis caused by a large unnamed piroplasm originally described in North Carolina. J Am Vet Med Assoc, in press.

23. Levine ND. Apicomplexa: the piroplasms. Veterinary protozoology. 1st edition. Ames (IA): Iowa State University Press; 1985. p. 291–328.

24. Groves MG, Yap LF. *Babesia gibsoni* (Patton, 1910) from a dog in Kuala Lumpur. Med J Malaya 1968;22:229.

25. Anderson JF, Magnarelli LA, Donner CS, et al. Canine *Babesia* new to North America. Science 1979;204:1431–2.

26. Farwell GE, Le Grand EK, Cobb CC. Clinical observations of *Babesia gibsoni* and *Babesia canis* infections in dogs. J Am Vet Med Assoc 1982;5:507–11.

27. Birkenheuer AJ, Correa MT, Levy MG, et al. Geographic distribution of babesiosis among dogs in the United States and association with dog bites: 150 cases (2000–2003). J Am Vet Med Assoc 2005;227:942–7.

28. Bostrom B, Wolf C, Greene C, et al. Sequence conservation in the rRNA first internal transcribed spacer region of *Babesia gibsoni* genotype Asia isolates. Vet Parasitol 2008;152(1/2):152–7.

29. Kjemtrup AM, Kocan AA, Whitworth L, et al. There are at least three genetically distinct small piroplasms from dogs. Int J Parasitol 2000;30:1501–5.

30. Zahler M, Rinder H, Zweygarth E, et al. '*Babesia gibsoni*' of dogs from North America and Asia belong to different species. Parasitology 2000;120:365–9.

31. Kjemtrup AM, Conrad PA. A review of the small canine piroplasms from California: *Babesia conradae* in the literature. Vet Parasitol 2006;138(1/2):112–7.

32. Meinkoth JH, Kocan AA, Loud SD, et al. Clinical and hematology effects of experimental infection of dogs with recently identified *Babesia gibsoni*-like isolates from Oklahoma. J Am Vet Med Assoc 2002;220:185–9.

33. Boozer AL, Macintire DK. Canine babesiosis. Vet Clin North Am Small Anim Pract 2003;33:885–904.

34. Birkenheuer AJ, Levy MG, Stebbins M, et al. Serosurvey of anti *Babesia* antibodies in stray dogs and American pit bull terriers and American Staffordshire terriers from North Carolina. J Am Anim Hosp Assoc 2003;39:551–7.

35. Birkenheuer AJ, Levy MG, Savary KC, et al. *Babesia gibsoni* infection in dogs from North Carolina. J Am Anim Hosp Assoc 1999;35:125–8.

36. Macintire DK, Boudreaux MK, West GD, et al. *Babesia gibsoni* infection among dogs in the southeastern United States. J Am Vet Med Assoc 2002;220:325–9.

37. Irizarry-Rovira AR, Stephens J, Christian J, et al. *Babesia gibsoni* infection in a dog from Indiana. Vet Clin Pathol 2001;30:180–8.

38. Kocan AA, Kjemtrup A, Meinkoth J, et al. A genotypically unique *Babesia gibsoni* –like parasite recovered from a dog in Oklahoma. J Parasitol 2001;87: 437–8.

39. Stegeman J, Birkenheuer AJ, Kruger JM, et al. Transfusion-associated *Babesia gibsoni* infection in a dog. J Am Vet Med Assoc 2003;222:959–63.
40. Matsuu A, Kawabe A, Koshida Y, et al. Incidence of canine *Babesia gibsoni* infection and subclinical infection among Tosa dogs in Aomori Prefecture, Japan. J Vet Med Sci 2004;66:893–7.
41. Higuchi S, Konno H, Hoshi F, et al. Observations of *Babesia gibsoni* in the ovary of the tick, *Haemaphysalis longicornis*. Kitasato Arch Exp Med 1993;65(Suppl): 153–8.
42. Higuchi S, Fujimori M, Hoshi F, et al. Development of *Babesia gibsoni* in the salivary glands of the larval tick, *Rhipicephalus sanguineus*. J Vet Med Sci 1995; 57(1):117–9.
43. Swaminath CS, Shortt HE. The arthropod vector of *Babesia gibsoni*. Indian J Med Res 1937;25(2):499–503.
44. Yamane I, Gardner IA, Telford SR III, et al. Vector competence of *Rhipicephalus sanguineus* and *Dermacentor variabilis* for American isolates of *Babesia gibsoni*. Exp Appl Acarol 1993;17:913–9.
45. Fukumoto S, Suzuki H, Igarashi I, et al. Fatal experimental transplacental *Babesia gibsoni* infections in dogs. Int J Parasitol 2005;35:1031–5.
46. Jefferies RR, Jardine UM, Broughton J, et al. Bull Terriers and Babesiosis: further evidence for direct transmission of *Babesia gibsoni* in dogs. Aust Vet J 2007; 85(11):459–63.
47. Inokuma H, Okuda M, Yoshizaki Y, et al. Clinical observations of *Babesia gibsoni* infection with low parasitaemia confirmed by PCR in dogs. Vet Rec 2005;156(4): 116–8.
48. Botros BAM, Moch RW, Barsoum IS. Some observations on experimentally induced infection of dogs with *Babesia gibsoni*. Am J Vet Res 1975;36:293–6.
49. Yamane I, Gardener I, Ryan C, et al. Serosurvey of *Babesia canis, Babesia gibsoni*, and *Ehrlichia canis* in pound dogs in California, USA. Prev Vet Med 1994; 18:293–304.
50. Conrad PA, Thomford J, Yamane I, et al. Hemolytic anemia caused by *Babesia gibsoni* infection in dogs. J Am Vet Med Assoc 1991;199:601–5.
51. Wozniak EJ, Barr BC, Thomford JM, et al. Clinical, anatomic, and immunopathologic characterization of *Babesia gibsoni* infection in the domestic dog (*Canis familiaris*). J Parasitol 1997;83(4):692–9.
52. Eaton P. *Piroplasma canis* in Florida. J Parasitol 1934;20:312–3.
53. Hauschild S, Shayan P, Schein E. Characterization and comparison of merozoite antigens of different *Babesia canis* isolates by serological and immunological investigations. Parasitol Res 1995;81:638–42.
54. Schetters THPM, Moubri K, Precigout E, et al. Different *Babesia canis* isolates, different diseases. Parasitology 1997;115:485–93.
55. Uilenberg G, Franssen FFJ, Perié NM, et al. Three groups of *Babesia canis* distinguished and a proposal for nomenclature. Vet Q 1989;11:33–40.
56. Zahler M, Schein E, Rinder H, et al. Characteristic genotypes discriminate between *Babesia canis* isolates of differing vector specificity and pathogenicity to dogs. Parasitol Res 1998;84(7):544–8.
57. Martinod S, Laurent N, Moreau Y. Resistance and immunity of dogs against *Babesia canis* in an endemic area. Vet Parasitol 1986;19:245–54.
58. Hill MWM, Bolton BL. Canine babesiosis in Queensland. Aust Vet J 1966;42:391–2.
59. Freeman MJ, Kirby BM, Panciera DL, et al. Hypotensive shock syndrome associated with acute *Babesia canis* infection in a dog. J Am Vet Med Assoc 1994; 204(1):94–6.

60. Breitschwerdt EB, Malone JB, MacWilliams P, et al. Babesiosis in the greyhound. J Am Vet Med Assoc 1983;182:978–82.
61. Hauschild S, Schein E. The subspecies specificity of *Babesia canis*. Berl Munch Tierarztl Wochenschr 1996;109:216–9.
62. Bansal SR, Kharole MU, Banerjee DP. Clinicopathological studies in experimental *Babesia canis* infection in dogs. J Vet Parasitol 1990;4(1):21–5.
63. Ristic M, Lykins JD, Smith AR, et al. *Babesia canis* and *Babesia gibsoni*: soluble and corpuscular antigens isolated from blood of dogs. Exp Parasitol 1971;30: 385–92.
64. Brown GK, Canfield PJ, Dunstan RH, et al. Detection of *Anaplasma platys* and *Babesia canis vogeli* and their impact on platelet numbers in free-roaming dogs associated with remote Aboriginal communities in Australia. Aust Vet J 2006;84(9):321–5.
65. Lehtinen LE, Birkenheuer AJ, Droleskey RE, et al. In vitro cultivation of a newly recognized *Babesia* sp. in dogs in North Carolina. Vet Parasitol 2008;151(2/4): 150–7.
66. Mehlhorn H, Schein E. The piroplasms: life cycle and sexual stages. Adv Parasitol 1984;23:37–103.
67. Anderson JF, Magnarelli LA, Sulzer AJ. Canine babesiosis: indirect fluorescent antibody test for a North American isolate of *Babesia gibsoni*. Am J Vet Res 1980;41:2102–5.
68. Jefferies R, Ryan UM, Irwin PJ. PCR-RFLP for the detection and differentiation of the canine piroplasm species and its use with filter paper-based technologies. Vet Parasitol 2007;144(1/2):20–7.
69. Vercammen F, De Deken R, Maes L. Prophylactic treatment of experimental canine babesiosis (*Babesia canis*) with doxycycline. Vet Parasitol 1996;66: 251–5.
70. Adeyanju BJ, Aliu YO. Chemotherapy of canine ehrlichiosis and Babesiosis with imidocarb dipropionate. J Am Anim Hosp Assoc 1982;18:827–30.
71. Penzhorn BL, Lewis BD, de Waal DT, et al. Sterilisation of *Babesia canis* infections by imidocarb alone or in combination with diminazene. J S Afr Vet Assoc 1995;66:157–9.
72. Matsuu A, Koshida Y, Kawahara M, et al. Efficacy of atovaquone against *Babesia gibsoni* in vivo and in vitro. Vet Parasitol 2004;124:9–18.
73. Birkenheuer AJ, Levy MG, Breitschwerdt EB. Efficacy of combined atovaquone and azithromycin for therapy of chronic *Babesia gibsoni* (Asian genotype) infections in dogs. J Vet Intern Med 2004;18:494–8.
74. Jefferies R, Ryan UM, Jardine J. *Babesia gibsoni*: detection during experimental infections and after combined atovoquone and azithromycin therapy. Exp Parasitol 2007;117:115–23.
75. Matjila PT, Penzhorn BL, Leisewitz AL, et al. Molecular characterisation of *Babesia gibsoni* infection from a pit-bull terrier pup recently imported into South Africa. J S Afr Vet Assoc 2007;78(1):2–5.
76. Wagner JE. Cytauxzoonosis in domestic cats (*Felis domestica*) in Missouri. J Am Vet Med Assoc 1975;167:874.
77. Wagner JE. A fatal cytauxzoonosis-like disease in cats. J Am Vet Med Assoc 1976;68:585–8.
78. Kier AB. The etiology and pathogenesis of feline cytauxzoonosis. 1979. PhD Dissertation, University of Missouri, Columbia, MO.
79. Bendele RA, Schwartz WL, Jones LP. Cytauxzoonosis-like disease in Texas cats. Southwestern Vet 1976;29:244–6.

80. Wightman SR, Kier AB, Wagner JE. Feline cytauxzoonosis: clinical features of a newly described blood parasite disease. Feline Pract 1977;7:23–6.
81. Hauck WN. Cytauxzoonosis in a native Louisiana cat. J Am Vet Med Assoc 1982; 180:1472–4.
82. Glenn BL, Stair EL. Cytauxzoonosis in domestic cats: report of 2 cases in Oklahoma, with review and discussion of the disease. J Am Vet Med Assoc 1984; 184:822–5.
83. Hoover JP, Walker DB, Hedges JD. Cytauxzoonosis in cats: 8 cases (1985–1992). J Am Vet Med Assoc 1994;205:455–60.
84. Ferris DH. A progress report on the status of a new disease of American cats: cytauxzoonosis. Comp Immunol Microbiol Infect Dis 1979;1:269–76.
85. Walker DB, Cowell RL. Survival of a domestic cat with naturally acquired cytauxzoonosis. J Am Vet Med Assoc 1995;206:1363–5.
86. Meinkoth J, Kocan AA, Whitworth L, et al. Cats surviving natural infections with *Cytauxzoon felis*: 18 cases (1997–1998). J Vet Intern Med 2000;14:521–5.
87. Greene CE, Latimer K, Hopper E, et al. Administration of diminazene aceturate or imidocarb dipropionate for treatment of cytauxzoonosis in cats. J Am Vet Med Assoc 1999;215(4):497–500.
88. Birkenheuer AJ, Le JA, Valenzisi AM, et al. *Cytauxzoon felis* infection in cats in the mid-Atlantic states: 34 cases (1998–2004). J Am Vet Med Assoc 2006; 228(4):568–71.
89. Haber MD, Tucker MD, Marr HS, et al. The detection of *Cytauxzoon felis* in apparently healthy free-roaming cats in the USA. Vet Parasitol 2007;146(3/4): 316–20.
90. Jackson CB, Fisher T. Fatal cytauxzoonosis in a Kentucky cat (*Felis domesticus*). Vet Parasitol 2006;139:192–5.
91. Kier AB, Wagner JE, Kinden DA. The pathology of experimental cytauxzoonosis. J Comp Pathol 1987;97:415–32.
92. Blouin EF, Kocan AA, Glenn BL, et al. Transmission of *Cytauxzoon felis* (Kier, 1979) from bobcats, *Lynx rufus* (Schreber), to domestic cats by *Dermacentor variabilis* (Say). J Wildl Dis 1984;20:241–2.
93. Reichard MV, Baum KA, Cadenhead SC, et al. Temporal occurrence and environmental risk factors associated with cytauxzoonosis in domestic cats. Vet Parasitol 2008;152:314–20.
94. Kier AB, Wagner JE, Morehouse LG. Experimental transmission of *Cytauxzoon felis* from bobcats (*Lynx rufus*) to domestic cats (*Felis domesticus*). Am J Vet Res 1982;43:97–101.
95. Glenn BL, Kocan AA, Blouin EF. Cytauxzoonosis in bobcats. J Am Vet Med Assoc 1983;183:1155–8.
96. Birkenheuer AJ, Mar HS, Warren C, et al. *Cytauxzoon felis* infections are present in bobcats (*Lynx rufus*) in a region where cytauxzoonosis is not recognized in domestic cats. Vet Parasitol 2008;153:126–30.
97. Meinkoth J, Cowell RL, Cowell AK. What is your diagnosis? 10-year-old vomiting, anorexic cat. Vet Clin Pathol 1996;25:48.
98. Birkenheuer AJ, Marr H, Alleman AR, et al. Development and evaluation of a PCR assay for the detection of *Cytauxzoon felis* DNA in feline blood samples. Vet Parasitol 2006;137:144–9.
99. Motzel SL, Wagner JE. Treatment of experimentally induced cytauxzoonosis in cats with parvoquone and buparvaquone. Vet Parasitol 1990;35:131–8.
100. Uilenberg G, Franssen FFJ, Perié NM. Relationships between *Cytauxzoon felis* and African piroplasmids. Vet Parasitol 1987;26:21–8.

Canine Chagas' Disease (American Trypanosomiasis) in North America

Stephen C. Barr, BVSc, PhD

KEYWORDS

• Dog • Trypanosomiasis • Chagas disease
• North America • Zoonosis

Chagas disease, or American trypanosomiasis, is caused by the hemoflagellated protozoan, *Trypanosoma cruzi* (class Zoomastigophorea and family Trypanosomatidae). The disease was first described by the Brazilian doctor and scientist Carlos Chagas in 1909.[1] The parasite is a zoonosis in the Americas, particularly in South and parts of Central America, and is the leading cause of dilated cardiomyopathy in man.[2] In dogs in North America, disease usually manifests as cardiac disease typified by arrhythmias or myocarditis (acute and chronic), and rarely, neurologic disease.[3–8] However, many infected dogs remain asymptomatic for life. Although the parasite usually requires a reduviid vector for transmission, there is evidence that some dogs may become infected without being bitten by vectors; they may eat infected vectors instead. Canine Chagas disease is of importance to veterinary practitioners because it can be difficult to diagnose and is a serious zoonosis, and there is a lack of therapeutic options.

ETIOLOGY AND LIFE CYCLE

The organism exists in three morphologic forms. The blood-form found in circulation in the host, the trypomastigote, is 15 to 20 μm long, with a flattened spindle-shaped body and a centrally placed vesicular nucleus. A single flagellum originates near the large subterminal kinetoplast (situated posterior to the nucleus) and passes along the body to project anteriorly (**Fig. 1**). The host intracellular or amastigote form is approximately 1.5 to 4.0 μm in diameter, roughly spheroid, and contains both nucleus and rodlike kinetoplast. With regular cytological staining, these structures have similar staining properties although the kinetoplast stains more densely. The small flagellum is rarely obvious under light microscopy. Epimastigotes, the third morphologic form, are found in the reduviid vector (subfamily Triatomae). In South America, these large

Department of Clinical Sciences, College of Veterinary Medicine, Cornell University, Ithaca, NY 14853, USA
E-mail address: scb6@cornell.edu

Vet Clin Small Anim 39 (2009) 1055–1064
doi:10.1016/j.cvsm.2009.06.004
0195-5616/09/$ – see front matter © 2009 Elsevier Inc. All rights reserved.

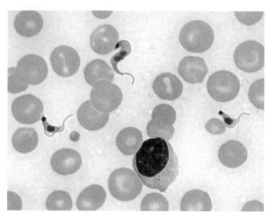

Fig. 1. Trypomastigotes of *T cruzi* in a blood smear of a dog (Wright-Giemsa stain, original magnification ×1000).

insects (adults can reach an inch in length) are commonly known as "kissing bugs." Epimastigotes are flagellated and spindle shaped with the kinetoplast situated anterior to the nucleus.

When the vector is involved, infection occurs when trypomastigotes are deposited in the insect vector's feces at the vector bite site, as occurs in human infections in South America, but this may not be the main route of infection for dogs in North America. Ingestion of infected insect vectors causing the parasite to be released into the mouth of the dog is probably more likely; certainly, opossums[9] and armadillos[10] fed infected vectors will become infected by this route. Blood transfusion and transplacental transmission can also occur, and transmission by ingestion of milk from infected lactating bitches has been proposed.[7] Ingestion of meat from infected reservoir hosts has also been suggested to occur in dogs, but transmission did not occur when infected meat was fed to armadillos.[10] After infection, trypomastigotes may enter macrophages, transform into amastigotes, which multiply by binary fission, or remain free in circulation to spread from the local site of infection. After hematogenous spread, myocardiocytes become infected with trypomastigotes which, after transforming into amastigotes, multiply and transform back into trypomastigotes before rupture of and release from the cell back into circulation. Parasitemia in dogs first appears as early as 3 days post infection (DPI), peaks at 17 DPI, and is usually subpatent by 30 DPI.[3] Clinical signs of acute myocarditis, should they occur, develop about 14 DPI with recovery occurring around 28 DPI.[3] Rapid intracellular multiplication cycles ensure a rapid rise in parasitemia before effective immunity develops. The vector becomes infected by ingesting circulating trypomastigotes, which transform to epimastigotes and multiply by binary fission. Transformation of the epimastigotes back into trypomastigotes occurs in the vector's hindgut before the trypomastigotes are passed in the feces.

EPIDEMIOLOGY

American trypanosomiasis is a major human health problem in South and Central America, and is becoming more recognized in Mexico[2,11] To date, there have been six human cases involving transmission by vectors reported in the United States. The last reported human case was detected in June 2006 in a 74-year-old woman residing in rural New Orleans, Louisiana, who experienced a large influx of vectors

(*Triatoma sanguisuga*) into her house after hurricane Katrina.[12] Of the 33 vectors found in her dwelling, 56% were found to contain *T cruzi*. However, by far the largest number of people (estimated to be 50,000 to 100,000) infected in the United States have emigrated from endemic regions. Consequently, reports of cases associated with transfusion transmission continue to increase in number,[13,14] and blood is now tested for *T cruzi* at blood banks. Most canine cases in the United States occur in Texas, especially within the southeastern quadrant.[15–17] Isolated canine cases have been reported in other southern states,[6,18–20] but also as far north in the east as Virginia.[7]

Transmission of *T cruzi* in endemic countries depends on the confluence of vectors, reservoirs, parasites, and hosts (both people and animals) in a single habitat. Only three Triatomae species (*Triatoma infestans*, *Triatoma dimidiata*, and *Rhodnius prolixus*) of the many that feed on humans in endemic regions in South America display the appropriate behavior that enables them to transmit *T cruzi* effectively. These parasites feed on blood from both people and domestic reservoir mammals (dog, cat, guinea pigs), reproduce prolifically while cohabiting close to people, and defecate soon after taking a blood meal, meaning that they are usually still on the host near the bite wound when they defecate.[21] Infection rates in these vectors can be as high as 100% south of the equator. By contrast, domestic transmission cycles probably do not occur in the United States, except in areas of southeastern Texas where there is evidence to suggest that the dog can be involved in domestic transmission cycles involving vectors and humans,[22] similar to what has been suggested across the boarder in Mexico[11] and endemic regions in South America.[21] In general, however, the two principal vectors in the United States (*Triatoma protracta* and *Triatoma sanguisuga*) have low infection rates (20%), display different feeding habits, and defecate about 20 minutes after feeding, often when they have long fled the host.[23] These factors and higher standards of housing in the United States are suggested to have contributed to a much lower rate of autochthonous transmission.

The principal sylvan reservoir hosts of *T cruzi* in the eastern seaboard states from Maryland south and most other southern states (Texas, Louisiana, Oklahoma, to name a few) are opossums and raccoons. Armadillos are also infected wherever they range.[24–31] Various mouse, squirrel, and rat species are the main sylvan hosts in New Mexico and California.[32] Isolates of *T cruzi* from infected vectors and animal reservoirs in North America are less pathogenic in mice than South American isolates despite showing similar in vitro characteristics.[24,33] Because inoculation of *T cruzi* isolates from opossums and armadillos into dogs experimentally produces a similar disease described in naturally acquired cases of acute and chronic canine trypanosomiasis, it is likely that dogs in nature are infected with the same isolates as these sylvan hosts.[3–7]

CLINICAL SIGNS AND PATHOGENESIS

As in humans, there are three distinct phases of Chagas myocarditis in dogs; acute, indeterminate (or latent), and chronic.[3–7] After infection, trypomastigotes enter cells (mainly macrophages) where they evade the immune system and spread throughout the body. Some do enter the circulation and can be detected cytologically as early as 3 DPI. The parasitemia steadily rises as more and more intracellular multiplication cycles add to the number of circulating trypomastigotes. Peak parasitemia occurs at about 17 DPI, roughly at about the time that clinical signs of generalized lymphadenopathy and acute myocarditis appear. The cause of the myocarditis is thought to be due to cell damage and the resulting inflammation as trypomastigotes rupture from myocardiocytes. Lethargy, generalized lymphadenopathy, slow capillary refill time with pale mucous membranes, and in some cases splenomegaly and hepatomegaly, are the main presenting signs in young puppies. In dogs older than 6 months, clinical signs are often much less severe and sometimes not apparent at all. Serum troponin I levels slowly increase in infected dogs to spike at 10 to 30 mg/mL at 21 DPI. Serum alanine aminotransferase, aspartate aminotransferase, creatinine, and urea nitrogen can be elevated, especially in dogs that are at risk of death from severe acute myocarditis. Dogs infected after 6 months of age may show no signs of acute disease other than slight depression and low-rising parasitemia. Serum troponin I levels are elevated in these dogs but usually not to high levels. The electrocardiogram (ECG) of dogs with severe myocarditis may show sinus tachycardia, decreased R-wave amplitude, prolonged P-R interval, axis shifts, T-wave inversion, and conduction abnormalities, including first- and second-degree atrioventricular block and right bundle branch block (**Fig. 2**). ECGs are usually within normal limits. Sudden death, presumably from cardiac muscle failure or conduction system failures leading to malignant arrhythmias, is not a common occurrence. Histopathologic findings include a severe diffuse granulomatous myocarditis, large numbers of parasitic pseudocysts, and minimal fibrosis (**Fig. 3**). Although less common than signs referable to cardiac abnormalities, neurologic signs referable to meningoencephalitis (as a direct result of parasitic invasion of the neurologic system) may also occur, and include weakness, pelvic limb ataxia, and hyperreflexive spinal reflexes suggestive of distemper.

Dogs that survive the acute phase enter the prolonged indeterminate phase typified by the lack of clinical signs. The parasitemia becomes subpatent at about 30 DPI and can only be demonstrated by blood culture or xenodiagnosis. The ECG is usually normal during this phase although ventricular-based arrhythmias can be induced by exercise.[4] Although not all dogs progress to develop chronic disease, some develop chronic myocarditis with cardiac dilatation over the next 8 to 36 months.[3,4] With the progressive development of cardiac dilation, ECG abnormalities become more prevalent and may even result in sudden death. Clinical signs referable to right-sided and eventually, in some, left-sided chamber failure occurs, and can include pulse deficits, ascites, pleural effusion, hepatomegaly, and jugular venous congestion.[3] Dogs

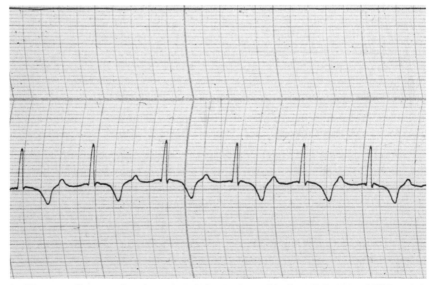

Fig. 2. Electrocardiogram showing second-degree heart block and depressed QRS complexes often present in dogs with acute Chagas disease.

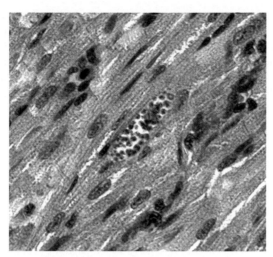

Fig. 3. Pseudocyst of *T cruzi* within a myocardiocyte of an infected dog (hematoxylin-eosin stain, original magnification ×1000).

diagnosed at an older age (mean of 9 years) survived between 30 to 60 months whereas dogs diagnosed at a younger age (mean of 4.5 years) survived only up to 5 months after diagnosis.[17] These cases are indistinguishable from chronic dilative cardiomyopathy seen in large breeds of dogs, and often are diagnosed as such until histology or immunohistochemistry findings are available.[5–7] Echocardiographic abnormalities include right ventricular dilation with progression to include a loss of left ventricular function with decreased fractional shortening, reduced ejection fraction, reduced left ventricular free wall thickness, and increase in end-systolic volume. The pathogenesis of the biventricular dilative cardiomyopathy is unknown, but possible mechanisms include immune-mediated mechanisms or toxic parasitic products directed against the myocardiocytes or autonomic nervous system, or microvascular disease coupled with platelet dysfunction.[34,35] Histopathology of the myocardium is characterized by multifocal interstitial mononuclear cellular infiltrates, perivasculitis, and marked fibrosis, and the rare presence, if any, of parasitic pseudocysts.[5,34] Cardiac dilatation occurs when fibrosis no longer permits efficient compensatory hypertrophy.[34,36] Some *T cruzi* isolates that infect dogs in the United States are not pathogenic but can produce a marked serologic response and a low parasitemia during times of stress or immunosuppression.[3,37]

DIAGNOSIS

The hallmark of making a diagnosis of Chagas disease is first to suspect the infection. Chagas disease should be considered in any dog with signs of myocarditis or cardiomyopathy, particularly if it lives or has lived at any time, even years before presentation, in an endemic region. During acute disease, trypomastigotes may be detected on examination of a blood smear during normal hematology examination (see **Fig. 1**). However, blood parasite counts may be so low that only a few parasites may be present on the entire slide, demanding diligent examination; some form of concentration technique may also be used. High-power (×400) examination of the buffy coat-plasma interface of a centrifuged microhematocrit tube may reveal characteristically motile parasites. Examination of a thick-film buffy coat smear stained with either

Wright's or Giemsa is more sensitive than examination of a blood smear preparation. A highly effective concentration technique involves pelleting trypomastigotes from plasma (obtained by centrifugation of 50 mL heparinized blood at 800 *g* for 10 minutes) by further centrifugation (8000 *g* for 15 minutes). The pellet from the final centrifugation may be examined microscopically after staining, be submitted for polymerase chain reaction (PCR) analysis, or used to inoculate liver infusion tryptose (LIT) growth media in which epimastigotes will grow over several weeks. Trypomastigotes may also be found on cytologic examination of lymph node aspirates and in abdominal effusions. Serology and PCR may also be extremely useful in the diagnosis of Chagas disease, especially during the indeterminate and chronic phases when trypomastigotes are extremely difficult to demonstrate.[38] The indirect fluorescent antibody assay, enzyme-linked immunosorbent assay, and radioimmunoprecipitation assay are most commonly used.[39] These tests confirm the presence of antibodies to *T cruzi* but most cross-react with antibodies to *Leishmania.* Further, in rare cases in dogs, the clinical signs of Chagas disease and leishmaniasis overlap to such a level that it is necessary to go to considerable lengths to establish a diagnosis.[40] Therefore, a detailed history of the likelihood of exposure to *Leishmania* must be known before an accurate interpretation of serologic results can be made.

A PCR assay, which detects DNA of the organism in various samples (blood, plasma, lymph node aspirates, or ascitic fluid may all be used), is highly specific for *T cruzi* but has low sensitivity unless multiple samples are examined.[38] Serology in association with clinical signs is considered the gold standard for the diagnosis of Chagas disease in dogs. The serum titer usually becomes positive by 21 DPI at the time when the parasitemia is declining, and persists for the life span of the animal irrespective of whether clinical signs develop.[37]

THERAPY

Treatment of dogs in the acute phase of disease is poorly reported as this phase is seldom recognized. Nifurtimox (Bayer 2502 or Lampit; Bayer, Leverkusen-Bayerwerk, Germany), usually in association with corticosteroids,[41] and benznidazole (Ragonil; Roche, Buenos Aires, Argentina) use have been reported in the dog (**Table 1**). However, the severe side effects of nifurtimox preclude its use. The drug of choice currently is benznidazole because it has less side effects, has been reported effective in treating acute canine infections,[42] and is available from the Centers for Disease Control (CDC) in Atlanta, Georgia. The main side effect of benznidazole is vomiting. After treatment with benznidazole, serum antibody titers usually remain elevated although they are reported to drop in people. Ketoconazole, gossypol, allopurinol, imidazole, and verapamil have shown promise in other species but are all ineffective in the treatment of Chagas disease in dogs. It is unknown if successful treatment

Table 1 Drug therapy for Chagas disease					
Drug[a]	Tablet Size (mg)	Dose (mg/kg)	Route	Interval (h)	Duration (mos)
Benznidazole (Ragonil)	100	5–10	PO	24	2
Nifurtimox (Lampit)	120	2–7	PO	6	3–5
Prednisone	Multiple	0.5	PO	12	1

[a] Ragonil and Lampit are available from the Centers for Disease Control, Atlanta, GA.

during the acute phase changes the likelihood of development, or outcome, of chronic disease in dogs.

Most cases of Chagas disease are diagnosed during the chronic stage. Unfortunately, treatments directed against the parasite at this stage rarely change the outcome of disease. Treatment should be directed toward the myocardial failure and ventricular arrhythmias, although the latter seem resistant to drug therapy.[39]

Unfortunately, medical treatments rarely result in a clinical cure. In severe cases of acute myocarditis coupled with high parasitemia, prognosis is poor and zoonotic risk higher (to those handling blood products), so euthanasia should be considered in these cases. If dogs survive acute disease, progression to the chronic stage tends to occur more quickly (in about 1 to 2 years) in dogs diagnosed at a younger age (<2 years) than dogs diagnosed at an older age (>4 years), which survive longer (3 to 5 years).[17]

PREVENTION

Limiting contact with vectors and possible reservoir hosts (raccoons, opossums, armadillos, and skunks) should reduce the risk of infection. Dogs should not be fed meat from reservoir hosts. Kennels and surrounding structures (chicken houses, wood piles) should be sprayed monthly with a residual insecticide such as benzene hexachloride. Dog housing should be upgraded to remove vector nesting sites. Applications of fipronil on the coats of dogs do not appear to prevent infections in dogs, or reduce the feeding of vectors,[43] but deltamethrin-treated collars do reduce *Tri infestans* feeding.[44,45] Dogs used as blood donors should be serologically screened to determine previous exposure to *T cruzi*. In highly endemic regions (southern Texas), bitches should be screened serologically and positive animals should not be bred.

PUBLIC HEALTH CONSIDERATIONS

Chagas disease is the most common cause of congestive heart failure in the world. Most cases in humans in the United States are acquired by blood transfusion or laboratory accident. There are probably several reasons why only 6 naturally acquired cases have been reported in the United States. First, North American vector species are poorly adapted to living in houses, and do not defecate on the host after a blood meal. Second, the high standard of housing in North America prevents vectors nesting in human dwellings. Third, it is possible that some human cases of Chagas disease in North America have not been identified because of a low level of suspicion.

Although the risk of acquiring infection from an infected dog is extremely low, the severity and difficulty of treating disease in humans makes this disease of considerable public health significance. Veterinarians should be particularly careful in handling blood samples from infected dogs, and warn laboratory staff of the potential infectivity of the samples. Accidental needle sticks when administering therapy to or withdrawing samples from infected dogs should be reported immediately to the CDC.

SUMMARY

Chagas disease mainly occurs in working dogs in southeastern Texas. The protozoan traditionally is transmitted in the feces of the vector, which defecates in the bite wound caused by vector feeding. However, it is likely that most dogs become infected by eating infected vectors, causing the release of the organisms into the mouth of the host. Soon after infection, an acute myocarditis results from organism multiplication in and rupture from myocardiocytes. This stage is rarely appreciated clinically. Most dogs are diagnosed during the chronic stage of the disease, which is typified by dilated cardiomyopathy and malignant ventricular-based arrhythmias. Although benznidazole is effective in removing parasites from circulation, supportive therapy to control the arrhythmias and cardiac dysfunction become the mainstay of treatment. Chagas disease is considered zoonotic, although infected dogs are of little risk to humans.

REFERENCES

1. Chagas C. Nova tripanosomiase humana. Estudos sobre a morfologia e o ciclo evolutivo do *Schizotrypanum cruzi* n. gen., n. sp., agente etiologico de nova entrade morbida do homen. Mem Inst Oswaldo Cruz 1909;1:1–9 [in Spanish].
2. Espinosa R, Carrasco HA, Belandria F. Life expectancy analysis in patients with Chagas' disease. Prognosis after one decade (1973–1983). Int J Cardiol 1985;8: 45–56.
3. Barr SC, Gossett KA, Klei TR. Clinical, clinicopathologic, and parasitologic observations of trypanosomiasis in dogs infected with North American *Trypanosoma cruzi* isolates. Am J Vet Res 1991;52:954–60.
4. Barr SC, Holmes RA, Klei TR. Electrocardiographic and echocardiographic features of trypanosomiasis in dogs inoculated with North American *Trypanosoma cruzi* isolates. Am J Vet Res 1992;53:521–7.
5. Barr SC, Schmidt SP, Brown CC, et al. Pathologic features of dogs inoculated with North American *Trypanosoma cruzi* isolates. Am J Vet Res 1991;52:2033–9.
6. Barr SC, Simpson RM, Schmidt SP, et al. Chronic dilatative myocarditis caused by *Trypanosoma cruzi* in two dogs. J Am Vet Med Assoc 1989;195:1237–41.
7. Barr SC, van Beek O, Carlisle-Nowak MS, et al. *Trypanosoma cruzi* infection in Walker hounds from Virginia. Am J Vet Res 1995;56:1037–44.
8. Berger SL, Palmer RH, Hodges CC, et al. Neurologic manifestations of trypanosomiasis in a dog. J Am Vet Med Assoc 1991;198:132–4.
9. Yaeger RG. Transmission of *Trypanasoma cruzi* infection to opossums via the oral route. J Parasitol 1971;57:1375–6.
10. Roellig DM, Ellis AE, Yabsley MJ. Oral transmission of *Trypanosoma cruzi* with opposing evidence for the theory of carnivory. J Parasitol 2009;95(2):360–4.
11. Estrada-Franco JG, Bhatia V, Diaz-Albiter H, et al. Human *Trypanasoma cruzi* infection and seropositivity in dogs, Mexico. Emerg Infect Dis 2006;12:624–30.
12. Dorn PL, Perniciaro L, Yabsley MJ, et al. Autochthonous transmission of *Trypanasoma cruzi*, Louisiana. Emerg Infect Dis 2007;13:605–7.
13. Kirchhoff LV. American trypanosomiasis (Chagas' disease) Ca tropical disease now in the United States. N Engl J Med 1993;329:639–44.
14. Schmunis GA. *Trypanosoma cruzi*, the etiologic agent of Chagas' disease: status in the blood supply in endemic and nonendemic countries. Transfusion 1991;31: 547–57.
15. Barr SC. Canine American trypanosomiasis. Compend Cont Educ Pract Vet 1991; 13:745–55.
16. Kjos SA, Snowden KF, Craig TM, et al. Distribution and characterization of canine Chagas disease in Texas. Vet Parasitol 2008;152:249–56.
17. Meurs KM, Anthony MA, Slater M, et al. Chronic *Trypanosoma cruzi* infection in dogs: 11 cases (1987–1996). J Am Vet Med Assoc 1998;213:497–500.
18. Bradley KK, Bergman DK, Woods JP, et al. Prevalence of American trypanosomiasis (Chagas disease) among dogs in Oklahoma. J Am Vet Med Assoc 2000;217: 1853–7.

19. Snider TG, Yaeger RG, Dellucky J. Myocarditis caused by *Trypanosoma cruzi* in a native Louisiana dog. J Am Vet Med Assoc 1992;177:247–9.
20. Tippit TS. Canine trypanosomiasis (Chagas' disease). Southwest Vet 1978;2: 97–104.
21. Carcavallo RU. The subfamily Triatominae (hemiptera, reduviidae): systematics and ecological factors. In: Brenner RR, Stoke A, editors. Chagas' disease vectors. Boco Rotan (FL): CRC Press; 1987. p. 13–8.
22. Beard CB, Pye G, Steurer FJ, et al. Chagas' disease in a domestic transmission cycle, southern Texas. Emerg Infect Dis 2003;9:103–5.
23. Yaeger RG. The present status of Chagas' disease in the United States. Bull Tulane Univ Med Fac 1961;21:6–13.
24. Barr SC, Brown C, Dennis VA, et al. The lesions and prevalence of *Trypanosoma cruzi* in opossums and armadillos from southern Louisiana. J Parasitol 1991;77: 624–7.
25. Burkholder JE, Allison TC, Kelly VP. *Trypanosoma cruzi* (Chagas) (protozoa: Kinetoplastida) in invertebrate, reservoir and human hosts of the lower Rio Grande Valley of Texas. J Parasitol 1980;66:305–11.
26. John DT, Hoppe KL. *Trypanosoma cruzi* from wild raccoons in Oklahoma. Am J Vet Res 1986;47:1056–9.
27. Karsten V, Davis C, Kuhn R. *Trypanosoma cruzi* in wild raccoons and opossums in North Carolina. J Parasitol 1992;78:547–9.
28. Pung OJ, Banks CW, Jones DN, et al. *Trypanosoma cruzi* in wild raccoons, opossums, and triatomine bugs in southeast Georgia, USA. J Parasitol 1995;81:324–6.
29. Walton BC, Bauman PM, Diamond LS, et al. The isolation and identification of *Trypanosoma cruzi* from raccoons in Maryland. Am J Trop Med Hyg 1958;7:603–10.
30. Yabsley MJ, Noblet GP. Seroprevalence of *Trypanosoma cruzi* in raccoons from South Carolina and Georgia. J Wildl Dis 2002;38:75–83.
31. Yaeger RG. The prevalence of *Trypanasoma cruzi* infection in armadillos collected at a site near New Orleans, Louisiana. Am J Trop Med Hyg 1988;38: 323–6.
32. Woody NC, Woody NB. American trypanosomiasis I. Clinical and epidemiologic background of Chagas' disease in California. J Pediatr 1961;58:568–80.
33. Barr SC, Dennis VA, Klei TR. Growth parameters in axenic and cell cultures, protein profiles, and zymodeme typing of three *Trypanosoma cruzi* isolates from Louisiana mammals. J Parasitol 1990;76:631–8.
34. Andrade ZA, Andrade SG, Correa R, et al. Myocardial changes in acute *Trypanosoma cruzi* infection: ultrastructural evidence of immune damage and the role of microangiopathy. Am J Pathol 1994;144:1403–11.
35. Andrade ZA, Andrade SG, Sadigursky M, et al. The indeterminate phase of Chagas disease: ultrastructural characterization of cardiac changes in the canine model. Am J Trop Med Hyg 1997;57:328–36.
36. Tanowitz HB, Kirchhoff LV, Simon D, et al. Chagas' disease. Clin Microbiol Rev 1992;5:400–19.
37. Barr SC, Dennis VA, Klei TR, et al. Antibody and lymphoblastogenic responses of dogs experimentally infected with *Trypanosoma cruzi* isolates from North American mammals. Vet Immunol Immunopathol 1991;29:267–83.
38. Araujo FM, Bahia MT, Magalhaes NM, et al. Follow-up of experimental chronic Chagas' disease in dogs: use of polymerase chain reaction (PCR) compared with parasitological and serological methods. Acta Trop 2002;81:21–31.
39. Barr SC. American trypanosomiasis. In: Greene CE, editor. Infectious diseases of the dog and cat. 2nd edition. Philadelphia: WB Saunders; 2006. p. 676–80.

40. Nabity MB, Barnhart K, Logan KS. An atypical case of *Trypanosoma cruzi* infection in a young English Mastiff. Vet Parasitol 2006;140:356–61.
41. Andrade ZA, Andrade SG, Sadigursky M. Experimental Chagas' disease in dogs. Arch Pathol Lab Med 1981;105:460–4.
42. Viotti R, Vigliano C, Armenti H, et al. Treatment of chronic Chagas' disease with benznidazole: clinical and serologic evolution of patients with long-term follow-up. Am Heart J 1994;127:151–62.
43. Gurtler RE, Ceballos LA, Stariolo R, et al. Effects of topical application of fipronil spot-on on dogs against the Chagas' disease vector *Triatoma infestans*. Trans R Soc Trop Med Hyg 2009;103(3):298–304.
44. Reithinger R, Ceballos L, Stariolo R, et al. Chagas disease control: deltamethrin-treated collars reduce *Triatoma infestans* feeding success on dogs. Trans R Soc Trop Med Hyg 2005;99:502–8.
45. Reithinger R, Ceballos L, Stariolo R, et al. Extinction of experimental *Triatoma infestans* populations following continuous exposure to dogs wearing deltamethrin-treated collars. Am J Trop Med Hyg 2006;74:766–71.

Canine Leishmaniasis in North America: Emerging or Newly Recognized?

Christine A. Petersen, DVM, PhD[a],*, Stephen C. Barr, BVSc, PhD[b]

KEYWORDS

• Canine • *Leishmania infantum* • Protozoa • Emerging
• Treatment • Diagnosis

Leishmania infantum, an obligate intracellular parasite, is the causative agent of visceral leishmaniasis (VL) in the Mediterranean Basin and more recently North America. Natural hosts include dogs and humans[1] and transmission is usually by way of a sand fly vector. Infected dogs are the primary reservoir for zoonotic visceral leishmaniasis in endemic regions (**Fig. 1**A), and are the most significant risk factor predisposing humans to infection.[2] Dogs have a wide range of clinical presentation caused by infection with *Le infantum*, ranging from asymptomatic to fatal visceralizing disease. Host factors which determine clinical outcome are poorly understood. When clinical signs in dogs occur, they include enlarged lymph nodes and hepato- and splenomegaly caused by parasitic invasion of the reticulo-endothelial system of phagocytic lymphocytes.[3] Visceral leishmaniasis symptoms often persist in canine patients for several weeks to months before patients seek medical care, and in the United States it may be even longer before a correct diagnosis is made. In the meanwhile these patients are at risk of death from bacterial co-infections, massive bleeding, severe anemia,[3] or renal failure.

TRANSMISSION OF *LEISHMANIA INFANTUM*

In endemic areas, the primary means of transmission is vector-borne by way of the sand fly (**Fig. 2**). Vector-borne transmission has not been shown in the United States to date.[4,5] Instead, vertical transmission appears to be the primary means of transmission in dogs in the United States without a travel history to an endemic region.[4] The

Dr Petersen is currently funded by AKC CHF grants 1159 and 1220 and NIH R21AI074711.
[a] Department of Veterinary Pathology, 2714 Vet. Med., Iowa State University, Ames, IA 50014, USA
[b] Department of Clinical Sciences, College of Veterinary Medicine, Cornell University, C2 502A Clinical Programs Center, Ithaca, NY 14853, USA
* Corresponding author.
E-mail address: kalicat@iastate.edu (C.A. Petersen).

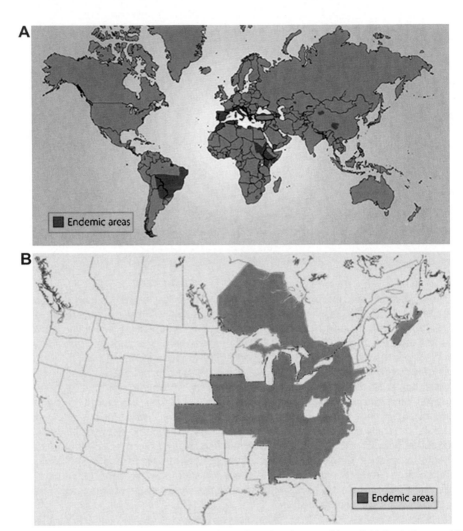

Fig. 1. Prevalence of canine visceral *Leishmaniasis* in the World and United States. (*A*) Global seroprevalence of Canine VL. (*Adapted from* Desjeux P. Disease watch focus: leishmaniasis. Nature Rev Microbiol 2004;2:692; with permission.) (*B*) Seroprevalence of CVL in Foxhounds in North America. (*Adapted from* Duprey ZH, Steurer FJ, Rooney JA, et al. Canine visceral leishmaniasis, United States and Canada, 2000–2003. Emerg Infect Dis 2006;12(3):440–6.)

frequency of vertical transmission in endemic areas is unknown because of the overwhelming likelihood of vector contact.[6]

A potential sand fly vector of *Le infantum*, *Lutzomyia shannoni*, is present within Southern and Southeastern United States.[4] *Lu shannoni* is known to bite dogs and other mammals and has been incriminated in the transmission of *Le brasiliensis* in South and Central America.[7] Anecdotal data indicate that United States species of *Lu shannoni* can become infected with *Le infantum*, but it is not known whether these flies permit *Le infantum* development into infectious metacyclic infectious parasites. Vector feeding preferences can importantly influence disease transmission. In the

A   Classical *Leishmania infantum* Lifecycle

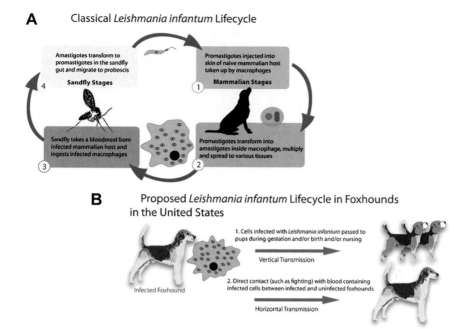

B   Proposed *Leishmania infantum* Lifecycle in Foxhounds in the United States

Fig. 2. The classical *Leishmania* life cycle (*A*) requires a sand fly and mammalian host. (*B*) A proposed *Leishmania infantum* life cycle in the United States Foxhound population with a prominent role for vertical transmission.

United States, *Lu shannoni* has also been shown to feed on dogs (Rowton, personal communication, 2006).

In many settings dogs have been shown to be a link between sylvatic and domestic cycles of visceral leishmaniasis. Dogs often cross forest-edge boundaries, thereby potentially bringing parasites to, or from, sylvatic systems, and to and from other potential mammal hosts, such as foxes and opossums. In the United States, because of frequent exchange of Foxhounds between kennels and these dogs' penchant for spending time in the woods, these dogs may be a primary focal point for transmission of *Le infantum* to continue transmission to sand flies. Thus, if *Lu shannoni* indeed prefers to feed on dogs in comparison to other mammals, infected dogs are more likely than other mammals to serve as a source of *Le infantum* to an uninfected fly.

EPIDEMIOLOGY OF CANINE VISCERAL LEISHMANIASIS IN THE UNITED STATES

A retrospective study performed by the Centers for Disease Control and Prevention, Division of Parasitic Diseases, employed sera samples that were collected between April 2000 and December 2003. Samples were taken from greater than 12,000 Foxhounds and other canids in the United States, and an 8.9% seroprevalence was observed in Foxhounds but not other randomly selected domestic dogs or wild canids.[4] Samples detected at 1:16 and 1:32 were considered suspect.[4] This study initially had participation from almost all registered Foxhound kennels in the United States, but after the first year participation greatly decreased, perhaps leading to a selection bias in further years of kennels with known clinical infection with *Le infantum*.

Between years 2000 and 2001, even though the number of participating kennels decreased, the number of *Leishmania* seropositive samples increased, most likely indicating that there was increased infection/incidence of disease in these participating kennels. In studies of Foxhound kennels, we observe a similar 9.8% overall seropositivity/seroprevalence in our current cohort of 10 kennels and over 500 dogs, but among high-risk kennels the seropositivity and presence of polysymptomatic disease is 13.5%. Infection in this cohort is greater than observed by serology as indicated by a 22.8% quantitative Polymerase Chain Reaction Assay (qPCR) positivity in the overall cohort. The percent qPCR positive dogs in high-risk kennels is 44.8%. Roughly half of the qPCR positive (infected) population was clinically asymptomatic (Petersen, unpublished data, 2008). In dog breeds from endemic countries, a higher sero- or PCR prevalence is also seen as compared with the overall canine population. This includes dog breeds from Southern Europe, such as Corsicas, Italian Spinones, and Neapolitan Mastiffs (Petersen, and CDC serologic unpublished data, 2008).

TRANSMISSION OF VISCERAL LEISHMANIASIS IN THE UNITED STATES

Visceral Leishmaniasis is classically transmitted to a suitable mammalian host by the bite of an infected sand fly after which the promastigote form of the parasite is phagocytosed by macrophages (**Fig. 2**).[1] Although endemic in many parts of the world, this disease has only recently been described in the United States.[8] Previously, sporadic cases have been reported in the United States, in canine travelers returning to the United States from endemic areas.[5] However, in 2000, a kennel in New York State reported four Foxhounds to be infected with *Le infantum*.[8] By 2005, 60 kennels in 22 states and two Canadian provinces had reported seropositive Foxhounds.[9] Nonvector based mechanisms postulated for transmission of canine visceral leishmaniasis in the United States include vertical transmission (transplacental or transmammary) and horizontal transmission by direct contact with infected cells in blood (**Fig. 2**).[4,5,10] Transmission has been documented by way of packed red blood cell transfusion from infected Foxhounds.[11] It is not known how frequently vertical transmission occurs naturally in endemic areas, although studies which used collars or topical insecticides to prevent transmission do not see transmission reduced below 4% in dogs.[2,12] There are reports of congenital transmission of visceral leishmaniasis in humans and during experimental *Le infantum* infection of beagles.[9] In spite of a possible change in primary suspected route of transmission, clinical signs and microscopic lesions of visceral leishmaniasis of United States Foxhounds is equivalent to that seen in dogs infected in endemic areas through sand fly transmission.[10] Whether vertical transmission itself is solely responsible for the focus of disease particularly in Foxhounds, Corsicas, Spinones, and Neapolitan Mastiffs in the United States or whether there are genetic factors predisposing particular breeds to disease has not been well investigated. In endemic areas all breeds of dogs are affected.

The genotype of *Le Infantum* isolated from Foxhounds in the United States is MON-1. The MON-1 genotype is isolated most frequently from dogs living in the Mediterranean basin suggesting that infected dogs may have originally been brought to the United States from this area. A Centers of Disease Control and Prevention (CDC) investigation indicated that it was most likely that these infected hounds first originated from Southern France, were then imported into Great Britain, and further brought to the United States. (Schantz and colleagues, unpublished data, 2005).

COMMON CLINICAL AND PATHOLOGIC FINDINGS WITH VISCERAL LEISHMANIASIS

Physical examination findings may include depression, loss of condition, particularly decreased muscle mass over shoulders, hips, and spine, with a mildly distended abdomen, serosanguineous nasal discharge, dull hair coat, splenomegaly, and generalized lymphadenopathy. About one third of cases have a fever. Other clinical signs may include diarrhea, vomiting, epistaxis, melena, dry brittle hair coat, and long brittle nails. Although officially categorized as a form of visceral leishmaniasis, cutaneous lesions including bilaterally symmetric nonpruritic alopecia, hyperkeratosis, excessive epidermal scale with thickening, depigmentation, and chapping of the muzzle and footpads, occur with some regularity. Abnormal clinical pathologic values often include decreased hematocrit, thrombocytopenia, and signs of renal failure including azotemia, increased blood urea nitrogen and creatinine, hyperphosphatemia, hypermagnesemia, and proteinuria. Signs of hepatic compromise are also common including elevated alkaline phosphatase (ALP), elevated alanine transferase (ALT), and hypercholesterolemia. Other common clinical chemistry abnormalities include hyperproteinemia observed with hypergammaglobulinemia and hypoalbuminemia.

Gross pathologic examination may find emaciation with minimal adipose tissue in body cavities and subcutaneous tissues. Many lymph nodes, including peripheral, mesenteric, and mediastinal, are often moderately to markedly enlarged. The liver and spleen will also be diffusely enlarged. Kidneys may be moderately enlarged and diffusely pale. Impression smears obtained at necropsy from the spleen, popliteal lymph node, liver stained with Diff-Quick, often will reveal widely scattered macrophages with intracellular amastigotes consistent with *Leishmania* species. Cytologically within the liver, spleen, bone marrow, and lymph nodes there will often also be amastigotes consistent with *Leishmania* species. These organisms are 1 to 3 µm in diameter, and have a round, deeply basophilic nucleus and a rod shaped kinetoplast (**Fig. 3**A). These can be specifically identified as *Leishmania* by immunohistochemistry (**Fig. 3**B.)

DIAGNOSIS OF VISCERAL LEISHMANIASIS

In humans and dogs, infection with *Le. infantum* frequently does not equate with clinical illness. The ratio of incident asymptomatic infection to incident clinical cases varies with location, vector and parasite. Ratios of 18:1 in Brazil and 50:1 in Spain have been observed in human populations[3] and is estimated to be 2:1 in high-risk United States' Foxhounds. We suggest that a different means of transmission, as observed in United States' Foxhounds, will also alter this ratio. At present, diagnosis and control of visceral leishmaniasis is difficult as humans and dogs can be infected but seronegative for years.[13] Various means of serology are the primary diagnostic tests used for surveillance of visceral leishmaniasis. For public health surveillance in the United States where this disease is not endemic in humans, testing is performed by way of an indirect fluorescent antibody assay (IFA) by the CDC. IFA is sufficient for screening purposes, but is found to cross react with antibodies to the kinetoplastid *Trypanosoma cruzi*. *T cruzi* infects dogs in the Southeastern United States, thus further testing is required to determine parasite specificity unless clinical signs are much more consistent with one infection over the other (eg, cardiomyopathy in the case of Chagas disease). Other serologic tests are available in the United States for detection of canine leishmaniasis including a highly sensitive and specific kinetic ELISA available through the Cornell University diagnostic laboratory and a K39-antigen based assay available through Heska. Positive serology in Foxhounds appears to more closely correlate with the appearance of clinical disease than incidence of infection. Reports have shown that qPCR performed by a well-regulated and stringently tested laboratory can be a more sensitive test for *Le infantum* infection in dogs and can detect asymptomatic dogs or dogs that have yet to seroconvert.[10] qPCR is available through Iowa State University and the CDC.

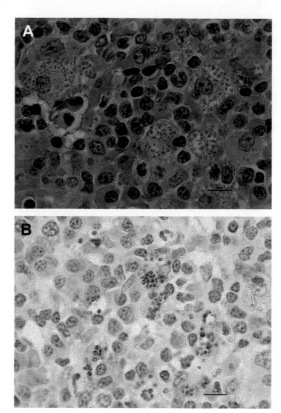

Fig. 3. Numerous *Leishmania infantum* amastigotes in a section of spleen from a U.S. Foxhound. Notice multiple amastigotes within macrophages. *(A)* Multiple amastigotes (H&E stain, original magnification ×40). *(B)* Immunohistochemistry for *Leishmania infantum* amastigotes *(red)*; bar = 20 μm.

IMMUNE ALTERATION AND PATHOGENESIS OF VISCERAL LEISHMANIASIS

Mammalian host responses which prevent progression to clinical VL has been shown to be dependent on promoting T helper-1 IFN-γ production-based immunity and parasiticidal activity within infected macrophages.[3] A key immunologic feature of late stage clinical VL in dogs is an inability to proliferate or to produce IFN-γ in response to *Leishmania* antigen,[14] (Petersen, unpublished data, 2008). Pharmacologically-cured individuals are resistant to reinfection and mount antigen-specific IFN-γ responses in vitro, indicating that there is not an inherent defect in host CD4+ T cell responses of clinical patients once they have reached this stage. High levels of TNF-α have been proposed to stimulate production of regulatory cytokines, specifically IL-10, as a homeostatic response to prevent further inflammation-mediated pathology. High leisonal IL-10 mRNA production is frequently found in human patients with VL,[15,16] and produced by polysymptomatic Foxhounds (Petersen, unpublished data, 2008). IL-10 can be produced by many cell types including T cells, B cells, and macrophages. One of the proposed mechanisms of IL-10 promotion of VL is by conditioning macrophages for parasite growth and survival versus killing of intracellular parasites.

In our surveillance studies, we have observed repeated cases where Foxhounds do not show clinical signs of VL until there is secondary immunosuppression caused by pregnancy, concomitant Lyme disease, or other tick-borne illness.[10] This clinical shift toward disease consistently appears upon a change from being seronegative to seropositive in these dogs. Further studies are required to determine the effects of immune alterations that lead to clinical disease in these dogs. Congenital infection secondary to vertical transmission may predispose to initial immune abnormalities, although by the time clinical signs of disease and seroconversion have appeared, evidence shows that CD4+ T cells from these dogs are able to respond normally to parasite antigen. In advanced disease it is not unusual to see immunosuppression including T-cell changes, in terms of reduced CD4+ T cell proliferation in response to whole *Le infantum* antigen or routine canine vaccines and decreased ability of these cells to produce IFN-γ in response to *Le infantum* antigen.

GENETIC FACTORS RELATED TO VISCERAL LEISHMANIASIS DISEASE SUSCEPTIBILITY

Although several genetic polymorphisms, including alterations in TNF-α and solute carrier family 11A1 (SLC11A1, formerly NRAMP1) allelic expression, have been indicated to predispose to disease,[17,18] causative factors of disease susceptibility in humans and dogs, specifically those associated with heritability, remain elusive. Breed type has also been shown to alter the response to therapy, suggesting that canine breed-related genetic factors modulate disease progression and are therefore prognostically significant.[19]

Numerous Foxhounds have tested positive for VL in the United States and infection appears to be endemic only within this breed here. If vertical transmission is indeed the primary route of transmission in these dogs, a particular genetic susceptibility is not absolutely necessary for widespread infection to occur in the Foxhound population. The observance of visceral leishmaniasis within specific families of Foxhounds and finding dogs that are *Leishmania* disease resistant suggests that it is highly likely that particular genetic traits of dogs at least in part determine which dogs develop visceral leishmaniasis versus remain clinically disease-free.

TREATMENT/PROGNOSIS

Treatment of canine visceral leishmaniasis (CVL) is rarely curative. Prognosis for emaciated chronically infected animals is very poor and in these cases euthanasia should be considered. It is critical to advise the owner of potential zoonotic transmission of organisms from lesions to humans before maintaining a *Leishmania*-infected dog in their household, particularly if there are immunosupressed people sharing the household. The owner should be informed that the organism will never be completely eliminated (ie, no sterile cure) and relapse occurs very frequently requiring retreatment. Treatment should be undertaken on an outpatient basis. Because of the chronic wasting that can occur with leishmaniasis, it is important to provide a good high-quality protein diet or a diet appropriate for renal insufficiency if this manifestation of leishmaniasis is present.

Because of difficulty obtaining certain drugs in the United States, treatment is recommended to begin with allopurinol (Zyloric). This drug is efficacious and nontoxic when used as a maintenance drug. Clinical remission is often achieved when used alone. Relapses are common when treatment ceases, complete cures are rare but survival occurs in 80% of cases over 4 years if renal insufficiency is not present when treatment is initiated. This drug is sometimes used in combination with pentavalent antimony (Glucantime), as drug resistance is seen for pentavalent antimony alone in endemic areas (France, Spain, and Italy). Pentavalent antimonials are not licensed for use in the United States and can only be obtained by way of an investigational drug

Table 1
First-line treatment options for canine visceral leishmaniasis.

Drug	Dose (mg/kg)	Route	Interval (Hrs)	Duration (Mos)
Allopurinol	7.0–20.0	PO	8–12	3–24[a]
Amphotericin B – Fungizone	0.25–0.5[b]	IV	48[c]	[d]
Meglumine antimoniate[e] – Glucantime	100.0	IV,	24	1
Sodium stibogluconate – Pentostam	30.0–50.0	IV, SC	24	1

Abbreviations: IV, intravenously; PO, orally; SC, subcutaneous.
[a] Or for rest of dog's life.
[b] Reconstituted in 5% dextrose (do not reconstitute in electrolyte solutions which precipitate the drug) and dilute to administer; if normal renal function, dilute in 60 to 120 mL 5% dextrose given over 15 minutes; if renal compromise, dilute in 0.5 to 1 L 5% dextrose given over 3 to 4 hours to reduce further renal toxicity.
[c] Or 3 times a week.
[d] Administer until a total cumulative dose of 5 to 10 mg/kg is reached.
[e] Not available in the United States.

use protocol from the CDC.[20,21] The two main drugs in this class are: (1) sodium stibogluconate (Pentostam, Wellcome Foundation Ltd, U.K.), which requires daily injection and has severe side effects, and (2) meglutamine antimoniate (Glucantime , Pfizer/ Merial, France), which has less side effects. Dosages have been listed (**Table 1**). Amphotericin B in the lipid emulsion or liposomal form is non-nephrotoxic and is effective against the organism, although it is not thought to be superior to allopurinol as it is still more costly and more toxic. Renal insufficiency must be treated before giving antimonial drugs or amphotericin B as prognosis is dependent on renal function at the onset of treatment. Treatment efficacy is best monitored by clinical improvement and presence of organisms in biopsy or as measured by rigorously controlled qPCR. Relapses occur a few months to a year after therapy, so dogs should be rechecked at least every 2 months after the end of treatment. Prognosis for a cure is very guarded, but therapy does provide infected dogs improved quality of life.

Second-line drugs, which require further clinical studies to understand their efficacy in dogs, include miltefosine (Impavido or Miltex) and paromomycin (Humantin). Paromymycin has been shown to have fewer side effects than other drugs in humans. Use of this drug has been primarily targeted to the cutaneous versions of *Leishmania*, less is known about its ability to remove organ-based infection. There is no effective vaccine against CVL available in the United States. A secreted parasite antigen-based vaccine has recently been licensed for use in dogs in Brazil. Sand fly vector control measures, including deltamethrin or permethrin-impregnated collars are useful to date to prevent disease.[22] In many countries, because of the tie of canine infection to human disease, culling of dogs is still used as a means to prevent human disease.[23,24]

SUMMARY

Canine of VL is endemic in the United States' Foxhound population. Current evidence indicates that vertical transmission may be a primary route of transmission of the parasite in this population, although *Lutzomyia* species in the United States may be involved in transmission. Further study is necessary to determine the likelihood of vector-borne transmission in the United States. There are two main diagnostic tools to characterize ongoing disease in this population: (1) qPCR to detect infection, and (2) IFA, ELISA or K39-based serology to indicate the onset or presence of clinical visceral leishmaniasis. Treatment options include allopurinol, glucantime, and newer less-toxic formulations of amphotericin B, but none of these drugs lead to life-long sterile cure and recrudescence of infection is common. Because of lack of surveillance and imperfect diagnosis in the United States, this disease may be present within at-risk canine populations before the more recently recognized outbreaks in Foxhounds.

REFERENCES

1. Roberts LJ, Handman E, Foote SJ. Science, medicine, and the future: Leishmaniasis. BMJ 2000;321(7264):801–4.
2. Gavgani AS, Hodjati MH, Mohite H, et al. Effect of insecticide-impregnated dog collars on incidence of zoonotic visceral leishmaniasis in Iranian children: a matched-cluster randomised trial. Lancet 2002;360(9330):374–9.
3. Chappuis F, Sundar S, Hailu A, et al. Visceral leishmaniasis: what are the needs for diagnosis, treatment and control? Nat Rev Microbiol 2007;5(11):873–82.
4. Duprey ZH, Steurer FJ, Rooney JA, et al. Canine visceral leishmaniasis, United States and Canada, 2000–2003. Emerg Infect Dis 2006;12(3):440–6.
5. Schantz PM, Steurer FJ, Duprey ZH, et al. Autochthonous visceral leishmaniasis in dogs in North America. J Am Vet Med Assoc 2005;226(8):1316–22.
6. Mancianti F, Gramiccia M, Gradoni L, et al. Studies on canine leishmaniasis control. 1. Evolution of infection of different clinical forms of canine leishmaniasis following antimonial treatment. Trans R Soc Trop Med Hyg 1988;82(4):566–7.
7. Travi BL, Ferro C, Cadena H, et al. Canine visceral leishmaniasis: dog infectivity to sand flies from non-endemic areas. Res Vet Sci 2002;72(1):83–6.
8. Gaskin AA, Schantz P, Jackson J, et al. Visceral leishmaniasis in a New York foxhound kennel. J Vet Intern Med 2002;16(1):34–44.
9. Rosypal AC, Troy GC, Duncan RB, et al. Utility of diagnostic tests used in diagnosis of infection in dogs experimentally inoculated with a North American isolate of Leishmania infantum. J Vet Intern Med 2005;19(6):802–9.
10. Gibson-Corley KN, Hostetter JM, Hostetter SJ, et al. Disseminated Leishmania infantum infection in two sibling American Foxhound dogs from potential vertical transmission. Can Vet J 2008;49:1005–8.
11. Owens SD, Oakley DA, Marryott K, et al. Transmission of visceral leishmaniasis through blood transfusions from infected English foxhounds to anemic dogs. J Am Vet Med Assoc 2001;219(8):1076–83.
12. Maroli M, Mizzon V, Siragusa C, et al. Evidence for an impact on the incidence of canine leishmaniasis by the mass use of deltamethrin-impregnated dog collars in southern Italy. Med Vet Entomol 2001;15(4):358–63.
13. Quinnell RJ, Courtenay O, Garcez LM, et al. IgG subclass responses in a longitudinal study of canine visceral leishmaniasis. Vet Immunol Immunopathol 2003; 91(3–4):161–8.
14. Sacks DL, Lal SL, Shrivastava SN, et al. An analysis of T cell responsiveness in Indian kala-azar. J Immunol 1987;138(3):908–13.
15. Nylen S, Maurya R, Eidsmo L, et al. Splenic accumulation of IL-10 mRNA in T cells distinct from CD4+CD25+ (Foxp3) regulatory T cells in human visceral leishmaniasis. J Exp Med 2007;204(4):805–17.
16. Nylen S, Sacks D. Interleukin-10 and the pathogenesis of human visceral leishmaniasis. Trends Immunol 2007;28(9):378–84.

17. Blackwell JM, Mohamed HS, Ibrahim ME. Genetics and visceral leishmaniasis in the Sudan: seeking a link. Trends Parasitol 2004;20(6):268–74.
18. Karplus TM, Jeronimo SM, Chang H, et al. Association between the tumor necrosis factor locus and the clinical outcome of Leishmania chagasi infection. Infect Immun 2002;70(12):6919–25.
19. Modiano JF, Breen M, Burnett RC, et al. Distinct B-cell and T-cell lymphoproliferative disease prevalence among dog breeds indicates heritable risk. Cancer Res 2005;65(13):5654–61.
20. Miro G, Cardoso L, Pennisi MG, et al. Canine leishmaniosis–new concepts and insights on an expanding zoonosis: part two. Trends Parasitol 2008;24(8):371–7.
21. Croft SL, Sundar S, Fairlamb AH. Drug resistance in leishmaniasis. Clin Microbiol Rev 2006;19(1):111–26.
22. Foglia Manzillo V, Oliva G, Pagano A, et al. Deltamethrin-impregnated collars for the control of canine leishmaniasis: Evaluation of the protective effect and influence on the clinical outcome of Leishmania infection in kenneled stray dogs. Vet Parasitol 2006;142(1-2):142–5.
23. Ashford DA, David JR, Freire M, et al. Studies on control of visceral leishmaniasis: impact of dog control on canine and human visceral leishmaniasis in Jacobina, Bahia, Brazil. Am J Trop Med Hyg 1998;59(1):53–7.
24. Moreira ED Jr, Mendes de Souza VM, Sreenivasan M, et al. Assessment of an optimized dog-culling program in the dynamics of canine Leishmania transmission. Vet Parasitol 2004;122(4):245–52.

Cestodes of Dogs and Cats in North America

Gary Conboy, DVM, PhD

KEYWORDS

- *Taenia* • *Echinococcus* • *Dipylidium* • *Mesocestoides*
- *Diphyllobothrium* • *Spirometra* • Cystic echinococcosis
- Alveolar echinococcosis

CESTODES

Cestodes are hermaphroditic flatworms consisting of a scolex, neck region, and repeating segments. Cestodes lack a mouth, intestine, and body cavity. Life cycles are indirect, with the definitive host acquiring the adult form of the tapeworm by the ingestion of the larval metacestode stage contained in an intermediate host. This process usually occurs in the form of a predator-prey relationship. Cestode infection in dogs and cats in North America is common, involving various species including cyclophyllidean (*Taenia, Dipylidium, Mesocestoides, Echinococcus*) and pseudophyllidean (*Diphyllobothrium, Spirometra*) tapeworms. Dogs and cats most often serve as definitive hosts (ie, carry the adult tapeworms in the small intestine) but on occasion are infected as intermediate hosts (ie, carry the immature metacestode stages in various tissues). The presence of adult tapeworms in the canine or feline small intestine is usually well tolerated, producing little or no clinical signs of disease. The major consequence of such infections is the shedding of eggs and proglottids which, at best, is aesthetically abhorrent and unacceptable to pet owners and, at worst, a serious economic or zoonotic health threat. The presence of the immature (metacestode) stages of tapeworms occurring in various tissues can result in life-threatening disease in dogs, cats, and humans.

Cyclophyllidean Tapeworms

In this group of tapeworms the scolex is characterized by the presence of muscular suckers, with or without an armed rostellum. Eggs pass out of the definitive host contained in a gravid proglottid (segment) that detaches from the tapeworm ribbon to pass to the outside.

Taenia spp

Although recent data are lacking, necropsy surveys in the past have indicated *Taenia* infection was fairly common in dogs and cats in North America, with a reported

Department of Pathology and Microbiology, Atlantic Veterinary College-UPEI, 550 University Avenue, Charlottetown, PEI C1A 4P3, Canada
E-mail address: conboy@upei.ca

Vet Clin Small Anim 39 (2009) 1075–1090
doi:10.1016/j.cvsm.2009.06.005
vetsmall.theclinics.com

prevalence as high as 35% in dogs and 33% in cats.[1–3] Fecal flotation surveys report much lower infection rates (0.5%–7.4%), but this reflects the poor detection sensitivity of this technique for cyclophyllidean tapeworm infection.[2,4–6] The scolex of *Taenia* has four muscular suckers and a rostellum armed with 2 rows of hooks. The segments have an irregularly alternating single lateral genital pore (**Fig. 1**). Species of *Taenia* that infect dogs include *Taenia pisiformis*, *Taenia crassiceps*, *Taenia hydatigena*, *Taenia multiceps*, *Taenia ovis*, and *Taenia serialis*. Cats may be infected with *Taenia taeniaeformis* and (rarely) *T pisiformis*. All of these species occur worldwide. In North America, *T pisiformis* is the most common, and *T multiceps* and *T ovis* are the least commonly encountered in dogs.[7,8] Adult *T taeniaeformis* are 15 to 60 cm and *T pisiformis* 60 to 200 cm in length.[9–11] Metacestode stages of *Taenia* include cysticerci (bladderworm, a single invaginated scolex inside a fluid-filled bladder), strobilocerci (scolex has evaginated and segmentation has begun), and coenuri (bladderworm contains multiple invaginated scolices).

Dogs acquire infection by the ingestion of cysticerci in the viscera of rabbits (*T pisiformis*), rodents (*T pisiformis*, *T crassiceps*), domestic and wild ruminants, horses, and pigs (*T hydatigena*), or the muscle of sheep (*T ovis*). Infection in dogs also occurs by the ingestion of coenuri in the brain or spine of sheep (*T multiceps*), or in subcutaneous and intramuscular connective tissues of rabbits and rodents (*T serialis*).[9–11] Cats acquire infection of *T taeniaeformis* by ingestion of strobilocerci contained in the tissues of rodents.[9–11] Hunting and freedom to roam are risk factors for acquiring infection with *T pisiformis*, *T crassiceps*, *T hydatigena*, and *T serialis* in dogs; proximity to a farm with livestock, particularly sheep, is a risk factor for *T hydatigena*, *T multiceps*, and *T ovis* infection in dogs.[12] Opportunity to roam and hunt is the sole risk factor for *Taenia* spp infection in cats. Infected animals pass gravid segments in the feces, or the actively motile segments may exit through the anus on their own. The prepatent period is 34 to 80 days for *T taeniaeformis* in cats and 42 to 56 days for *T pisiformis* in dogs.[13,14] Proglottid shedding tends to be irregular and persists for months to years.[14–16] The eggs contain a hexacanth embryo and are immediately

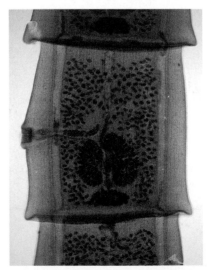

Fig. 1. Mature *Taenia* sp segment showing a single lateral genital pore (Semichon's acetic-carmine stain, original magnification ×18.5).

infective. Intermediate hosts become infected by ingesting eggs, which then develop into metacestodes in various tissues. Eggs remain viable for up to a year at low temperatures and high humidity, and less than 1 week at high temperatures and low humidity.[17]

Clinical signs are usually not associated with infection. Anal pruritus and irritation from the release of actively motile tapeworm segments, resulting in scooting behavior in dogs, has been cited to occur in some animals. However, other causes (ie, anal sac impaction) are more likely for this behavior.[18] Metacestode infection can have serious consequences in the intermediate host. Severe central nervous system disease due to coenuri in the brain or spinal chord (*T multiceps*), or condemnation at slaughter of the liver (*T hydatigena*) or the entire carcass (*T ovis*) due to the presence of cysticerci can occur in sheep and goats. In rare instances, dogs and cats can become infected with the metacestode stages of *Taenia*. To date, seven cases of fatal cerebral coenurosis due to *T serialis* infection have been reported in cats in North America.[19] Infected cats develop signs of severe central nervous system disease, and diagnosis is invariably by detection of the coenuri in the brain at necropsy. Fatal cerebral cysticercosis has also been reported in a cat due to infection with *T crassiceps*.[20] Subcutaneous cysticercosis due to *T crassiceps* and hepatic cysticercosis due to *T pisiformis* have been reported in dogs.[21] A fatal case of disseminated thoracic and abdominal cysticercosis due to *T crassiceps* has been reported in a dog.[22] The severity of the infection was attributed to a state of immunosuppression in the dog coupled with the ability of *T crassiceps* cysticerci to undergo asexual reproduction by external budding. Infection in humans with metacestodes of *T crassiceps*, *T multiceps*, *T serialis*, and *T taeniaeformis* have all been reported; however, the risk of zoonotic infection in North America seems to be very low.[23]

Diagnosis of *Taenia* infection is based on detection and identification of passed segments or by the detection of eggs on fecal flotation examination. Eggs are only present in fecal samples if the segments are damaged in transit or after fecal deposit. Therefore, fecal flotation is often negative in an animal infected with *Taenia*.[2] Segments collected by clients and brought in for identification may be dehydrated. Placement of the desiccated segments in water for 10 to 30 minutes will facilitate examination. Examination of the intact segment may show evidence of a single lateral genital pore; however, this can be difficult to visualize in unstained segments. Proglottids can be examined for the presence of eggs and identified based on egg size and morphology. Care should be taken when handling the segments during examination (gloves should be worn and strict laboratory practices observed) due to the danger of potential exposure to the eggs. The eggs are brown in color and 25 to 40 microns in diameter.[24] The eggs contain a hexacanth embryo (ie, embryo has six hooks) (**Fig. 2**). The shell wall is thick and has radial striations. Eggs detected on fecal flotation cannot be differentiated from those of *Echinococcus* spp. Eggs recovered from grossly visible tapeworm segments (10–12 mm in length) allow for a diagnosis to the level of genus (*Taenia* spp).

Infection in dogs and cats can be controlled by the administration of anthelmintics, and reducing the risk of reexposure by curbing the animal's opportunity to roam and hunt. Reinfection is likely to occur in cases in which the lifestyle of the pet remains unchanged. Praziquantel (5 mg/kg, oral or subcutaneously) is approved for use and highly effective in the treatment of *T hydatigena*, *T pisiformis*, and *T ovis* infection in dogs, as well as *T taeniaeformis* in cats. Epsiprantel is approved for use, and highly effective for the treatment of cats (2.75 mg/kg, oral) infected with *T taeniaeformis* and in dogs (5.5 mg/kg, oral) infected with *T pisiformis*. Fenbendazole (50 mg/kg,

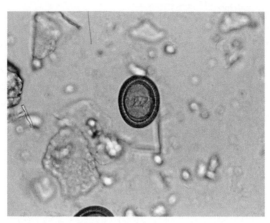

Fig. 2. A taeniid egg (*Taenia* or *Echinococcus* spp) with three of the six hooks visible in this plane of focus (original magnification ×400).

once a day for 3 days, oral) is approved for use and is effective against *T pisiformis* in dogs.[8]

Echinococcus granulosus/Echinococcus multilocularis

Echinococcus granulosus, the cause of cystic echinococcosis, and *Echinococcus multilocularis*, the cause of alveolar echinococcosis, are serious zoonotic parasites in humans.[25] *Echinococcus* spp are similar in morphology to *Taenia* with respect to the scolex and segments, but are much smaller in size (**Fig. 3**). *Echinococcus granulosus* occurs in the small intestine of dogs and various wild canids, is 2 to 7 mm in length, and consists of three to four segments. *E granulosus* occurs as two strains in North America, a sylvatic (wild canid-cervid) strain endemic in Alaska and parts of

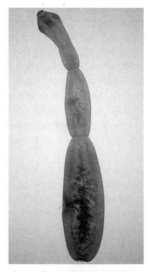

Fig. 3. Adult *Echinococcus granulosus* (Semichon's acetic-carmine stain, original magnification ×18.5).

Canada, and a pastoral (dog-sheep) strain that has a sporadic distribution in parts of Utah, Arizona, New Mexico, and California.[25] Dogs acquire infection by the ingestion of unilocular hydatids contained in the organs of infected sheep. A unilocular hydatid is a fluid-filled cyst that contains hundreds to thousands of protoscolices. The unilocular hydatid may subdivide due to internal budding of the germinal layer, but the entire cyst is contained within a host fibrous capsule as a single mass that in domestic animals may be several centimeters in diameter. The prepatent period is 34 to 53 days, and segments are shed in an irregular pattern for 5 to 29 months.[26] The proglottids are 1 to 2 mm in length and contain about 600 eggs.

People are also susceptible to infection with the dog-sheep strain of E granulosus by the ingestion of eggs, resulting in potentially life-threatening disease (cystic echinococcosis). Hydatids most often occur in the liver and lungs, and grow to a large size in people (1–15 cm in diameter or larger). Presence of the hydatid can cause pressure atrophy and impair organ function of the surrounding tissues, and usually requires surgical or medical intervention. Human infection with the sylvatic strain results in a less serious disease condition.[27]

Echinococcus multilocularis occurs in the small intestine of dogs, cats, foxes, and coyotes, is 1.2 to 4.5 mm in length, and consists of four to five segments.[9,28] Previously the E multilocularis endemic range in North America was restricted to the subarctic tundra region of Alaska and Canada. Following an expansion in the geographic distribution that has occurred over the last 4 decades, it is now endemic in three Canadian provinces (Alberta, Manitoba, Saskatchewan) and 14 states (Alaska, Illinois, Indiana, Iowa, Michigan, Minnesota, Missouri, Montana, Nebraska, North Dakota, Ohio, South Dakota, Wisconsin, Wyoming).[29,30] Dogs and cats acquire infection from predating on microtine rodents infected with alveolar hydatids. Alveolar (multilocular) hydatids are highly invasive in the tissues of the infected intermediate host due to external budding. In this respect, they mimic malignant metastatic neoplasms. Infection in red fox and coyote is common in some parts of the endemic region, and may be as high as 75%.[31] Prevalence of infection (1%–5%) is much lower in dogs and cats, and has been reported in North Dakota, Minnesota, and Saskatchewan.[29,32–34] Dogs are equal to the fox in susceptibility to infection as definitive hosts. Cats develop patent infections but seem to be less suitable hosts than canids.[32] The prepatent period is about 26 to 29 days, and gravid segments containing about 300 eggs are shed irregularly over a period of 1 to 4 months. Infected foxes may shed as many as 100,000 eggs per day.[35]

Humans are susceptible to infection with E multilocularis by the ingestion of eggs shed by infected canids or cats. Alveolar echinococcosis is a potentially fatal disease in people due to the tissue-invasive nature of the multilocular hydatid. For reasons unknown, the dramatic expansion in the endemic range that has occurred in North America, resulting in a high prevalence of infection in the wild red fox and coyote populations, has not led to widespread human infection in the provinces and states where E multilocularis occurs.[26,32,33]

Antemortem diagnosis in dogs and cats is difficult. As with Taenia, eggs are found free in the feces only if segments are damaged in transit or released after fecal deposit. The eggs cannot be differentiated from those of Taenia spp and the small (1–2 mm) gravid segments are unlikely to be detected grossly. Appropriate as an epidemiologic research tool but not in clinical practice, adult tapeworms can be induced to pass by arecoline bromide purging of dogs. Coproantigen and copro-DNA/polymerase chain reaction (PCR) detection tests have been developed recently, which show promise as accurate and safe diagnostic methods.[36]

Praziquantel (5 mg/kg, oral or subcutaneously) is approved for use and is effective in the treatment of both *E granulosus* and *E multilocularis* infections in dogs and cats. Epsiprantel (7.5 mg/kg, oral) was effective against *E multilocularis* infection in dogs.[8] Treatment results in the release of a large number of viable infective eggs, so great care should be taken in the handling and disposal of fecal matter from the animal in the 72-hour posttreatment period.[32] In regions of high exposure risk in the dog-sheep pastoral cycle, preventive dewormings at 6-week intervals were reported to be effective in the control of *E granulosus*.[37] Monthly preventive deworming for the control of *E multilocularis* in dogs and cats that have the opportunity to roam and hunt would be appropriate in endemic regions.[32] Additional control measures are prevention of access of dogs to feed on sheep offal for *E granulosus* and restriction of hunting activities of dogs or cats for *E multilocularis*.

Dipylidium caninum

Exposure risk for *Dipylidium caninum* infection in dogs and cats exists wherever the flea (*Ctenocephalides felis*, *Ctenocephalides canis*, *Pulex irritans*) or chewing louse (*Trichodectes canis*) intermediate hosts occur. As such, infection in dogs and cats is very common, with reported prevalence rates based on necropsy surveys from the older literature as high as 62% in dogs and 22% in cats.[38,39] The scolex has a protrusible rostellum armed with 30 to 150 small hooks and 4 muscular suckers, and the segments have bilateral genital pores (**Fig. 4**). Adult worms are 15 to 70 cm in length.[40] Gravid segments (10–12 mm) are narrowed at both ends giving a similar appearance to cucumber seeds (hence the common name cucumber seed tapeworm).[18] Eggs are contained in egg packets with 2 to 63 eggs per packet. Animals acquire infection by the ingestion of the metacestode stage (cysticercoids) contained in fleas or, less frequently, lice. Flea and lice larvae become infected by feeding on segments shed by infected dogs and cats. Dogs and cats shed segments in as little as 17 days after ingestion of infected fleas.[40] Infections are well tolerated with signs, if present, similar to those cited for *Taenia* infection. Human infection can occur, mainly in young children, resulting in minimal clinical signs of disease.[41] Diagnosis is by detection and

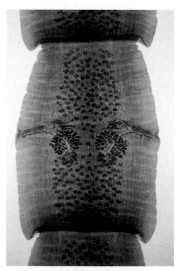

Fig. 4. Mature segment of *Dipylidium caninum* showing the bilateral genital pores (Semichon's acetic-carmine stain, original magnification ×18.5).

identification of grossly visible segments passed by animals. Bilateral genital pores may be visualized on examination of the segments. Identification can also be based on recovering egg packets from segments. Fecal flotation has poor detection sensitivity but may demonstrate eggs or egg packets.[2] Egg packets are 120 to 200 μm in length and usually contain 25 to 30 eggs (**Fig. 5**). Eggs are 35 to 60 microns in size and contain a hexacanth embryo.[24] Treatment of infected dogs and cats occurs by praziquantel (5 mg/kg, oral or subcutaneously) or epsiprantel at 2.75 mg/kg in cats and 5.5 mg/kg in dogs.[8] Treatment with cestocidal anthelmintics in the absence of concurrent flea control will most likely result in reexposure.

Mesocestoides spp

Infrequently, dogs and cats may be infected with *Mesocestoides* spp. The taxonomy of *Mesocestoides* is confused as to the number of species involved.[42] Adult tapeworms are about 30 to 70 cm in length, the scolex has 4 muscular suckers but no rostellum, and the genital pore opens on the ventral surface of the segments. Eggs are contained in a muscular parauterine organ that lies along the central longitudinal midline of the segment (**Fig. 6**).[43] Fecal and necropsy surveys both report a low prevalence (0%–1%) of infection in dogs and cats in North America. *Mesocestoides* may be more common in the southeastern and western states than elsewhere in North America.[4,5,38]

The life cycle is unknown. Dogs and cats acquire infection by the ingestion of the metacestode stage (tetrathryridium) contained in the abdominal cavity of various vertebrate intermediate hosts. Gravid segments are passed about 3 weeks after infection. Tetrathyridia have been reported in more than 200 species of reptiles, amphibians, mammals, and birds.[43] Speculation has posed a cysticercoid stage in an arthropod, perhaps ants, as a first intermediate host, but experimental infections have failed to confirm this.[44,45] In one species, *Mesocestoides corti* (also known as *Mesocestoides vogae*), both the adult tapeworm and tetrathyridia can undergo asexual reproduction.[46]

No clinical signs are associated with the presence of adult tapeworms in the small intestine of the host. However, in rare cases dogs and cats may become infected with the tetrathyridial stage of the parasite and develop a life-threatening peritoneal cestodosis. The route of exposure leading to tertrathyridia infection in the peritoneal cavity as opposed to adult tapeworms in the small intestine is unknown. In North America, most cases of peritoneal cestodosis due to *Mesocestoides* have been reported in

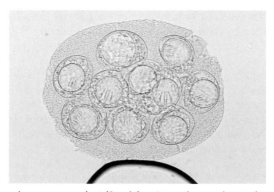

Fig. 5. *Dipylidium caninum* egg packet (Semichon's acetic-carmine stain, original magnification ×200).

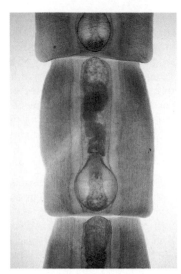

Fig. 6. Mature segment of *Mesocestoides* with the muscular paraterine organ lying in the central longitudinal midline of the segment (Semichon's acetic-carmine stain, original magnification ×18.5).

dogs in California.[47–49] Single cases have also been reported in dogs from New Mexico, Washington, and British Columbia.[48–50] Cases in cats have been reported in Europe.[51] Affected animals present with signs that may include a combination of: anorexia, vomiting, depression, diarrhea, ascites, and abdominal distension. Peritonitis occurs due to the asexually dividing metacestodes. Viable tetrathyridia or nonviable acephalic metacestodes may be produced. Ages of dogs involved in these cases have ranged from 4 to 12 years. Several cases reported finding tetrathyridia in the scrotum of dogs.[52]

Diagnosis of *Mesocestoides* infection involving adult tapeworms in the small intestine is by detection of passed segments by gross observation, or eggs on fecal flotation. Fecal flotation is presumed to have poor detection sensitivity for the same reasons given for *Taenia, Echinococcus,* and *Dipylidium*. Gravid segments are 3 to 4 mm in size. The parauterine organ can be visualized by flattening the segments between two glass slides. Segments can also be teased apart to release eggs and identified based on egg morphology. Eggs are thin-walled, 30 to 40 microns in size, and contain a hexcanth embryo (**Fig. 7**).[24] Diagnosis of peritoneal cestodosis is by clinical signs and detection of tetrathyridia or calcareous corpuscles on abdominal fluid cytology collected by centesis or exploratory laparoscopy.[47] Identification of acephalic metacestodes should be confirmed by PCR-restriction fragment length polymorphism.[48]

Praziquantel (5 mg/kg, oral or subcutaneously) is approved for use and is effective in the treatment of dogs and cats infected with adult *Mesocestoides*.[8] Treatment of dogs infected with the tetrathyridial stage of the parasite involves long-term administration of a high dose of fenbendazole (100 mg/kg, twice a day for 28 days) combined with peritoneal lavage to remove as many tetrathyridia as possible.[48] Posttreatment follow-up should be long term due to the possibility of reoccurrence, and the prognosis is guarded.

Human infection with adult *Mesocestoides* in the small intestine has rarely been reported. Infections appeared to be well tolerated and are diagnosed based on the passage of segments. Treatment with praziquantel is effective.[53]

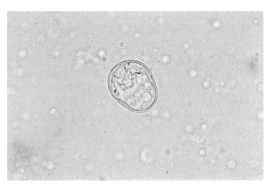

Fig. 7. *Mesocestoides* sp egg (original magnification ×400).

Hymenolepis diminuta/Choanotaenia atopa

On rare occasion dogs may be infected with the rodent tapeworm *Hymenolepis diminuta* by ingestion of cysticercoids contained in various insects.[18] There is a single report of infection of a cat in Kansas with *Choanotaenia atopa*, also a tapeworm of rodents.[54]

Pseudophyllidean Tapeworms

In contrast to the cyclophyllideans, the hold-fast organ on the scolex in this group of tapeworms consists of bothria (liplike longitudinal grooves), and eggs are released from the tapeworm segment through a uterine pore to pass free in the feces of the infected host. In addition, the eggs are operculate and undeveloped when released.[55]

Diphyllobothrium/Spirometra

Diphyllobothrium latum occurs in the small intestine of fish-eating mammals including humans, dogs, and cats. In North America it is endemic in the Great Lakes region of the United States and Canada. *Diphyllobothrium dendriticum* also occurs in North America, infecting piscivorous birds (gulls, pelicans, ravens, herons, and others) and mammals (including humans, dogs, and cats). *D dendriticum* has been reported in Alaska, Maine, Michigan, Minnesota, Montana, Nevada, Oregon, Wyoming, British Columbia, Manitoba, Newfoundland-Labrador, Northwest Territories, Ontario, and Quebec.[56] Many of the *D latum* cases reported in humans in the United States were probably due to infection with *D dendriticum*.[56] Animals acquire infections by the ingestion of the metacestode stage (plerocercoids) in perch, pike, burbot, sauger, and walleye (*D latum*) or salmonids, three-spine sticklebacks, and osmerids (*D dendriticum*).[56] *D latum* grow to an adult length of 3 to 25 m, and *D dendriticum* to more than 2 m in length.[56,57] Operculate eggs are released through the uterine pore to the lumen of the intestine and are passed in the feces about 24 days after infection.[58] Eggs that are deposited in water develop and hatch ciliated coracidia, which are then eaten by the first intermediate host, free-living copepods. Procercoids develop inside the copepods and these are in turn eaten by the second intermediate host, fish. Plerocercoids survive for prolonged periods of time in the tissue of fish, as well as surviving transfer from freshwater to marine environments and fish to fish predation.[58]

Most infections reported in North America have been in dogs, but infection in cats has also been reported.[3,59–62] No clinical signs of infection have been associated with infection in dogs and cats. Pernicious anemia due to tapeworm absorption of vitamin B-12 and various clinical signs have been reported in human infections. Diagnosis is by the detection of operculate eggs in the feces by sedimentation techniques or by the identification of varying lengths of segments that may be passed. Fecal flotation may detect eggs but is less reliable than sedimentation. Eggs are operculate, 58 to 76 by 40 to 51 microns in size, light brown in color, and undifferentiated (**Fig. 8**).[24] Eggs of *D latum* cannot be differentiated from those of *D dendriticum*; specific diagnosis may be inferred from the type of fish most likely to have been the source of infection (ie, perch, pike and so forth versus salmonids and so forth). Passed segments have a darkened central area due to the uterus filled with eggs (**Fig. 9**). Treatment in dogs is with praziquantel (7.5 mg/kg, oral) either as a single treatment or daily for 2 days.[8,60] A single oral dose of praziquantel at 35 mg/kg has been recommended for treatment of cats.[8]

The adult tapeworms of *Spirometra* spp are similar in morphology to *Diphyllobothrium*. Adult worms reach a length of up to 1.5 m in the definitive host.[63] *Spirometra mansonoides* occurs in the small intestine of cats, bobcats, raccoons and, rarely, dogs in North America. Infection seems to be most common in the southeastern and Gulf coast states (Florida, Georgia, Louisiana, North Carolina, South Carolina, Texas, West Virginia) but has also been reported in Hawaii, New Jersey, New York, and Pennsylvania.[64] A prevalence of 3% was reported in the stray cat population of Syracuse, New York and 1% in cats in New Jersey.[63–65] It is presumed that a higher prevalence would occur in cats in the southeastern and Gulf coast states.

Animals acquire infections by the ingestion of plerocercoids (spargana) contained in the tissues of a wide variety of vertebrate intermediate hosts (except fish) including amphibians, reptiles, birds, and mammals.[63,64] The prepatent period is 10 to 30 days and infections persist for up to 3.5 years.[63,64] Eggs are released through the uterine pore to pass free in the feces. Eggs shed into water develop and hatch ciliated coracidia, which are eaten by free-living copepods. Procercoids develop in the copepods. The second intermediate host accidentally ingests the copepod while drinking water. Spargana develop, mostly in muscle and connective tissue, in the second intermediate host. The sparganum is highly paratenic, continuing in the sparganum stage in tissues if ingested by an unsuitable host.[63]

Infection with adult *S mansonoides* in the small intestine of dogs and cats is usually well tolerated, although diarrhea, weight loss, and vomiting have been reported in some natural infections.[64–67] Infection with the plerocercoid stage (sparganosis)

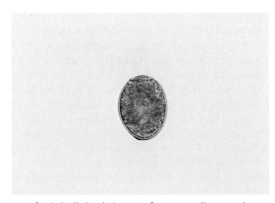

Fig. 8. Operculate egg of *Diphyllobothrium* sp from a sedimentation examination of feces (original magnification ×250).

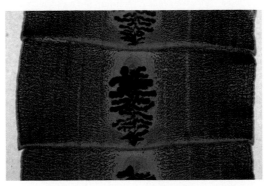

Fig. 9. Mature segment of *Diphyllobothrium* sp (Semichon's acetic-carmine stain, original magnification ×6).

occasionally occurs in cats, dogs, and humans and, depending on the tissue involved, can be serious.[68,69] Usually infection in cats and dogs involves a single sparganum.[70] Speculation as to probable exposure routes have included ingestion of procercoids in copepod contaminated drinking water or plerocercoids in second intermediate/paratenic hosts. In some cases spargana may migrate from intermediate/paratenic host tissue into an open wound. Consumption of undercooked meat from Florida feral hogs was considered a potential source of spargana for human exposure.[71,72]

A more serious but rarely diagnosed condition occurs with infection of the newly named *Sparganum proliferum*, causing a proliferative sparganosis in humans, dogs, cats, and feral hogs.[70,73–75] Infection usually ends in death. The spargana proliferate asexually in the abdominal and thoracic cavities and subcutaneous tissues affecting multiple organs (stomach, lungs, spleen, liver). Septic peritonitis and pleuritis were reported as a complication in a case involving a dog.[70] The spargana are acephalic and nonviable (ie, adult tapeworms do not develop when spargana are fed to a susceptible definitive host).[75] Molecular characterization of the spargana has led to the description of *S proliferum* as a new species.[70,76,77] The routes of exposure for dogs and cats as well as the adult stages and natural definitive hosts for *S proliferum* are unknown. Proliferative sparganosis infection is rare in both animals and humans, but has been reported in widespread geographic locations including parts of South America, Asia, Australia, and the USA.[70,74–76]

Diagnosis of definitive host infection is by detection of eggs in feces on sedimentation or fecal flotation. Fecal sedimentation is presumed to be the more reliable technique. Eggs are yellow-brown, 55 to 76 by 30 to 43 microns, and have an operculum at one end (**Fig. 10**).[68] The eggs are narrowed at both ends, in slight contrast to those of *Diphyllobothrium*. Segments may also be passed or vomited, and could be identified as pseudophyllidean tapeworms by the presence of a uterine pore and operculate eggs. Diagnosis of sparaganosis in dogs and cats is rare and occurs by clinical signs, history, and detection of spargana in tissues. Clinical signs are dependent on the organ location of the sparganum. Subcutaneous tissue involvement may appear as nonpainful swellings.[64] Proliferative sparganosis is even less common, and animals show signs of chronic disease that may present as abdominal distension, abdominal pain, and abdominal mass or masses; in one dog the presenting sign was lameness.[64,70–74]

Treatment of animals infected with the adult form of the parasite is with praziquantel at 7.5 mg/kg or 25 mg/kg, oral or subcutaneously, daily for 2 days.[8,64] Medical

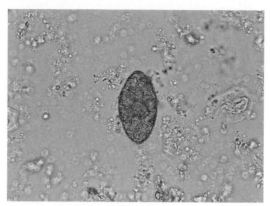

Fig. 10. Operculate *S mansonoides* egg from a sedimentation examination of feces (original magnification ×250).

treatment of proliferative sparganosis using praziquantel and mebendazole, combined with abdominal cavity lavage to remove as many spargana as possible, could be tried; however, the prognosis is guarded. Alternating 3 week courses of mebendazole (20 mg/kg, oral, daily for 21 days) and praziquantel (5 mg/kg, oral or subcutaneously, daily for 21 days) for 3 months was reported as a successful treatment in the only dog reported to survive proliferative sparganosis.[74] The effect of substituting other benzimidazoles for mebendazole, which is no longer available for use, in the afore-mentioned treatment regimen is unknown.

SUMMARY

Tapeworm infection is common in dogs and cats in North America. Most infections are due to *D caninum* (dogs and cats), *T pisiformis* (dogs), and *T taeniaeformis* (cats). Infection rarely results in clinical disease; however, for reasons of owner discomfort and potential economic or public health concerns, animals infected with tapeworms should be treated. Infrequently, life-threatening disease can occur in dogs or cats due to infection with the metacestode stages of *Mesocestoides*, *Taenia*, and *Spirometra*. Echinococcosis, though infrequently diagnosed, remains a serious human health threat in North America.

REFERENCES

1. Kazacos KR. Gastrointestinal helminths in dogs from a humane shelter in Indiana. J Am Vet Med Assoc 1978;173:995–7.
2. Lillis WG. Helminth survey of dogs and cats in New Jersey. J Parasitol 1967;53: 1082–4.
3. Unruh DHA, King JE, Eaton RDP, et al. Parasites of dogs from Indian settlements in north-western Canada: a survey with public health implications. Can J Comp Med 1973;37:25–32.
4. Blagburn BL, Lindsay DS, Vaughn JL, et al. Prevalence of canine parasites based on fecal flotation. Comp Cont Educ Pract Vet 1996;18:483–509.
5. Jordan HE, Mullins ST, Stebbins ME. Endoparasitism in dogs: 21,583 cases (1981–1990). J Am Vet Med Assoc 1993;203:547–9.

6. Streitel RH, Dubey JP. Prevalence of sarcocystis infection and other intestinal parasitisms in dogs from a humane shelter in Ohio. J Am Vet Med Assoc 1976;168:423–4.
7. Becklund WW. Current knowledge of the gid bladder worm, *Coenurus cerebralis* (*Taenia multiceps*), in North American domestic sheep, *Ovis aries*. Proc Helminthol Soc Wash 1970;37:200–3.
8. Bowmann DD. Helminths. In: Georgis' parasitology for veterinarians. 9th edition. St. Louis (MO): Saunders Elsevier; 2009. p. 115–239.
9. Abuladze KI. Taeniata of animals and man and diseases caused by them. In: Skrjabin KI, editor. Essentials of cestodology, vol. IV. (translated from Russian by M. Raveh, A. Storfer). Jerusalem: Israel Program for Scientific Translations Ltd.; 1970. p. 1–547.
10. Loos-Frank B. An up-date of Verster's (1969) taxonomic revision of the genus Taenia Linnaeus (cestoda) in table format. Syst Parasitol 2000;45:155–83.
11. Verster A. A taxonomic revision of the genus Taenia Linnaeus, 1758 S. str. Onderstepoort J Vet Res 1969;36:3–58.
12. Carbrera PA, Parietti S, Haran G, et al. Rates of reinfection with *Echinococcus granulosus*, *Taenia hydatigena*, *Taenia ovis* and other cestodes in a rural dog population in Uruguay. Int J Parasitol 1996;26:79–83.
13. Bowmann DD, Lin DS, Johnson RC, et al. Effects of nitroscanate on adult *Taenia pisiformis* in dogs with experimentally induced infections. Am J Vet Res 1991;52: 1542–4.
14. Williams JF, Shearer AM. Longevity and productivity of *Taenia taeniaformis* in cats. Am J Vet Res 1981;42:2182–3.
15. Jones A, Pybus MJ. Taeniasis and echinococcosis. In: Samual WM, Pybus MJ, Kocan AA, editors. Parasitic diseases of wild mammals. Ames (IA): Iowa State University Press; 2001. p. 150–92.
16. Rickard MD, Coman BJ, Cannon RM. Age resistance and acquired immunity to *Taenia pisiformis* infection in dogs. Vet Parasitol 1977;3:1–9.
17. Coman BJ. The survival of *Taenia pisiformis* eggs under laboratory conditions and in the field environment. Aust Vet J 1975;51:560–5.
18. Georgi JR. Tapeworms. Vet Clin North Am Small Anim Pract 1987;17(6):1285–305.
19. Huss BT, Miller MA, Corwin RM, et al. Fatal cerebral coenurosis in a cat. J Am Vet Med Assoc 1994;205:69–71.
20. Wunschmann A, Garlie V, Averbeck G, et al. Cerebral cysticercosis by *Taenia crassiceps* in a domestic cat. J Vet Diagn Invest 2003;15:484–8.
21. Chermette R, Bussieras J, Mialot M, et al. Subcutaneous *Taenia crassiceps* cysticercosis in a dog. J Am Vet Med Assoc 1993;203:263–5.
22. Hoberg EP, Ebinger W, Render JA. Fatal cysticercosis by *Taenia crassiceps* (cyclophyllidea: taeniidae) in a presumed immunocompromised canine host. J Parasitol 1999;85:1174–8.
23. Hoberg EP. Taenia tapeworms: their biology, evolution and socioeconomic significance. Microbes Infect 2002;4:859–66.
24. Zajac AM, Conboy GA. Veterinary clinical parasitology. 7th edition. Ames (IA): Blackwell; 2006. p. 3–148, Chapter 1.
25. Bryan RT, Schantz PM. Echinococcosis (hydatid disease). J Am Vet Med Assoc 1989;195:1214–7.
26. Miyazaki I. Echinococciasis-echinococcosis. Helminthic zoonoses. Tokyo: International Medical Foundation of Japan; 1991. p. 247–67.
27. Finlay JC, Speert DP. Sylvatic hydatid disease in children: case reports and review of endemic *Echinococcus granulosus* infection in Canada and Alaska. Pediatr Infect Dis J 1992;11:322–6.

28. Thompson RCA, McManus DP. Aetiology: parasites and life-cycles. In: Eckert J, Gemmell MA, Meslin F-X, Pawlowski ZS, editors. WHO/OIE manual on echinococcosis in humans and animals: a public health problem of global concern. Paris: World Organisation for Animal Health; 2002. p. 1–19.

29. Kazacos KR, Storandt ST. Echinococcus multilocularis in North America. [abstract 131] In: Proceedings of the 42nd Annual Meeting of the American Association of Veterinary Parasitologists. Reno, Nevada, July 19–22, 1997.

30. Storandt ST, Virchow DR, Dryden MW, et al. Distribution and prevalence of *Echinococcus multilocularis* in wild predators in Nebraska, Kansas and Wyoming. J Parasitol 2002;88:420–2.

31. Hildreth MB, Sriram S, Gottstein B, et al. Failure to identify alveolar echinococcosis in trappers from South Dakota in spite of high prevalence of *Echinococcus multilocularis* in wild canids. J Parasitol 2000;86:75–7.

32. Hildreth MB, Johnson MD, Kazacos KR. *Echinococcus multilocularis*: a zoonosis of increasing concern in the United States. Comp Cont Educ Pract Vet 1991;13: 727–40.

33. Eckert J, Schantz PM, Gasser RB, et al. Geographic distribution and prevalence. In: Eckert J, Gemmell MA, Meslin F-X, Pawlowski ZS, editors. WHO/OIE manual on echinococcosis in humans and animals: a public health problem of global concern. Paris: World Organisation for Animal Health; 2002. p. 101–43.

34. Wobesor G. The occurrence of *Echinococcus multilocularis* (Leukart, 1863) in cats near Saskatoon, Saskatchewan. Can Vet J 1971;12:65–8.

35. Eckert J, Rausch RL, Gemmell MA, et al. Epidemiology of *Echinococcus multilocularis*, *Echinococcus vogeli* and *Echinococcus oligarthrus*. In: Eckert J, Gemmell MA, Meslin F-X, Pawlowski ZS, editors. WHO/OIE manual on echinococcosis in humans and animals: a public health problem of global concern. Paris: World Organisation for Animal Health; 2002. p. 164–75.

36. Eckert J. Predictive values and quality control of techniques for the diagnosis of *Echinococcus multilocularis* in definitive hosts. Acta Trop 2003;85:157–63.

37. Carbrera PA, Lloyd S, Haran G, et al. Control of *Echinococcus granulosus* in Uruguay: evaluation of different treatment intervals for dogs. Vet Parasitol 2002; 103:333–40.

38. Amin OM. Helminth and arthropod parasites of some domestic animals in Wisconsin. Wisc Acad Sci Arts Letters 1980;68:106–10.

39. Rubin R. A survey of internal parasites of 100 dogs in Oklahoma county, Oklahoma. J Am Vet Med Assoc 1951;121:30–3.

40. Boreham RE, Boreham PFL. *Dipylidium caninum*: life cycle, epizootiology, and control. Comp Cont Educ Pract Vet 1990;12:667–75.

41. Gleason NN. Records of human infections with *Dipylidium caninum*, the double-pored tapeworm. J Parasitol 1962;48:812.

42. Crosbie PR, Nadler SA, Platzer EG, et al. Molecular systematics of *Mesocestoides* spp. (cestoda: mesocestoididae) from domestic dogs (*Canis familiaris*) and coyotes (*Canis latrans*). J Parasitol 2000;86:350–7.

43. Rausch RL. Family mesocestoididae. In: Khalil LF, Jones A, Bray RA, editors. Keys to the cestode parasites of vertebrates. Wallingford (CT): CAB International; 1994. p. 309–14.

44. Loos-frank B. One or two intermediate hosts in the life cycle of Mesocestoides (cyclophyllidea, mesocestoididae)? Parasitol Res 1991;77:726–8.

45. Padgett KA, Boyce WM. Ants as first intermediate hosts of Mesocestoides on San Miguel Island, USA. J Helminthol 2005;79:67–73.

46. Conn DB. The rarity of asexual reproduction among *Mesocestoides tetrathrydia* (Cestoda). J Parasitol 1990;76:453–5.
47. Caruso KJ, James MP, Fisher D, et al. Cytologic diagnosis of peritoneal cestodiasis in dogs caused by *Mesocestoides* sp. Vet Clin Pathol 2003;32:50–60.
48. Crosbie PR, Boyce WM, Platzer EG, et al. Diagnostic procedures and treatment of eleven dogs with peritoneal infections caused by *Mesocestoides* spp. J Am Vet Med Assoc 1998;213:1578–83.
49. Parker MD. An unusual cause of abdominal distention in a dog. Vet Med 2002;97: 189–95.
50. Barsanti JA, Jones BD, Bailey WS, et al. Diagnosis and treatment of peritonitis caused by a larval cestode *Mesocestoides* spp. in a dog. Cornell Vet 1979;69: 45–53.
51. Eleni C, Scaramozzino P, Busi M, et al. Proliferative peritoneal and pleural cestodiasis in a cat caused by metacestodes of *Mesocestoides* sp. anatomohistopathological findings and genetic identification. Parasite 2007;14:71–6.
52. Rodriguez F, Herraez P, Espinosa A, et al. Testicular necrosis caused by *Mesocestoides* species in a dog. Vet Rec 2003;153:275–6.
53. Fuentes MV, Galan-Puchades MT, Malone JB. A new case report of human *Mesocestoides* infection in the United States. Am J Trop Med Hyg 2003;68:566–7.
54. Rausch RL, McKown RD. *Choanotaenia atopa* n sp. (cestoda: dilepidiae) from a domestic cat in Kansas. J Parasitol 1994;80:317–20.
55. Bray RA, Jones A, Andersen KI. Order pseudophyllidea carus, 1863. In: Khalil LF, Jones A, Bray RA, editors. Keys to the cestode parasites of vertebrates. Wallingford (CT): CAB International; 1994. p. 205–47.
56. Andersen K, Ching HL, Vik R. A review of freshwater species of Diphyllobothrium with redescriptions and the distribution of *D. dendriticum* (Nitzsch, 1824) and *D. ditremum* (Creplin, 1825) from North America. Can J Zool 1987;65:2216–28.
57. Miyazaki I. Diphyllobothriasis. In: Helminthic zoonoses. Tokyo: International Medical Foundation of Japan; 1991. p. 201–7.
58. Vik R. The genus *Diphyllobothrium* an example of the interdependence of systematics and experimental biology. Exp Parasitol 1964;15:361–80.
59. Desrochers F, Curtis MA. The occurrence of gastrointestinal helminths in dogs from Kuujjuaq (Fort Chimo), Quebec, Canada. Can J Public Health 1987;78:403–6.
60. Kirkpatrick CE, Knochenhauer AW, Jacobson SI. Use of praziquantel for treatment of *Diphyllobothrium* sp infection in a dog. J Am Vet Med Assoc 1987;190:557–8.
61. Salb AL, Barkema HW, Elkin BT, et al. Dogs as sources and sentinels of parasites in humans and wildlife, northern Canada. Emerg Infect Dis 2008;14:60–3.
62. Cameron TWM. Fish-carried parasites in Canada (1) parasites carried by freshwater fish. Can J Comp Med 1945;9:245–54, 283–6, 302–11.
63. Mueller JF. The biology of Spirometra. J Parasitol 1974;60:3–14.
64. Little S, Ambrose D. *Spirometra* infection in cats and dogs. Comp Cont Educ Pract Vet 2000;22:299–305.
65. Lillis WG, Burrows RB. Natural infections of *Spirometra mansonoides* in New Jersey cats. J Parasitol 1964;50:680.
66. Kirkpatrick CE, Sharninghausen F. *Spirometra* sp in a domestic cat in Pennsylvania. J Am Vet Med Assoc 1983;183:111–2.
67. Ugarte CE, Thomas DG, Gasser RB, et al. *Spirometra erinacei/S. erinaceieuropaei* in a feral cat in Manawatu with chronic intermittent diarrhea. New Zeal Vet J 2005;53:347–51.
68. Miyazaki I. *Spirometriasis*. In: Helminthic zoonoses. Tokyo: International Medical Foundation of Japan; 1991. p. 207–14.

69. Schmidt RE, Reid JS, Garner FM. Sparganosis in a cat. J Small Anim Pract 1968; 9:551–3.

70. Drake DA, Carreno AD, Blagburn BL, et al. Proliferative sparganosis in a dog. J Am Vet Med Assoc 2008;233:1756–60.

71. Bengtson SD, Rogers F. Prevalence of sparganosis by county of origin in Florida feral swine. Vet Parasitol 2001;97:239–42.

72. Gray ML, Rogers F, Little S, et al. Sparganosis in feral hogs (*Sus scrofa*) from Florida. J Am Vet Med Assoc 1999;215:204–8.

73. Buergelt CD, Greiner EC, Senior DF. Proliferative sparganosis in a cat. J Parasitol 1984;70:121–5.

74. Beveridge I, Friend SCE, Jeganathan N, et al. Proliferative sparganosis in Australian dogs. Aust Vet J 1998;76:757–9.

75. Mueller JF, Strano AJ. *Sparganum proliferum*, a sparganum infected with a virus? J Parasitol 1974;60:15–9.

76. Miyadera H, Kokaze A, Kuramochi T, et al. Phylogenetic identification of *Sparganum proliferum* as a pseudophyllidean cestode by the sequence analyses on mitochondrial CO1 and nuclear sdhB genes. Parasitol Int 2001;50:93–104.

77. Okamoto M, Iseto C, Shibahara T, et al. Intraspecific variation of *Spirometra erinaceieuropaei* and phylogenetic relationship between *Spirometra* and *Diphyllobothrium* inferred from mitochondrial CO1 gene sequences. Parasitol Int 2007; 56:235–8.

Intestinal Nematodes: Biology and Control

Christian Epe, Dr Med Vet

KEYWORDS

• *Toxocara* • *Toxascaris* • *Ancylostoma* • *Uncinaria* • *Trichuris*

A variety of nematodes occur in dogs and cats. Several nematode species inhabit the small and large intestines. Important species that live in the small intestine are roundworms of the genus *Toxocara* (*T canis, T cati*) and *Toxascaris* (ie, *T leonina*), and hookworms of the genus *Ancylostoma* (*A caninum, A braziliense, A tubaeforme*) or *Uncinaria* (*U stenocephala*). Parasites of the large intestine are nematodes of the genus *Trichuris* (ie, whipworms, *T vulpis*).

After a comprehensive description of their life cycle and biology, which are indispensable for understanding and justifying their control, current recommendations of nematode control are presented and discussed thereafter.

BIOLOGY OF INTESTINAL NEMATODES
Ascaridae

Toxocara canis
Life cycle The most frequent and important roundworm of dogs is the zoonotic parasite *Toxocara canis*. The adult stages live in the lumen of the small intestine. Eggs produced by mature female worms pass through the intestine and are deposited in the environment via feces as unembryonated and not infective eggs.

Depending on soil type and climatic conditions, such as temperature and humidity, eggs will develop to an infective stage (L3) within a period ranging from 3 weeks to several months. These embryonated and infective eggs can survive for several years under optimal conditions. After oral uptake of these stages, development continues during and after a typical blood-liver-lung migration pathway. A few hours after infection, L3 reach the liver, and pass on to the lungs where they molt to the L4 stage. These larvae penetrate the blood-air-barrier, migrate upward to the trachea, pass the larynx and pharynx, and are swallowed down the esophagus, to reach the lumen of the duodenum as immature adults or, in older descriptions, the fifth larval stage.[1,2]

Alternatively, infective larvae (L3) as somatic stages can also be transmitted via paratenic hosts or vertically between dam and puppies. When paratenic hosts ingest infective eggs, development occurs only to a resting L3 in various tissues, so that

Companion Animal Parasiticides Research Group, Novartis Centre de Recherche Santè Animale SA, CH-1566 St Aubin FR, Switzerland
E-mail address: christian.epe@novartis.com

Vet Clin Small Anim 39 (2009) 1091–1107
doi:10.1016/j.cvsm.2009.07.002
0195-5616/09/$ – see front matter © 2009 Elsevier Inc. All rights reserved.

the L3 are protected from the environment and can wait until the host, usually prey of canids like rodents, will be eaten by the definitive host, the dog.

After ingestion of infective *Toxocara* eggs, larval development depends on the immune status of the host. Either adults form in the duodenum after tracheal migration, or in older immunocompetent animals, somatic larvae are found after passive hematogenic distribution to various peripheral organs like the musculature, kidneys, liver, and the central nervous system.

These dispersing and later resting (hypobiotic) somatic larvae—still L3—were shown to have epidemiologic importance in the pregnant dam. These stages are released and reactivated in the last third of pregnancy, when they migrate transplacentally into the fetuses' organs as vertical infection. This host-finding strategy of *Toxocara* is further enhanced by lactogenic transmission of larvae to newborn puppies. Both transmission types happen independently of whether the dam is patently infected or not. Additionally, infective larvae can infect paratenic hosts where they are stored for infection after predation of *Toxocara*-infected paratenic hosts by dogs. There, the larvae develop in most cases directly to adult worms in the intestinal tract without further migration.

Pathogenesis The larval migration through the liver leads to an increase of specific enzymes such as glutamate dehydrogenase (GLDH) and alanine aminotransferase (ALT).[3] Also, pneumonia caused by the migration of larvae in the lung is described within the first days of life. Severe infections cause signs beginning in the second week of life including ascites, anorexia, and anemia and a dilatation of the proximal duodenum is reported. On necropsy, multiple petechiae and intestinal ruptures or perforations were seen with parasites penetrating the small intestinal wall into the peritoneal cavity, followed by peritonitis or massive blood loss into the peritoneal cavity.[3-5]

Clinical signs Clinical signs are dependent on the age of the animal and on the number, location, and stage of development of the worms.[1,6,7] After birth, puppies can get acute toxocarosis from pneumonia owing to tracheal migration and die within 2 to 3 days. At an age of 2 to 3 weeks, puppies can show digestive disturbances and emaciation, caused by mature worms in the stomach and intestine. They can show diarrhea, vomiting, coughing, constipation, and nasal discharge at clinical examination. Distension of the abdomen ("potbelly") can occur as a result of a heavy worm burden but more probably from gas formation caused by dysbacteriosis. Mortality is possible because of obstruction of the gall bladder, bile duct, and pancreatic duct and rupture of the intestine, but is rather rare in this stage.

Toxocara cati

Toxocara cati is the most common gastrointestinal helminth of the cat worldwide. It plays an important role not only by infecting young kittens but also as a zoonotic parasite that can cause human toxocarosis.[8-10] Following the oral uptake of eggs containing infective L3, these undergo a tracheal migration via the liver and lungs until they finally reach the small intestine. During and after this migration the larvae develop to the adult stage, and patency starts 8 weeks post infection. Some of the larvae reach the muscle tissue where they are encysted and retain infectivity.[11,12] Although the life cycle is very similar to that of *T canis*, a different adaptation of the host-parasite-relationship can be observed: lactogenic transmission of larvae occurs only after acute infection of the queen during late pregnancy but not during chronic natural infection. There is no evidence for the existence of arrested somatic larvae in the adult cat as an important host-finding strategy in the life cycle of *T cati*. Following milk-borne infections, most larvae seem to undergo direct development in the intestine without tracheal migration. Only a small number of larvae were found in other organs.[13]

Toxocarosis in cats can be seen as catarrhal enteritis with diarrhea, vomiting, dehydration, anemia, and anorexia after heavy infection.[14]

Toxascaris leonina

The ascarid nematode *Toxascaris leonina* is a parasite of the dog and cat, and cross-infection between the two species has been described.[15] However, there are anecdotal reports of a dog isolate that could not infect cats and vice versa. This has been confirmed with one dog isolate in Hannover, Germany (Institute of Parasitology, Hannover Vet School), which definitely could not produce a patent infection in cats.

Eggs of *T leonina* are not infective when passed in feces. Embryonation to the infective L3 stage can occur within 8 to 9 days at +27°C, but normally needs 3 to 4 weeks. Infection occurs by ingestion of embryonated eggs or L3 in paratenic hosts. After hatching in the duodenum, further development continues in the wall of the small intestine, until preadults return to the gut lumen to reach patency after 7 to 10 weeks.[16] A small fraction can also perform somatic migration to the liver, lung, musculature, and other organs.[16] Vertical infection of pups or kittens is not described or experimentally proven.

Pathogenic effects on the host are less dramatic than for *Toxocara*, although sometimes enteritis can be observed.

Ancylostomatidae

Ancylostoma caninum
Life cycle The canine hookworm species *Ancylostoma caninum* is among the most prevalent canine helminths[17] and can be responsible for developmental disturbances, severe clinical signs, and increased death rate in young animals.[18] Besides this importance for canids, *A caninum* is also pathogenic in humans, causing cutaneous larva migrans (CLM) or "creeping eruption"[19] and "eosinophilic enteritis."[20,21]

Infective stages are either ingested by the definitive host as free-living third-stage larvae, lactogenically, or via paratenic hosts. However, the L3 also are able to penetrate percutaneously after complex neurohormonal actions that are triggered by skin conditions. A prenatal infection as with *T canis* can be excluded. Similar to roundworms, a blood-lung migration pathway is described; however, most ingested larvae enter the gut mucosa, where they show a relatively short histotropic phase before returning to the lumen and reaching maturity. Other larvae, either from direct migration or through passive distribution by the blood stream, reach peripheral organs like musculature and fat tissue where they can survive for several years as infective larvae capable of completing development.[16,22] Patent infection with *A caninum* often occurs in puppies after vertical transmission of third-stage larvae with the milk, either during dissemination of larvae following an acute infection or after reactivation of arrested larvae in late pregnancy. In contrast to puppies, older dogs often show a prolonged prepatency and shortened patency of infection, which is expected to be based on partial immunity or age resistance.

Thus, control measures should especially focus on arrested, somatic larvae of *A caninum* in the female dog, which provide a reservoir for transmission to neonates for up to three following litters.[23–25] These larvae are reactivated during oestrus[18] and in the last third of pregnancy.[6,25] After reactivation they either cause an autoinfection of the dam or they infect the dam's offspring lactogenically via the mammary gland.[25–27] The resulting patent infections in the puppies not only lead to a risk of disease for puppies and their dam, but they also contaminate the environment, being a major source for human infection, especially children.[28–30]

Clinical signs Diseased pups, but also parasite-naïve older animals during infection, occasionally show occult blood in feces, bloody diarrhea (melena), and symptoms of a beginning anemia. During lung migration, coughing, nasal discharge, fever, or other signs of pneumonia may occur. After heavy infection, pups can die after massive blood loss and diarrhea. Diagnostically, similar problems as for roundworm infection are present: only after final development and reaching patency can parasite stages be detected in fecal examination, ie, after approximately 2 to 3 weeks post infection. The presence of hookworm eggs in the feces of the dam is unreliable owing to partial immunity and highly variable shedding of hookworm stages.

Ancylostoma braziliense and Uncinaria stenocephala

Compared with *A caninum*, the development of *Ancylostoma braziliense* and *Uncinaria stenocephala* is less pathogenic. For *Uncinaria*, larvae develop in the glands of the duodenum primarily after oral infection. After experimental percutaneous infection only very few larvae reach the intestine.[15] Two days post infection larvae are back in the lumen of the small intestine, where L4 and immature adults complete the development with a prepatency of approximately 14 to 18 days.[16] So far, no proof of prenatal or lactogenic infection has been published.[31]

Both species show less dramatic signs than *A caninum;* in most cases, the infection is not pathogenic or chronic. Heavy infections can cause some signs of diarrhea, but are less severe than with *A caninum;* blood in feces is rare for an uncinariosis.

Ancylostoma tubaeforme

The cat hookworm *Ancylostoma tubaeforme*, shows similar development to *A caninum*: infection can occur percutaneously or orally leading to similar worm burdens.[32] After oral infection, the hookworm directly colonizes the small intestine; after percutaneous infection, migration occurs, which leads to slightly differing prepatencies of 19 to 28 days. Transmammary infections are not described, but literature is scarce.[15] Paratenic hosts like mice and other rodents can harbor L3 for several months and may play a major epidemiologic role.

Pathogenesis of the cat hookworm is similar to that of *A caninum* in dogs, blood loss in feces, anemia, diarrhea, and cachexia can be symptoms and consequences of a cat hookworm infection.

Whipworms—Trichuris Vulpis

The whipworm of dogs, *Trichuris vulpis*, passes single-celled, uninfective eggs into the environment. Development to the infective first-stage larva requires approximately 1 month, but the larvae do not hatch unless the egg is swallowed by a suitable host. This egg is very resistant and can survive several months in the environment if conditions are favorable. After ingestion, development to adult worms occurs within the epithelium of the intestine. Adults colonize the large intestine after a prepatency of approximately 70 to 90 days.[33]

Most infections do not provoke clinical signs, and only heavy infections can cause diarrhea (often alternating with diarrhea-free periods), with mucus and sometimes blood in the feces.

Trichuris infections in cats are rare and of no major clinical importance.

Other Nematodes

Other nematode species that can be found in the intestine of dogs and cats are rare and are of little clinical importance. These include *Ollulanus triscuspis*, a parasite of felidae causing gastritis, and *Strongyloides stercoralis* infections, mainly a parasite of humans, which causes gastrointestinal symptoms after heavy infections, predominantly occurring in puppies. Respiratory signs are also often observed in those cases.[34] Finally, spirurids occur, mainly of the genus *Physaloptera,* which cause chronic vomiting, and *Gnathostoma,* which can infect carnivores (and therefore, dogs and cats), causing mainly liver lesions and complications when the cystic nodules break open into the peritoneal cavity.[35]

CONTROL OF INTESTINAL NEMATODES: CURRENT RECOMMENDATIONS
Diagnostic Options

Patent nematode infections in dogs and cats can be tentatively diagnosed from the medical history, particularly when the absence of an appropriate anthelmintic schedule is accompanied by clinical signs. More likely, the infection will be diagnosed with a fecal examination and microscopic detection of eggs in a fecal sample. Different techniques can be applied; usually centrifugal flotation techniques, which have an increased sensitivity compared with more simple flotation methods, are used for fecal examination.[36] An enzyme-linked immunosorbent assay (ELISA) test, using TES antigens for *T canis* detection, was described as a sensitive technique for determining whether or not a bitch is carrying somatic larvae[37] but is not used in routine diagnosis because of problems with reliable results on an individual basis in connection with a relatively low prevalence of patent infections.

Benefits of a chemotherapeutic intervention are (1) in the case of a diseased animal where a classical curative treatment, particularly for pups, prevents a severe course of disease by eliminating parasites; or (2) as a prophylactic or preventive measure where the benefit is the interruption or prevention of environmental contamination. This has to be explained to the pet owner, who may be concerned about cost. Owners need to be informed about invisible beneficial effects of routine treatment.

Rationale for Chemotherapeutic Treatment

There are two reasons to control nematode infections. Besides curative treatment of heavily infected and diseased animals, the risk of infection to pets is reduced. In addition, human infection with zoonotic species is prevented. Because the eggs of *Toxocara* and *Trichuris* are very resistant to environmental conditions, they may remain infective for years. There are no practical methods to reduce the environmental contamination with eggs; prevention of initial contamination is still the most important tool.[2,38,39] Prevention includes elimination of patent infections in dogs and cats with treatment, but preventing defecation by pets in public areas and education of owners are also required.

Therapies and Regimes

The major classes of anthelmintics used for small animals are the (pro-) benzimidazoles (fenbendazole, febantel, flubendazole, febendazole), the tetrahydropyrimidines (pyrantel), and the macrocyclic lactones (ivermectin, selamectin, milbemycin oxime, moxidectin). Recently a new class of compounds, the cyclic octadepsipeptides, such as emodepside, has become available.

The principal mode of action of benzimidazoles (BZ) is based on the complete reduction of microtubulin polymerization inside the parasite's cells leading to disintegration of the hypodermis, muscle layer, and intestine.[40] Also, formation of gametocytes and gametes is prevented.[41] Because of their very low toxicity and their excellent tolerance, overdosing of most of the marketed formulations is practically impossible.[42] The range of parasite species and stages that are affected is dependent on the pharmacokinetics of the single compound. This leads to individual differences within the group of available BZ formulations. The half-life is approximately 10 hours.

The tetrahydropyrimidines are represented by pyrantel; at the moment the only available and marketed compound for companion animals of this group. Pyrantel as a pamoate formulation with low solubility is used for oral application as a broad-spectrum anthelmintic. The pharmacodynamic effect is direct to the m- and n-cholin receptors in parasympathetic organs and vegetative ganglions. In higher concentrations, inhibition of ACE (acetylcholinesterase) also occurs. This leads to neuromuscular blockade and, therefore, death of the parasite as a result of spastic paralysis. Although this mechanism is also seen in the vertebrate host, there is no expected effect because of the very low bioavailability.[42] The half-life is approximately 4 to 8 hours.

Within the macrocyclic lactones (MLs), fermentation products of fungi of the genus *Streptomyces* spp, ivermectin, selamectin, moxidectin, and milbemycin oxime are registered for application in companion animals. The mode of action of these very lipophilic molecules is directed against the glutamate- and γ-aminobutyric acid (GABA)-receptor-mediated chloride channels, which are found in a range of nematodes as well as in different ectoparasites (leading to the designation of these products as "endectocides"). Cestodes and trematodes show a natural resistance because of the lack of these GABA- and glutamate-controlled channels. The result of this mode of action is a hyperpolarization of these channels followed by paralysis of the parasite. Because the vertebrate blood-brain-barrier prevents the penetration of the molecule and because the glutamate receptor is not existent in the vertebrate host, the tolerance and safety interval are very broad. Exceptions are some Scottish sheepdog breeds that do not prevent the penetration of MLs through the blood-brain-barrier and can show similar effects as in the target species. Registered for veterinary use in dogs are ivermectin in an oral dosage of 0.006 mg/kg body weight (bw) (only for heartworm prevention in this dosage), selamectin at 6 mg/kg bw as a spot-on application, and milbemycin-oxime with 0.5 mg/kg bw as an oral application. Moxidectin is also available in the United States at 2.5 mg/kg as a spot-on application (in combination with imidicloprid 10 mg/kg) and as a sustained release subcutaneous injection at 0.17 mg/kg bw. Studies also show that MLs such as moxidectin and doramectin are able to interrupt a vertical infection of *T canis* from bitch to pups.[43,44]

Finally, the cyclic octadepsipeptides (CO), developed in the1990s, have shown promising results in terms of efficacy and safety. Only a feline product so far is on the veterinary market (Profender, combination of emodepside and praziquantel). The proposed mode of action is a neuropharmacological effect on a new heptahelical transmembrane receptor (HC110R) with similarity to human, bovine, and rodent lactrophilin.[45] Data from rodent endoparasites[46] and results from a recent study show efficacy against *T cati* in cats.[47] Because this class of compounds shows, so far, nematocide efficacy, there may also be a new anthelmintic for dogs in the future.

Table 1 provides an overview of the different compounds registered for dogs and cats, including treatment application, dosage, and regimen. For regular strategic anthelmintic treatment, numerous recommendations are known, some of them are discussed in the following sections.

Chemoprophylaxis

Chemoprophylaxis is better described as "regular deworming" or "worming" (which is inaccurate; however, it is very common in daily language nowadays). Often, complicated regimens are recommended, which were not always accepted or understood by owners and practitioners. So, in the last years more simple and easy-to-digest recommendations were promoted, which contain the problem that they do not always fit to individual cases. In the following, suggestions as "categories" are presented, including a description of what they can do and what they cannot.

Category 1: infected dam ("contaminated breeder")

The most serious and investigated source of infection is the nursing bitch with puppies aged between 3 weeks and 6 months.[48] A major aim of long-term prophylactic anthelmintic programs is to prevent any environmental contamination in suppressing roundworm and hookworm egg-output throughout the whole puppy period with multiple dosing. The anthelmintic treatment should be started before the age of 3 weeks, as a shortened prepatency period of vertically infected pups is known.[49] Because lactogenic transmission can occur continuously for up to 5 weeks postpartum, repeated treatments are necessary. Immature adult worms that reach the intestine need at least 2 weeks to mature and start shedding ova; therefore, the treatment should cover this period depending on the pharmacokinetics of the compounds used.

Because reinfection of the bitch can occur throughout the suckling period, bitches should always be included in the treatment at the same time as the puppies[50] for the first 2 to 3 months. Control in older dogs can be realized by periodic treatments with anthelmintics whose efficacy can be limited to the intestinal stages, or by treatments prescribed based on the results of periodic diagnostic fecal examinations. But with these measures, the potential of environmental infection and, therefore, new contamination cannot be excluded if a schedule is not used that interrupts any prepatency period before egg shedding starts.

Elimination of the larvae from the tissues and therefore prevention of vertical intrauterine and transmammary transmission would have a significant effect on the parasite population.[51] Deworming of bitches during pregnancy is sometimes advised in anthelmintic schedules, but this advice is questionable. Efficacy of nearly all licensed anthelmintics against somatic larvae in experimental animals and bitches at various dosages and treatment periods has been intensively investigated.[5,43,52–54] In general it can be concluded that anthelmintics at the recommended doses are not effective against inhibited somatic larvae[17] and treatment of bitches before mating and 2 weeks before the anticipated whelping date had no useful effect on prenatal transmission.[55] Prenatal infection can be substantially reduced by daily treatments with fenbendazole (25 mg/kg) given to the bitch from the 40th day of pregnancy until 2 days postpartum, but this treatment regimen is too expensive for general use,[56] and it seems to be difficult to explain a daily chemotherapeutic treatment in pregnancy to the owner and to get compliance in the treatment. An alternative for interrupting the vertical infection with less-frequent applications of macrocyclic lactones is known to be effective,[17,43,57,58] either once around day 50 to 55 of pregnancy or twice on day 55 of pregnancy and day 5 postpartum. Although no label claim is registered so far for the different macrocyclic lactones, this indication may lead to increased compliance of the owner because of the less frequent application.

Comment If done strictly and conscientiously, an interruption of the cycle can be achieved. Often, in practice, a heavy contamination of the environment—particularly in runs with natural soil—complicates the situation and leads to reinfection and backslides of a control program. Be cautious to promise too much.

Category 2: reducing environmental contamination ("dog/cat in family with small kids")

There are two reasons for *Toxocara* or *Ancylostoma* control: to prevent human infection and to reduce the risk of infection of pets. Because *Toxocara* eggs are very resistant to adverse environmental conditions and may remain infective for years, and

Table 1
List of available anthelmintics for treatment of intestinal nematodes

Compound Class and Compound	Trade Name[a]	Dosage [mg/kg bw × Days of Application]	Application	SI[b]	Contraindication[c]	Comments
Benzimidazoles						
Fenbendazole	Panacur	D/C: 50 × 3d	po	D: >10, C: >3	Not known[j]	
Febantel (Pro-Benzimidazole)	Drontal Plus[e]	D: 5.0–10.0 × 1	po	D: >10	Not known[j]	
Tetrahydropyrimidines						
Pyrantel	Drontal[e] Drontal Plus[e] Nemex Heartgard Plus[i] Iverhart Plus Flavored Chew.[i] Iverhart Max Chew. Tab.[i,k] Tri-Heart Chew. Tab.[i,k]	C: 20.0 × 1 D: 5.0–10.0 × 1 D: 5.0 × 1 (monthly)	po	D: >10	Not known[j]	Cave: Combinations with Ivemectin: with certain Scottish sheepdog breeds (Collie breeds) and others adverse effects are reported in dosages >0.006
Isothiocyanates						
Nitroscanate	Lopatol[f]	D: 50 × 1	po	D: >10	Not known[j]	

		Dosage	Route	Safety Index[b]	Comments[a,c]
Macrocyclic lactones					
Ivermectin	Heartgard chewables for cats	C: 0.024 × 1 (monthly)	po	Not known[j]	Cave: with certain Scottish sheepdog breeds (Collie breeds) and others adverse effects are reported in dosages >0.006
Milbemycin oxime	Interceptor Flavor Tabs Sentinel[g]	D: 0.5–1.0 × 1; C: 2 × 1 (monthly)	po	>20[d]	Not known[j]
Selamectin	Revolution	D/C: 6.0 × 1 (monthly)	Spot-on	>10[d]	Not known[j]
Moxidectin	Advantage Multi[h]	D: 2.5–6.5 × 1; C: 1–2 × 1 (monthly)	Spot-on	>10[d]	Not known[j]
	ProHeart[f]	D: 0.17 × 1 (6-monthly)	Injectable	>10[d]	Not known[j]
Cyclic octadepsipeptides					
Emodepside	Profender[e]	C: 3	Spot-on	C: >5	Not known[j]	Also during lactation and pregnancy

Abbreviations: bw, body weight; C, cat; D, dog; po, orally.

a As available, please check in your country presence of generic compounds and other/additional trade names.

b Safety Index.

c As far as listed in registration, usual warning comments such as "do not use for pups <6 weeks" or similar, which are requested by law in case of missing documentation of such an application, are not listed, as these comments are not pharmacologic contraindications.

d Collie breeds: >2.5 for Selamectin, 5 for Moxidectin; 18 for pups.

e Combination product, combination with Praziquantel (Cestocide).

f Canada only, not United States.

g Combination product, combination with Lufenuron.

h Combination product, combination with Imidacloprid.

i Combination product, combination with Ivermectin.

j No others known beside hypersensitivity against this class.

k Combination product, combination with Praziquantel.

because no practical methods exist for reducing environmental egg burdens in soil, prevention of initial contamination of the environment is the most important tool. This can be achieved by taking measures such as preventing defecation by pets in public areas, hygiene, and education of the public, but also by eliminating patent infections in dogs and cats with curative and strategic, ie, regular anthelmintic treatment.

Prevention of or a decrease in contamination can be achieved by methods including the following:

- restriction of uncontrolled dogs and cats
- cleaning up feces from soil and on pavements by dog owners
- preventing access of dogs and cats to public places (especially children's playgrounds)
- strategic anthelmintic treatment of dogs and cats with emphasis on puppies and nursing bitches.[59]

Because of their resistance, *Toxocara* eggs can survive sewage treatment and are not destroyed by composting. Infective eggs can therefore be present in soil produced out of sewage plant material. Here, we have to keep in mind that the presence of infected wild and stray canines can be a complicating factor in the prevention of environmental contamination.

Hygienic measures include removal of feces and thorough cleaning of kennels with a high-pressure steam cleaner and ascarid-effective disinfectants (eg, cresol formulations). Expelled worms must be destroyed. Dog owners should prevent contamination of the environment with *Toxocara* eggs and the exposure of other persons to unnecessary risks of *Toxocara* infection. There is a need for proper owner information about this zoonosis and the responsibility of pet ownership, in which pet owners have to be advised about deworming schemes, effective anthelmintics, and the need of preventing their animals from defecating on children's playgrounds.

Veterinarians are the most appropriate and asked source of information for their clients regarding the dangers and the control of zoonosis in general and toxocarosis in particular.[60,61]

Toxocara worms should be eliminated in the host by treatment with an effective and, if possible, larvicidal anthelmintic. For this purpose, benzimidazoles, pyrantel, and newer generation macrocyclic lactones (eg, selamectin, milbemycine, moxidectin) are recommended (see **Table 1**).

Comment If all measures are performed correctly, success is likely. However, although being correct and complete in an academic way, some of these measures are difficult to "sell," ie, to get the owner's compliance for and, therefore, trust in their effectiveness. Most often, the strategic anthelmintic treatment is the only measure that is applied (see next paragraph).

Category 3: chemoprophylaxis for reducing environmental contamination ("dog/cat in family with small kids")

A more recent approach of parasite control is presented for North America by the Companion Animal Parasite Council (http://www.capcvet.org/), which has established a World Wide Web platform containing defined "guidelines" for control principles. They were established mainly for the situation in North America but also serve as a possible control regimen for other areas as well against zoonotic endoparasites like *Toxocara*. There, a lifelong preventative treatment is suggested to exclude any zoonotic infection risk for the dog owner family. This is recommended, depending on the pharmacokinetic abilities of the anthelmintic used, as a 4-week interval ("monthly treatment"). The risk of safety and toxicologic side effects is seen as minor. Emphasis is made on the regular treatment not allowing a new environmental contamination with roundworm ova (see "The Case for Year-Round Parasite Control" by D. Bowman at http://www.capcvet.org/articles/article02.html).

This reflects an approach of interrupting the parasite's cycle within the definitive host, as no effective measures can be taken to eliminate the infectious stages in the environment. To date, no increase in anthelmintic resistance has been reported for dog nematodes as a result of routine, frequent deworming as has developed in other nematode species in small ruminants and in horses.[62,63] One hypothetical explanation will lie in the role of the refugium of the parasite. The larger the refugium is, ie, the larger the part of the parasite population that is not exposed to chemotherapy, the lower the selection pressure for resistant worms will be. This leads to a slower development of resistance. For dogs and cats it can be assumed that even frequent treatment of the individual dog does not affect the whole parasite population in a given area, because very likely not all hosts are treated simultaneously. Therefore, most of the *Toxocara* population will escape the treatment, remaining in the refugium either as anthelmintic-susceptible or at least heterozygous semisusceptible.

Comment This is a pragmatic and convenient approach, interrupting the cycle and preventing any potential contamination with regular anthelmintic treatment within or, for hookworms, just after the prepatent period. With no described resistance so far, this is, at least for certain scenarios, the way to go to exclude environmental contamination. Regular diagnostic surveillance with fecal samples is advisable to confirm the usefulness of the regimen (and to know if something is overlooked). However, it pays tribute to an easy-to-memorize (and easy to control) regimen, accepting that many animals are treated unnecessarily that do not have any parasites, because it is tough to convince the animal owner to pay for diagnosis AND treatment (which used to be the traditional way of healing, diagnose first and treat specifically)—still ethically an unsatisfying compromise.

Category 4: regular anthelmintic treatment—a European compromise (European Specialist Counsel Companion Animal Parasites recommendations)
Rationale In the recently published European recommendation, called ESCCAP (for European Specialist Counsel Companion Animal Parasites, see http://www. esccap.org/index.php/fuseaction/download/lrn_file/001-esccap-guidelines-ukfinal. pdf), a more diverse approach is undertaken to address the parasiticide treatment for dogs and cats. All categories described previously are also described in those recommendations; however, a more general approach is recommended to communicate with the pet owner. First, as a condition for successful anthelmintic treatment, central goals are defined as follows:

1. Control of acute worm infestation of the patient
2. Prevention of clinical manifestation of prepatently infected patient
3. Prevention of a (re-)infection of the patient
4. Prevention of infection of other animals in environment of the patient
5. Prevention of infection of humans in environment of the patient
6. Reduction of contamination of environment, a. a. as part of point 3.-5.

Each patient is individual! Of course it is organizationally impossible to consider all details in daily routine, but one should know that many factors can influence parasite infestation. Certain factors have certain consequences; all factors can help to categorize patients to different options for anthelmintic treatment. The following factors can be considered for judging special risks:

1. Zoonosis risk
   - eg, in families with small kids, households of grandparents, and environment of pregnant, chronically ill, or immune-compromised persons. Here, as intensive as possible treatment frequency is advised, to prevent a potential transmission and infection of parasites to humans (zoonoses).
2. Pups and dams
   - special consideration of a potential parasite transmission (round- or hookworms) to puppies
3. Flea infestation
   - consideration of transmission of tapeworms with fleas (optionally include flea control)
4. Nutrition
   - Example: Access to carcasses from slaughterhouses with potential parasite contamination, hunting dogs, and so forth
5. Endemic regions
   - Regions with high prevalence of certain parasites (example: fox tapeworm *Echinococcus multilocularis*)
6. Housing conditions
   - Dogs and cats in same household, groups with mutual infections, outdoor run possible or not, "dog greens," indoor cat, and so forth

Because all these factors have influence, each patient has an individual risk of parasite infection. With categorization in animal practice, a pragmatic containment can help to adapt recommendations during consultation.

Recommendation for regular anthelmintic treatment If regular deworming, at least four times a year or at intervals not exceeding 3 months.

In a questionnaire investigating *Toxocara*-positive cats, a deworming frequency of less than three to four times per year did not show any influence on parasite prevalence. Only the group with three or four or more treatments per year showed significantly fewer positive cases.[64] This correlation was confirmed by another investigation from Switzerland where a defined dog population was tested throughout 1 year. A treatment frequency of more than two treatments per year reduced the helminth frequency from 33% (no treatment) to 17% in this dog population.[65] Therefore, as a compromise (and not to exclude any infection and contamination!), a deworming four times per year is recommended, if no other categories as listed above are applicable!

Comment Somehow a typical European approach—more complicated than the pragmatic Companion Animal Parasite Council recommendations, but if applied accordingly, it helps practitioners to offer different regimens for different scenarios—and for different clienteles. In summary, it is the combination of all categories listed previously. But if it is not applied correctly, it may cause confusion and, therefore, contains some risks of unsound usage.

SUMMARY AND FUTURE DIRECTIONS

Before further advances in vaccine knowledge and development are described, there are no alternatives for prevention measures to chemoprophylaxis in the near future. Therefore, strategic control will be the tool for controlling zoonotic risks of intestinal nematodes. Summarizing recent information on all aspects of prevention and control, some recommendations are listed as suggestion for animal owners, veterinarians, physicians, and specialists:

Chemoprophylaxis

- A year-round treatment program can be recommended because there are broad-spectrum anthelmintics with activity against parasites with zoonotic potential. A year-round preventative program eliminates the need to predict potential transmission seasons, may improve compliance,[66] and covers pets that may travel to regions where transmission is active. Dogs and cats may be exposed to and become infected with roundworms (and hookworms) throughout the year. Consequently, stages capable of transmitting parasites can be shed into the environment, regardless of season or climate. Adult dogs and cats as well as puppies and kittens may develop patent infections leading to environmental contamination.
- In addition to routine treatment, a thorough physical examination and complete history are important for diagnosis, treatment, and control of most parasites and should be performed at least annually by a qualified veterinarian. Pets should not be fed raw meat but cooked or prepared food and provided fresh, potable water. Fecal examinations should be performed two to four times during the first year of life (may be associated with vaccine schedule), and one to two times per year in adult pets, depending on patient health and lifestyle factors. This allows monitoring of compliance with monthly preventive medication while facilitating diagnosis and treatment of parasites probably not covered by broad-spectrum preventives such as cestode or trematode infection, and also ectoparasites such as ear mites.

Intestinal parasite infections in puppies may cause serious illness or even death before a diagnosis is possible by fecal examination. Therefore, puppies require more frequent anthelmintic administration than adult animals. They often are serially reinfected via nursing and from the environment, and they often already harbor parasite larvae in migration or arrested development that later mature and commence egg laying.

Puppies and their mothers should be treated with appropriate anthelmintics either on a monthly coverage or when puppies are 2, 4, 6, and 8 weeks of age, then put on a monthly preventive. Nursing bitches should be treated concurrently with their offspring because they often develop patent infections along with their youngsters, presumably because of immunologic stress during the nursing period and the close proximity to the patent pups.

Because factors as geography, season, and life style, eg, parks and public greens used by pets and children, and close contact with pets in households, substantially affect parasite prevalence, veterinarians should tailor prevention programs to fit the needs of individual patients

Environmental Control of Parasite Transmission

Environmental control is an integral component of parasite prevention and control to minimize environmental stages (eggs, larvae). Parasite eggs are long lived in the environment and responsible for infection of pets as well as zoonotic transmission. Ascarid eggs are highly resistant to environmental conditions and may persist in the soil for years. Extreme measures are needed for decontamination, including heat (boiling water, steam, propane gun, burning straw, and so forth) to kill the eggs, removal of contaminated substrate (eg, 10–20 cm/6 in of soil properly disposed of) and/or entombment of eggs under concrete or asphalt. These methods are often not realizable because of costs and individual situation.

Therefore, it is most important to prevent initial environmental contamination with parasite stages, for instance through the comprehensive parasite control program mentioned previously. Parasitized animals should be treated and monitored by fecal examination to confirm treatment efficacy. At least weekly (preferably daily) fecal cleanup/removal should be conducted by the owner with proper disposal and sanitation from the environment. Feces can be bagged and put in the trash, burned, or flushed down a toilet. Following treatments, any worms passed should be disposed of similarly. Children 's sandboxes should be covered when not in use.

Education of Owner, Staff, and Community

Education of clients about the health risk to pets and people associated with parasitic infections and methods is essential to minimize risk. It can be realized with brochures, posters, and staff in practices to convey educational messages to pet owners. When potential zoonotic infections are diagnosed in pets, owners have to be advised of their risks and referred to a physician when appropriate. People in contact with animals that may transmit zoonotic parasites should be advised of the risks and made aware that risks are increased by pregnancy, underlying illness, or immune suppression. Advice should be provided, as the veterinarian is known to be a more important source of information for pet owners about zoonosis than the physician.[60] Precautions to prevent infections and occupationally acquired zoonoses in the veterinary hospital itself have to be taken. Veterinarians should be encouraged to interact with local physicians to increase physician awareness and understanding of pet-associated zoonotic infections and the value of preserving the human/animal bond.

REFERENCES

1. Parsons JC. Ascarid infections of cats and dogs. Vet Clin North Am Small Anim Pract 1987;17:1307–39.
2. Overgaauw PAM. Aspects of Toxocara epidemiology: toxocarosis in dogs and cats. Crit Rev Microbiol 1997;23:233–51.
3. Vossmann T, Stoye M. [Clinical, hematologic and serologic findings in puppies after prenatal infection with Toxocara canis Werner 1782 (Anisakidae)]. Journal of Veterinary Medicine Series B 1986;33:574–85 [in German].
4. Dade JW, Williams JF. Hepatic and peritoneal invasions by adult ascarids (Toxocara canis) in dog. Vet Med Small Anim Clin 1975;70:947–9.
5. Bosse M, Stoye M. [Effect of various benzimidazole carbamates on somatic larvae of Ancylostoma caninum Ercolani 1859 (Ancylostomidae) and Toxacara canis Werner 1782 (Anisakidae). 2. Studies of pregnant bitches]. Zentralbl Vet B 1981;28:265–79 [in German].
6. Stoye M. [Galactogenic and prenatal Toxocara canis infections in dogs (Beagle)]. Deutsche Tierärztl Woch 1976;83:107–8 [in German].
7. Zimmermann U, Löwenstein MD, Stoye M. [Migration and distribution of Toxocara canis Werner 1782 (Anisakidae) larvae in the definitive host (beagle) following primary infection and reinfection]. Zentralbl Veterinarmed B 1985;32:1–28 [in German].
8. Kinceková J, Reiterová K, Dubinský P. Larval toxocariasis and its clinical manifestation in childhood in the Slovak Republic. J Helminthol 1999;73:323–8.
9. Dubinsky P. New approaches to control larval toxocarosis. Helminthologia 1999; 36:159–65.

10. Janitschke K. Toxocarosis. 1: risk factors and detection. MMW Fortschr Med 1999;141:44–6.
11. Sprent JF. Observations on the development of *Toxocara canis* (Werner, 1782) in the dog. Parasitology 1958;48:184–209.
12. Swerczek TW, Nielsen SW, Helmboldt CF. Transmammary passage of *Toxocara cati* in the cat. Am J Vet Res 1971;32:89–92.
13. Coati N, Schnieder T, Epe C. Vertical transmission of *Toxocara cati* Schrank SCHRANK 1788 (Anisakidae) in the cat. Parasitol Res 2004;92:142–6.
14. Hendrix CM. Helminth infections of the feline small and large intestine: diagnosis and treatment. Vet Med 1995;90:456–76.
15. Anderson RC. Nematode parasites of vertebrates. 2nd edition. Wallingford, Oxon (UK): CAB International; 2000.
16. Stoye M. [Ascarid and Ancylostomatid infections of the dog]. Tieraerztl Prax 1983;11:229–43 [in German].
17. Epe C, Schnieder T, Stoye M. [Opportunities and Limitations of chemotherapeutic control of vertical infections of *Toxocara canis* and *Ancylostoma caninum* in the dog]. Der Praktische Tierarzt 1996;6:483–90 [in German].
18. Stoye M. [Biology, pathogenicity, diagnosis and control of *Ancylostoma caninum*]. Dtsch Tierarztl Wochenschr 1992;99:315–21 [in German].
19. Brenner MA, Patel MB. Cutaneous larva migrans: the creeping eruption. Cutis 2003;72:111–5.
20. Dowd AJ, Dalton JP, Loukas AC, et al. Secretion of cysteine proteinase activity by the zoonotic hookworm *Ancylostoma caninum*. Am J Trop Med Hyg 1994;51:341–7.
21. Croese J, Loukas A, Opdebeeck J, et al. Occult enteric infection by *Ancylostoma caninum*: a previously unrecognized zoonosis. Gastroenterology 1994;106:3–12.
22. Stoye M. [Round- and Hookworms of the dog - Development, Epidemiology, Control]. Berl Muench Tieraerzt. Wschr 1979;92:464–72 [in German].
23. Clapham PA. Canine hookworm disease. J Small Anim Pract. 1962;3:133–6.
24. Stoye M. [Studies on the possibility of prenatal and galactogenic infections with Ancylostoma caninum Ercolani 1859 (Ancylostomidae) in the dog]. Zbl Vet Med B 1973;20:1–39 [in German].
25. Bosse M, Manhardt J, Stoye M. [Epidemiology and Control of neonatal Helminth Infections of the dog]. Fortschr Vet Med 1980;30:247–56 [in German].
26. Stone WM, Girardeau MH. Transmammary passage of *Ancylostoma caninum* larvae in dogs. J Parasitol 1968;54:426–9.
27. Stoye M, Schmelzle HM. [Method of the spread of larvae of Ancylostoma caninum Ercolani 1859 (Ancylostomidae) in the definitive host (beagle)]. J Vet Med B 1986;33:273–83 [in German].
28. Nunes CM, Pena FC, Negrelli GB, et al. [Presence of larva migrans in sand boxes of public elementary schools, Brazil]. Rev Saúde Pública 2000;34:656–8 [in Portuguese].
29. Guimarães AM, Alves EGL, Ferreira de Rezende G, et al. [*Toxocara* sp. eggs and *Ancylostoma* sp., larva in public parks, Brazil]. Rev Saúde Pública 2005;39:293–5 [in Portuguese].
30. Macpherson CNL. Human behaviour and the epidemiology of parasitic zoonoses. Int J Parasitol 2005;35:1319–31.
31. Walker MJ, Jacobs DE. Pathophysiology of *Uncinaria stenocephala* infections of dogs. Vet Annual 1985;25:263–71.
32. Arasu P. In vitro reactivation of *Ancylostoma caninum* tissue-arrested third stage larvae by transforming growth factor-β. J Parasitol 2001;87:733–8.

33. Ruckstuhl N, Deplazes P, Reusch C. [Symptoms and Course of Disease of dogs infected with *Trichuris vulpis*]. Kleintierpraxis 2002;47:19–26 [in German].
34. Dillard KJ, Saari SA, Anttila M. *Strongyloides stercoralis* infection in a Finnish kennel. Acta Vet Scand 2007;49:37.
35. Bowman DD. Helminths. In: Georgis' parasitology for veterinarians. 9th edition. Bowman D, editor. MO: Saunders Elsevier; 2009. p. 209–11.
36. Lindsay DS, Blagburn BL. Practical treatment and control of infections caused by canine gastrointestinal parasites. Vet Med 1995;5:441–55.
37. Scheuer P. Sensitivity and specifity of IFAT and ELISA for determination of impatent infections with ascarides and ancylostomides in the dog [Thesis]. Dr Med Vet. Veterinary University Hannover, Foundation, 1987.
38. Overgaauw PAM. Aspects of *Toxocara* epidemiology: human toxocarosis. Crit Rev. Microbiol. 1997;23:215–31.
39. Overgauuw PAM. Prevalence of intestinal nematodes of dogs and cats in The Netherlands. Vet Q 1997;19:14–7.
40. Lacey E. The role of the cytoskeletal protein tubulin in the mode of action and mechanism of drug resistance to benzimidazoles. Int J Parasitol 1988;18: 885–936.
41. Hanser E, Mehlhorn H, Hoeben D, et al. In vitro studies on the effects of flubendazole against *Toxocara canis* and *Ascaris suum*. Parasitol Res 2003;89:63–74.
42. Ungemach FR. Antiparasitika. In: Loescher W, Ungemach FR, Kroker R, editors. Pharmakotherapie bei Haus- und Nutztieren. Berlin: Parey; 2002. p. 248–51.
43. Ungemach FR. [Antiparasitica]. In: Loescher W, Ungemach FR, Kroker R, editors. [Pharmaco-Therapy of Companion and Livestock Animals]. Berlin: Parey; 2002. p. 248–51 [in German].
44. Bowman DD, Legg W, Stansfield DG. Efficacy of moxidectin 6-month injectable and milbemycin oxime/lufenuron tablets against naturally acquired *Toxocara canis* infections in dogs. Vet Ther 2002;3:281–5.
45. Harder A, Schmitt-Wrede HP, Krucken J, et al. Cyclooctadepsipeptides—an anthelmintically active class of compounds exhibiting a novel mode of action. Int J Antimicrob Agents 2003;22:318–31.
46. Harder A, Samson-Himmelstjerna G. Activity of the cyclic depsipeptide emodepside (BAY 44-4400) against larval and adult stages of nematodes in rodents and the influence on worm survival. Parasitol Res 2001;87:924–8.
47. Harder A, Samson-Himmelstjerna G. Cyclooctadepsipeptides—a new class of anthelmintically active compounds. Parasitol Res 2002;88:481–8.
48. Jacobs DE, Pegg EJ, Stevenson P. Helminths of British dogs: *Toxocara canis*, a veterinary perspective. J Small Anim Pract 1977;18:79–92.
49. Yutuc LM. The incidence and prepatent period of *Ancylostoma caninum* and *Toxocara canis* in prenatally infected puppies. J Parasitol 1954;40:18–9.
50. Jacobs DE. Control of *Toxocara canis* in puppies: a comparison of screening techniques and evaluation of a dosing programme. J Vet Pharmacol Ther 1987;10:23–9.
51. Kassai T. Chemotherapy of larval toxocarosis: progress and problems. Overview from veterinary aspects. Helminthologia 1995;32:133–41.
52. Burke TM, Roberson EL. Fenbendazole treatment of pregnant bitches to reduce prenatal and lactogenic infections of *Toxocara canis* and *Ancylostoma caninum* in pups. J Am Vet Med Assoc 1983;183:987–90.
53. Lloyd S, Soulsby EJL. Prenatal and transmammary infections of *Toxocara canis* in dogs: effect of benzimidazole-carbamate anthelmintics on various developmental stages of the parasite. J Small Anim Pract 1983;24:763–8.

54. Fok E, Kassai T. *Toxocara canis* infection in the paratenic host: a study on the chemosusceptibility of the somatic larvae in mice. Vet Parasitol 1998;74:243–59.
55. Fisher MA, Jacobs DE, Hutchinson MJ, et al. Studies on the control of *Toxocara canis* in breeding kennels. Vet Parasitol Vet Parasitol 1994;55:87–92.
56. Barriga OO. A critical look at the importance, prevalence and control of toxocariasis and the possibilities of immunological control. Vet Parasitol 1988;29: 195–234.
57. Epe C, Pankow WR, Hackbarth H, et al. A field study on the prevention of prenatal and galactogenic *Toxocara canis* infections in puppies by treatment of impatently infected bitches with ivermectin or doramectin. Appl Parasitol 1995;36:115–23.
58. Samson-Himmelstjerna G, Epe C, Schimmel A, et al. Larvicidal and adulticidal efficacy of an imidacloprid and moxidectin topical formulation against endoparasites in cats and dogs. Parasitol Res 2003;90:114–5.
59. Schantz PM. Zoonotic toxocariasis: dimensions of the problem and the veterinarian's role in prevention. Proc US Anim Health Assoc 1981;85:396–8.
60. Harvey JB, Roberts JM, Schantz PM. Survey of veterinarians' recommendations for treatment and control of intestinal parasites in dogs: public health implications. J Am Vet Med Assoc 1991;199:702–7.
61. Overgaauw PAM. Effect of a government educational campaign in the Netherlands on awareness of *Toxocara* and toxocarosis. Prev Vet Med 1996;28: 165–74.
62. Wolstenholme AJ, Fairweather I, Prichard R, et al. Drug resistance in veterinary helminths. Trends Parasitol 2004;20:469–76.
63. Kaplan RM. Drug resistance in nematodes of veterinary importance: a status report. Trends Parasitol 2004;20:477–81.
64. Coati N, Hellmann K, Mencke N, et al. Recent investigation on the prevalence of gastrointestinal nematodes in cats from France and Germany. Parasitol Res 2003; 90:146–7.
65. Sager H, Moret CS, Grimm F, et al. Coprological study on intestinal helminths in Swiss dogs: temporal aspects of anthelminthic treatment. Parasitol Res 2006;98: 333–8.
66. Bowman DD. Alternatives, a veterinary clinical update: total parasite management in dogs. Compendium on Continuing Education for the Practicing Veterinarian 2003;25:1–12.

Helminth Parasites of the Canine and Feline Respiratory Tract

Gary Conboy, DVM, PhD

KEYWORDS

- *Eucoleus boehmi* • *Eucoleus aerophilus* • *Crenosoma vulpis*
- *Angiostrongylus vasorum* • *Aelurostrongylus abstrusus*
- *Oslerus osleri* • *Filaroides hirthi* • *Filaroides milksi*
- *Paragonimus kellicotti*

The helminth parasites of the respiratory tract of dogs in North America consist of two capillarids (*Eucoleus aerophilus*, *Eucoleus boehmi*), five metastrongyloids (*Angiostrongylus vasorum*, *Crenosoma vulpis*, *Filaroides hirthi*, *Filaroides milksi*, *Oslerus osleri*), and a trematode (*Paragonimus kellicotti*). Those infecting the cat include a capillarid (*E aerophilus*), a metastrongyloid (*Aelurostrongylus abstrusus*), and a trematode (*P kellicotti*). Diagnosis of these parasitic infections is infrequent in most parts of North America. Necropsy data on infection prevalence in North America is lacking for most of the lungworms. The results of fecal flotation examination surveys, some involving thousands of samples, have indicated a low prevalence for the various lungworms.[1–5] However, as acknowledged by the investigators of the studies, fecal flotation is not the technique of choice for most of the lungworm parasites and therefore these may have been underestimated. Fecal flotation is probably the most widely used diagnostic technique for the detection of parasitic infection in veterinary private practice, and appropriately so.[6,7] However, veterinary clinicians should bear in mind the limitations of fecal flotation as a diagnostic tool in the detection of operculate eggs and nematode larvae, which complicate the detection of most of the helminth lungworm parasites of dogs and cats. Clinical impressions that helminth parasites play little or no role as causative pathogens in canine and feline respiratory disease in a practice area may be inaccurate if based on fecal flotation as the primary or sole screening technique. The potential for missing lungworm cases that occur, whether they represent a significant number of animals or very few, exists due to the diagnostic challenge involved in the detection of most of these parasites. Never having had a case involving lungworm infection and never having diagnosed one may be two different things.

Department of Pathology and Microbiology, Atlantic Veterinary College-UPEI, 550 University Avenue, Charlottetown, PEI, C1A 4P3, Canada
E-mail address: conboy@upei.ca

Vet Clin Small Anim 39 (2009) 1109–1126
doi:10.1016/j.cvsm.2009.06.006
vetsmall.theclinics.com
0195-5616/09/$ – see front matter Crown Copyright © 2009 Published by Elsevier Inc. All rights reserved.

CANINE NASAL *EUCOLEOSIS*/CANINE AND FELINE TRACHEOBRONCHIAL *EUCOLEOSIS*

Eucoleus aerophilus (= *Capillaria aerophila*) occurs in the trachea, bronchi, and bronchioles, infects dogs, cats, and various wild carnivores, and has a worldwide distribution.[8] At one time, *E aerophilus* was also thought to sometimes occur in the nasal passages and sinuses of dogs and wild canids, but it is now recognized that this was a second species, *Eucoleus boehmi*.[9] Interpretation of study results from some of the older literature is complicated by the uncertainty of which of the two species the researchers may have been dealing with.

E boehmi occurs in the nasal passages and sinuses of wild and domestic canids in Europe, North America, and South America.[9] The worms are long, thin (22–43 mm × 0.08–0.15 mm), and are found embedded in the epithelial lining of the nasal turbinates, frontal sinuses, and paranasal sinuses.[9,10] The life cycle and routes of transmission are unknown. Earthworms may serve as intermediate hosts but further study is required to confirm this.[9] Clinically affected dogs show signs of sneezing and muco-purulent nasal discharge that may contain blood.

Fecal flotation survey results usually do not differentiate between capillarid species, therefore little is known on prevalence and distribution of *E boehmi* infection in canids in North America. Only 0.4% of 6458 canine fecal samples tested in a national fecal flota-tion survey in the United States were positive for capillarid eggs, most of which were *E boehmi*. Positive samples were recorded from each of the regions sampled.[4] A fecal flotation survey of greyhounds in Kansas detected eggs of *E boehmi* in 2% (4 of 230) of the samples.[11] Diagnosis is based on detection of eggs in feces by fecal flotation. Egg shedding may be cyclical, therefore multiple fecal examinations may be needed to detect infection.[11] Eggs may also be detected by microscopic examination of nasal discharge. The eggs are bipolar plugged, contain a multicelled embryo, and are 54 to 60 by 30 to 35 microns in size (**Fig. 1**).[12,13] The eggs of *E boehmi* resemble those of *Trichuris vulpis* (**Fig. 2**) and the other capillarids that may be present in canine fecal samples (*Eucoleus aerophilus*, *Pearsonema plica*, and *Callodium hepaticum*).[12,13] Eggs of *E boehmi* can be differentiated from those of *T vulpis* based on size and morphology. *Trichuris* eggs are 72 to 90 by 32 to 40 microns in size and the shell wall surface is smooth. The bipolar plugs tend to be more prominent, and have ridges that give the appearance that they are threaded into the shell wall. The bipolar plugs of

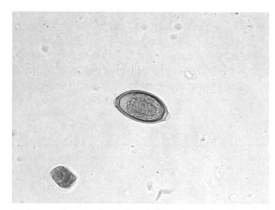

Fig. 1. *Eucoleus boehmi* egg detected on fecal flotation of a dog (original magnification ×400).

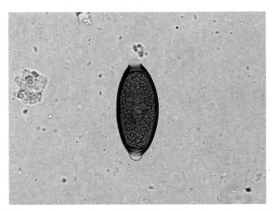

Fig. 2. *Trichuris vulpis* egg detected on fecal flotation of a dog (original magnification ×400).

capillarid eggs lack ridges, and the shell wall surface has a pattern unique for each of the species. The shell surface pattern of *E boehmi* consists of fine pitting (**Fig. 3**).[13]

Treatment using an oral dose of ivermectin at 0.2 mg/kg (this dose is not safe for use in collie-type breeds) appeared to be effective in a naturally infected dog.[14] Similar results were reported using milbemycin oxime (2.0 mg/kg, oral).[15] Failure to control an *E boehmi* infection in 2 dogs has been reported using ivermectin (0.2–0.3 mg/kg, oral) and fenbendazole (50 mg/kg, oral, once a day for 10 days).[16,17]

Eucoleus aerophilus are long and thin measuring 16 to 40 by 0.06 to 0.18 mm.[10] Reports of prevalence in North America have ranged from 0% to 5% in dogs and 0.2% to 9% in cats.[1–4] The life cycle is considered direct; however, there is some speculation that earthworms serve as a paratenic or intermediate host.[9,13] Eggs are long-lived in the environment and the prepatent period has been reported as 40 days.[8] Infection in dogs and cats is usually well tolerated; however, chronic cough can develop that may also lead to loss of weight and body condition, and rarely ends in death.[9,13] Definitive diagnosis is by detection of eggs on fecal flotation. The eggs are bipolar plugged and 58 to 79 by 29 to 40 microns in size (**Fig. 4**).[12] The shell wall surface has a series of anastomosing ridges forming a netlike pattern (**Fig. 5**). Eggs may also be detected in bronchoalveolar lavage samples.[18,19] Other diagnostic

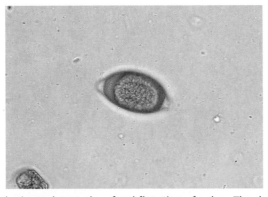

Fig. 3. *Eucoleus boehmi* egg detected on fecal flotation of a dog. The shell wall surface is in focus, showing the finely pitted surface (original magnification ×450).

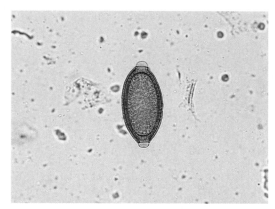

Fig. 4. *Eucoleus aerophilus* egg detected on fecal flotation of a dog (original magnification ×400).

tests, suggestive of but nonspecific for *E aerophila* infection, include radiographs indicating a diffuse interstitial lung pattern and transtracheal wash cytology showing an eosinophilic inflammatory response.[20]

Fenbendazole (30 mg/kg, oral, once a day for 2 days repeated every 2 weeks for a total of four treatments) was reported to be safe and effective in the treatment of clinically affected arctic foxes.[21] Use of fenbendazole (50 mg/kg, oral, once a day for 14 days) in a dog and abamectin (0.3 mg/kg, subcutaneous, repeated in 2 weeks) in a cat were also reported to be effective treatments for *E aerophilus* infection.[18,19] Anthelmintics with apparent efficacy against *E boehmi* (ivermectin, milbemycin oxime) may also be useful in cases of *E aerophilus* infection.

CANINE CRENOSOMOSIS (*CRENOSOMA VULPIS*)

Crenosoma vulpis, the fox lungworm, occurs in the trachea, bronchi, and bronchioles of wild and domestic canids in the temperate regions of North America and Europe.[22] Crenosomosis has recently been recognized as an important cause of chronic respiratory disease in dogs in parts of Canada and Europe.[23–25] Adult worms are 5 to 10 mm in length, and the anterior end is marked by a characteristic series of 18 to 26 ringlike cuticular folds.[22] In North America, the geographic distribution of *C vulpis*

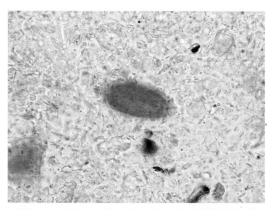

Fig. 5. *Eucoleus aerophilus* egg detected on fecal flotation of a dog. The shell wall surface is in focus, showing the network of anastomosing ridges (original magnification ×400).

seems to be mainly in the northeastern portion of the continent including parts of the United States and Canada.[23,25] The North American natural definitive hosts are species of wild canids including foxes and coyotes.[22,26] Excepting the Atlantic Canadian provinces (New Brunswick, Newfoundland-Labrador, Nova Scotia, Prince Edward Island), infection in dogs seems to be infrequent in North America. There are several case reports involving C vulpis infection in dogs in New York, Quebec, and Ontario.[27–29] In Atlantic Canada, crenosomosis has been found to be a frequent cause of chronic respiratory disease in dogs with C vulpis infection, occurring in 21% of dogs showing signs of chronic cough.[25] Canids acquire infection by the ingestion of terrestrial snail and slug gastropod intermediate hosts.[23] The prepatent period is 19 to 21 days, and the adult worm life-span is about 10 months.[25] Infection induces chronic bronchitis-bronchiolitis, which results in clinical signs consisting primarily of chronic cough sometimes accompanied by gagging.[30] Definitive diagnosis is by detection of first-stage larvae in feces or transtracheal wash samples. Larvae are detected in feces by Baermann examination, $ZnSO_4$ centrifugal flotation (CF), or FLOTAC device. The Baermann technique seems to be the most sensitive method for diagnosis.[24,25] Crenosomosis was diagnosed in a dog in Italy using the FLOTAC device, recently developed and available in Europe.[31] This method was considered superior in larval recovery when compared with the Baermann technique; however, this was based on the examination of fecal samples from a single dog. As with other metastrongylids, fecal larval shedding may be intermittent and appears to become more so on reinfection.[32] Therefore, examination of multiple fecal samples (three collected over 7 days) may increase detection sensitivity.[23] Larvae are 264 to 340 by 16 to 22 microns in size (Fig. 6).[12] There is a narrowing at the anterior-end of the larva (= cephalic button) and the tail lacks a kink or dorsal spine, but has a slight deflection that is best seen in a lateral view of a larva that has been killed with iodine, heat, or formalin.[12] Febantel (14 mg/kg, oral, once a day for 7 days), fenbendazole (25 to 50 mg/kg, oral, once a day for 3 to 14 days), and milbemycin oxime (0.5 mg/kg, oral, single dose) have all been used to treat dogs naturally infected with C vulpis, with a clinical cure occurring within 7 to 10 days of treatment.[23–25,27–30,33,34] A treatment efficacy of 98% to 99% was reported for milbemycin oxime (0.5 mg/kg, oral) used in the treatment of dogs experimentally infected with C vulpis.[34] Crenosomosis may be misdiagnosed as allergic respiratory disease, and dogs will show a positive clinical response due to the symptomatic relief of corticosteroid therapy.[30]

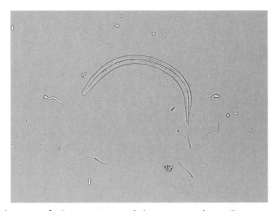

Fig. 6. First-stage larvae of Crenosoma vulpis recovered on Baermann examination of a canine fecal sample (original magnification ×200).

CANINE VERMINOUS NODULAR BRONCHITIS (*OSLERUS OSLERI*)

Oslerus osleri is a parasite found in the trachea and bronchi of dogs, dingoes, coyotes, and wolves,[22] and has a worldwide distribution. In North America, infection is fairly common and widespread in wild canids, particularly coyotes.[22] However, wild canids do not seem to serve as an infection reservoir for dogs; dogs exposed to infective larvae derived from coyotes failed to develop *O osleri* infections.[35] Infection in dogs is infrequent, but isolated cases have been reported throughout the United States and Canada.[36]

Adult worms are 6.5 to 13.5 mm long, and reside coiled inside wartlike nodules that are attached to the mucosal epithelium in the lumen of the trachea and bronchi.[37] The nodules are clustered at the bifurcation of the trachea. Individual nodules range in size from 1 to 20 mm and can become confluent when present in large numbers.[38,39] Nodules from naturally infected coyotes contained 1 to 105 worms per nodule.[40]

Atypical for metastrongyloid parasites, the life cycle for *O oslerus* is direct and the first-stage larva is the infective stage. Adult females lay thin-shelled larvated eggs (80 × 50 microns) that hatch, and the first-stage larvae migrate up the bronchial system to pass either in saliva or in the feces. Larvae recovered from the feces tend to be sluggish, and are often found to be dead and degenerating. Transmission in wild canids is thought to occur mainly by exposure of weanling pups by the dam through regurgitative feeding.[41] Transmission in dogs is thought to be mainly through saliva from the dam cleaning her pups through licking. Exposure can also be through ingestion of larvae from fecal contamination, but this is of lesser importance.[37,41] Immature worms arrive in the trachea about 70 days after exposure, and nodules are visible soon after. The prepatent period is about 92 to 126 days.[41,42]

Diagnosis of infections tends to occur in young dogs, 6 months to 2 years old,[39,43,44] which is consistent with exposure at an early age. Clinical signs consist of chronic cough, which may be worse with exercise. In some cases wheezing and dyspnea occur.[43] Weight loss, emaciation, and collapse may be observed in the most severely affected dogs.[45] Pneumothorax was reported in one case of *O osleri* infection.[46] Infections may be subclinical in some dogs.

Definitive diagnosis is by visualization of the nodules at the bifurcation of the trachea with bronchoscopy followed by recovery of first-stage larvae in bronchial mucus, or less commonly, in feces. Larvae recovered from bronchial mucus are 233 to 267 microns in length, and the tail ends in a distinctive sinus wave-shaped kink.[37] Transtracheal wash samples or bronchial mucus collected during bronchoscopy are superior for larval recovery to fecal detection. Zinc sulfate centrifugal fecal flotation ($ZnSO_4$ CF) has greater detection sensitivity than Baermann examination; however, false-negative results are a problem with both methods.[44] Larvae when recovered from feces are 326 to 378 microns in size (**Fig. 7**).[37] Evidence of tracheobronchial nodules may also be detected by radiographs in some cases.[43]

Fenbendazole and ivermectin have been used in naturally infected dogs, with variable results.[43,44,47] Fenbendazole (50 mg/kg, oral, once a day for 7 to 14 days) was reported to be effective in the treatment of 20 dogs with clinical *O osleri* infections.[43] One severely affected dog required two 14-day courses of the fenbendazole treatment. Ivermectin (0.4 mg/kg, subcutaneous, repeated every 3 weeks for four treatments) was reported to be effective in the treatment of four dogs, resulting in a clinical cure and resolution of tracheobronchial nodules.[47]

CANINE VERMINOUS PNEUMONIA (*FILAROIDES* SPP)

There are two closely related species, *Filaroides hirthi* and *Filaroides milksi*, occurring in the lung parenchyma of dogs.[22] *Filaroides milksi* (= *Andersonstrongylus milksi*) was

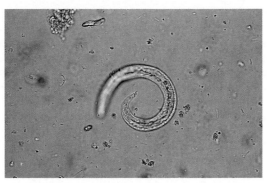

Fig. 7. First-stage larvae of *Oslerus osleri* detected on ZnSO₄ centrifugal flotation of a fecal sample from a coyote (original magnification ×400).

first reported as an incidental finding from the necropsy of a 10-year-old Boston terrier.[48] Adult worms (3.4 to 10.9 mm in length) were found in bronchioles and coiled in nests in the lung parenchyma. *Filaroides hirthi* was first reported, also as an incidental finding at necropsy, in the bronchioles and lung parenchyma of purpose bred research beagles.[49,50] Adult worms are 2.3 to 13 mm in length. The two species are differentiated from each other based on subtle differences in adult worm size, and male spicule morphology and length.[51] The validity of *F milksi* and *F hirthi* as two separate species has been questioned, resulting in some debate.[51–53] Prevalence of *F hirthi* infection as high as 78% in individual research dog colonies has been reported.[54] Diagnosis is rare in nonresearch colony dogs. Infections in client-owned dogs in the United States have been reported in Alabama, Georgia, New York, Pennsylvania, Texas, and Washington.[55–60]

There are fewer reports of *F milksi* infection. Diagnosis in dogs based on histopathology has been reported in Australia, Canada, and the United States; however, differentiation between *F hirthi* and *F milksi* is not possible based on histopathology and therefore, these may have been *F hirthi*.[49,53] In addition to the original species description, there is only one other report of a diagnosis in a dog based on identification of adult male worms.[61] Reports of *F milksi* infection in the skunk and in a dog from Belgium have been disputed.[53]

The life cycle is unknown for *F milksi*. Transmission of *F hirthi* occurs by ingestion of infective L1 larvae, usually through coprophagia of fresh fecal material. In research beagle colonies this is thought to occur in puppies by 4 to 5 weeks of age through exposure to feces from infected dams.[62] The prepatent period is 35 days.[63] Infections appear to be long-lived, and this is probably due to reexposure to infective first-stage larvae through autoinfection.

Most infections appear to be subclinical. *F hirthi* infection in research dogs can compromise or invalidate study results depending on the nature of the project.[49] Studies involving immunosuppression may induce a fatal hyperinfection.[64] Fatal hyperinfection secondary to immunosuppression or some predisposing state of stress has also been reported in client-owned dogs. Long-term corticosteroid therapy, neoplasia, severe trauma, and distemper infection have been cited as predisposing factors.[55,56,59,60,65] Most reports involve young (<3 years), small toy breeds such as Chihuahua, West Highland terrier, toy poodle, and Yorkshire terrier. Fatal infections have also occurred in dogs up to 10 years old and in such breeds as the King Charles spaniel and Dalmatian.[58,59] Clinically affected dogs show signs of dyspnea, cough, and cyanosis, and may be depressed. Diagnosis is by detection of first-stage larvae in bronchial mucus or feces. The larvae of *F hirthi* and *F milksi* cannot be differentiated from each other or those of *O osleri*. Larvae are 240 to 290 microns in length and have a kinked tail.[66] Also in common with *O osleri*, detection sensitivity of *Filaroides* larvae by Baermann examination is poor.[63] Larvae are best detected by examination of bronchial mucus. Fecal detection is best achieved by ZnSO$_4$ CF; however, false-negative results are common.[63] Additional diagnostics might include radiographs, showing interstitial linear and focal nodular pulmonary infiltrates.[67]

Albendazole, fenbendazole, and ivermectin have been used to treat dogs infected with *F hirthi*. Control in research dog colonies by treating breeding animals using albendazole (25 mg/kg, oral, twice a day for 5 days; repeated in 2 to 4 weeks) and ivermectin (1 mg/kg, subcutaneous, repeated in 1 week) has been reported.[54,68] Fenbendazole (50 mg/kg, oral, once a day for 14 to 21 days or 100 mg/kg, oral, once a day for 7 days) appeared to be an effective treatment in three dogs.[57,69,70] Corticosteroids were used in one of the dogs as an adjunct therapy due to severe posttreatment dyspnea that was attributed to an inflammatory response to dead worms.[57] Ivermectin (0.034 mg/kg, oral, single dose) followed by fenbendazole (50 mg/kg, oral, once a day for 14 days) appeared to be an effective treatment in one dog.[60]

FELINE AELUROSTRONGYLOSIS (*AELUROSTRONGYLUS ABSTRUSUS*)

Aelurostrongylus abstrusus occurs in the terminal respiratory bronchioles and alveolar ducts in the lung parenchyma of domestic cats, and has a worldwide distribution.[22] In North America it has been reported in the United States in the eastern (Connecticut, New York, Maryland, New Jersey, Pennsylvania), southeastern (Alabama, Georgia, North Carolina, South Carolina, Tennessee, Virginia), southwestern (Texas), and west coast (California, Oregon, Washington) states, and Hawaii.[1,2,5,36,71] In Canada, it has been diagnosed in cats in Ontario, Newfoundland-Labrador, and Nova Scotia[72] (Gary Conboy, DVM, unpublished data, 2003). Fecal flotation surveys have indicated *A abstrusus* infection rates in cats of 0.1% to 1.1%.[1,2,5] A Baermann fecal examination survey found 18.5% prevalence in cats in Alabama.[73] Results of experimental infections have indicated that dogs are not a susceptible host.[74] Coprophagia rather than patent infection may explain the occasional finding of *A abstrusus* larvae in canine fecal surveys.

Cats acquire infection by the ingestion of infective third-stage larvae contained in terrestrial gastropod intermediate hosts (slugs, land snails) or a wide range of paratenic hosts (amphibians, reptiles, birds, small rodents).[71] Adult worms are 4 to 10 mm in length.[74] Mature females produce undifferentiated eggs, which develop and hatch first-stage larvae. The larvae are coughed up, swallowed, and passed in the feces. The prepatent period is about 5 to 6 weeks, and infected cats shed L1 larvae in the feces for a period that usually lasts 2 to 7 months with a peak in shedding 10 to 17 weeks after infection.[71,75,76] In some cats, the period of larval shedding may last 1 to 2 years.[75,76] There is a delayed onset of patency, less larval shedding, and a more erratic shedding pattern after reexposure in cats that have been infected previously.[75,76]

Infections are usually subclinical.[71,77] Heavy infections can result in severe, potentially fatal, respiratory disease. Severe clinical disease was reproduced experimentally in kittens given 800 L3 larvae, with cough developing 6 weeks after exposure.[78] Clinically affected cats often show signs of cough, dyspnea, and fever, and may suffer anorexia and emaciation. As with *C vulpis* infection in dogs, *A abstrusus* infection may be misdiagnosed as allergic respiratory disease, and show a positive response to administration of corticosteroids and bronchodilators.[79] Infection occurs more often in younger cats (3 months to 3 years) and outdoor cats.[77,80] Pneumothorax and pyothorax secondary to *A abstrusus* infection has been reported in a kitten. It was speculated that third-stage larvae became contaminated with *Salmonella typhimurium* in the lumen of the intestine and carried it to the lungs.[81]

Diagnosis is by detection of L1 larvae in feces, bronchial mucus, or pleural fluid. False-negative results in larval detection can occur due to sporadic shedding patterns.[71] Fecal detection occurs by Baermann examination, fecal flotation, direct smear, and FLOTAC device. The Baermann is considered the most sensitive method for larval detection.[73] The FLOTAC device was considered more effective in larval recovery than the Baermann technique when compared on samples collected from a single *A abstrusus*-infected cat.[82] The larvae are 360 to 400 microns in length, and the tail ends in a distinctive sinus wave-shaped kink with a dorsal spine (**Fig. 8**).[12] A nested polymerase chain reaction assay for *A abstrusus* infection used on Baermann sediment, feces, and pharyngeal swabs has recently been developed in Europe, and shows great promise; it had a reported specificity of 100% and sensitivity of 96.6%.[83] Additional diagnostic testing options would involve radiography, transtracheal wash, and bronchoalveolar lavage. Radiographic changes tends to show a mixed pattern, with an alveolar pattern predominating during the period of heaviest larval shedding (5 to 15 weeks post-infection) followed by bronchial and interstitial patterns.[83] Computed tomography images may also be useful in assessing lesions in *A abstrusus*-infected cats.[84]

Options currently available for treating cats infected with *A abstrusus* include abamectin, fenbendazole, ivermectin, moxidectin, and selamectin. One to two applications of selamectin (6 mg/kg, topical) were reported to be effective in the treatment of 1 of 3 cats.[79] Ivermectin (0.4 mg/kg, subcutaneous, repeated in 2 weeks) has been reported to be effective in the treatment of several cats.[85-87] Fenbendazole (20 mg/kg, oral, once a day for 5 days or 50 mg/kg, oral, once a day for 15 days) was reported to be effective in the treatment of *A abstrusus* infection in cats.[79,88] One to three topical applications of 1 mg/kg moxidectin (in combination with imidacloprid) appeared to be effective in the treatment of eight cats infected with *A abstrusus*.[89] Abamectin (0.3 mg/kg, subcutaneous, repeated in 2 weeks) appeared to be effective in the treatment of one cat.[90]

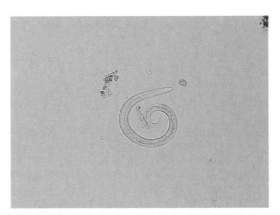

Fig. 8. First-stage larvae of *Aelurostrongylus abstrusus* recovered on Baermann examination of a feline fecal sample (original magnification ×200).

CANINE ANGIOSTRONGYLOSIS (*ANGIOSTRONGYLUS VASORUM*)

Angiostrongylus vasorum, the French Heartworm, is a metastrongyloid that occurs in the pulmonary arteries and right heart of wild and domestic canids in Europe, Africa, and South America, and in a single focus in North America in Canada (Newfoundland-Labrador).[22,25,91] The natural definitive hosts are various species of foxes. The risk of infection to dogs in North America is currently restricted to those animals living within this small endemic range. However, recent studies have indicated an alarming trend toward expansion in the geographic distribution of *A vasorum*, and an increased exposure risk of infection to dogs within the various endemic ranges.[92] Given the ease and frequency of travel within North America coupled with the presence of a large red fox population and the abundance of gastropod intermediate hosts, it seems highly likely that the endemic range of *A vasorum* will spread from Newfoundland to other parts of North America. Canids acquire infection by the ingestion of L3 larvae contained in intermediate hosts (terrestrial gastropods, frogs). The prepatent period is 28 to 108 days.[93] Adult worms are 14 to 20.5 mm in length (about one-tenth the size of *Dirofilaria immitis*) and males are bursate.[91] Infections result in potentially fatal cardiopulmonary disease with clinical signs consisting of chronic cough, dyspnea, exercise intolerance, anorexia, gagging, and weight loss.[91,93] Secondary coagulopathies (disseminated intravascular coagulation, immune-mediated thrombocytopenia) can also occur, resulting in subcutaneous hematomas or occasionally in fatal cerebral, spinal, or abdominal hemorrhage. Ascites, syncope, vomiting, and signs of central nervous system disease may also occur. On rare occasions sudden death after an acute onset of clinical disease can occur, usually in younger dogs.[91,93] Definitive diagnosis is by the detection of L1 larvae in feces or bronchial mucus.[91,94] Larvae are 310 to 399 microns in length and have a cephalic button at the anterior end, and the tail terminates in a sinus wave-shaped kink with a dorsal spine (**Figs. 9** and **10**).[12] The method of choice for fecal detection of L1 larvae is the Baermann technique.[25,93] Although not yet commercially available, a sandwich enzyme-linked immunosorbent assay detecting circulating antigens of *A vasorum* has recently been developed, and shows promise as a diagnostic test. A test specificity of 100% and sensitivity of 92% was reported.[95] The presence of radiographic changes, reduced serum levels of fructosamine, or calcemia may also aid in diagnosis.[93]

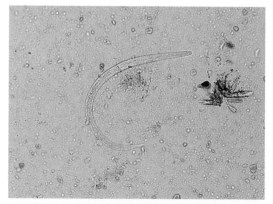

Fig. 9. First-stage larvae of *Angiostrongylus vasorum* recovered on Baermann examination of a canine fecal sample (original magnification ×200).

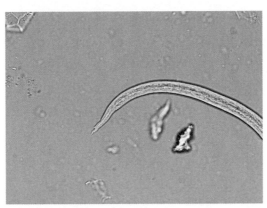

Fig. 10. First-stage larvae of *Angiostrongylus vasorum* recovered on Baermann examination of a canine fecal sample. Close-up view of the tail morphology showing the kink and dorsal spine (original magnification ×450).

Fenbendazole, ivermectin, milbemycin oxime, and moxidectin have all been used to treat angiostrongylosis in dogs, with apparent success. Irrespective of the choice of anthelmintic, posttreatment complications that may involve severe dyspnea or ascites can occur.[91] Administration of bronchodilators and diuretics are indicated in these cases. Fenbendazole (20 to 25 mg/kg, oral, once a day for 20 to 21 days or 50 mg/kg, oral, once a day for 5 to 21 days) has been widely used in naturally infected dogs.[93] Milbemycin oxime (0.5 mg/kg, oral) given once a week for 4 weeks has also been used in naturally infected dogs.[25] The same therapeutic protocol used to treat dogs experimentally infected with *A vasorum* had an efficacy of 85%. This study also reported an efficacy of 85% when experimentally infected dogs were given two doses of milbemycin oxime (0.5 mg/kg) at 1 month and 2 months after exposure (ie, as used in *Dirofilaria immitis* prevention).[96] A single topical application of moxidectin (2.5 mg/kg) was used to treat naturally infected dogs and an efficacy of 85% was reported.[97]

LUNG FLUKE (*PARAGONIMUS KELLICOTTI*)

Paragonimus kellicotti is a trematode that occurs in the lung parenchyma infecting dogs, cats, pigs, goats, and various wildlife species in an endemic area that includes much of the eastern half of North America.[36,98] Infections are most common in the north-central and southeastern states of the United States.[99] Fecal examination surveys have indicated a low prevalence of infection (<1%) however, these results are likely an underestimate due to suboptimal detection sensitivity of the flotation technique for fluke eggs.[2–4] Infection with *P kellicotti* was found to be the cause of disease in 8% (3 of 37) of cats showing signs of chronic respiratory disease in Louisiana.[100]

Adult flukes are 10 to 13 by 4 to 6 mm in size, occur inside capsules situated in the lung parenchyma, and rarely occur in other tissues.[99,101] These flukes are easily differentiated from the nematode lungworms of dogs and cats by the body shape and presence of oral and ventral suckers. Capsules are 2 to 5 cm in diameter with walls 1 to 4 mm thick, usually contain two or more flukes, and are connected to the bronchioles.[102] Capsules occur most often in the caudal lung lobes (right > left). Eggs passed in feces that are deposited into water develop and hatch ciliated miracidium, which

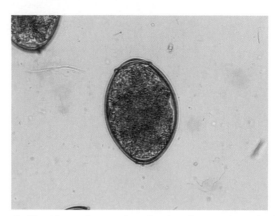

Fig. 11. *Paragonimus kellicotti* egg detected on fecal sedimentation of a feline fecal sample (original magnification ×400).

infect the first intermediate host, aquatic snails (*Pomatiopsis lapidaria; Pomatiopsis cincinnatiensis*).[99,103] Animals acquire infection by the ingestion of metacercaria contained in the tissues of the second intermediate host, crayfish (*Cambarus* spp, *Orconectes* spp). Prevalence of infection in crayfish can be as high as 94% in a stream in the late summer peak period.[104] In addition, rodents predating on infected crayfish can serve as paratenic hosts.[105] The prepatent period is 5 to 7 weeks. Infections have been reported to last as long as 4 years.[106]

The most common clinical sign of infection is cough that is sometimes accompanied by sneezing, exercise intolerance, hemoptysis, and dyspnea.[99,105] Infections can be subclinical to fatal. Subclinical and clinical pneumothorax may develop due to the rupture of the fluke capsule through the pleura, allowing air to pass from the bronchial system to the pleural space. Infected animals may suffer chronic cough for prolonged periods or die acutely, with no history of clinical disease.[99,107]

Definitive diagnosis is by detection of the distinctive operculate eggs of *P kellicotti* in feces or bronchial mucus. Fecal detection is best achieved through sedimentation.[12,108] Eggs may be found by fecal flotation; however, detection sensitivity in samples with low levels of eggs is poor. The eggs are 75 to 118 by 42 to 67 microns in size, yellow-brown in color, and have an operculum at one end (**Fig. 11**).[12] The eggs can be differentiated from those of other trematode or pseudophyllidean tapeworms by the thickened ridge in the shell wall highlighting the opercular line.[12] In addition, fluke capsules can be visualized radiographically as multiloculated cystic structures 2 to 5 cm in size in dogs.[102,109] Lesions in cats are smaller and have a greater density.[102,108]

Current treatment options include extra-label usage of albendazole, fenbendazole, or praziquantel. Albendazole (25 mg/kg, oral, twice a day for 14 days), fenbendazole (50 mg/kg, oral, once a day for 10 to 14 days), and praziquantel (23 mg/kg, oral, three times a day for 3 days) are recommended as effective in the treatment of *P kellicotti* infected dogs and cats.[98]

SUMMARY

The helminth parasite infection of the canine and feline respiratory tract, excepting aelurostrongylosis in cats in the southeastern United States, crenosomosis in dogs in Atlantic Canada and eucoleosis in dogs and cats throughout North America, is uncommon. As such, a veterinary clinician may be hesitant to include several fecal examination methods (fecal flotation: *E boehmi. E aerophilus*; $ZnSO_4$ CF: *O osleri, F hirthi, F milksi*; Baermann examination: *C vulpis, A vasorum, A abstrusus*; sedimentation: *P kellicotti*) when conducting a diagnostic investigation in cases involving animals with respiratory disease. However, these techniques are inexpensive, noninvasive, and if positive they indicate a clear course of action. An argument could be made, even in areas where prevalence seems to be low, for the inclusion of at least one of the aforementioned tests ($ZnSO_4$ CF) to be included as part of the baseline data collection in the diagnostic workup of all cases involving respiratory disease.

REFERENCES

1. Lillis WG. Helminth survey of dogs and cats in New Jersey. J Parasitol 1967;53: 1082–4.
2. Nolan T, Smith G. Time series analysis of the prevalence of endoparasitic infections in cats and dogs presented to a veterinary teaching hospital. Vet Parasitol 1995;59:87–96.
3. Jordan HE, Mullins ST, Stebbins ME. Endoparasitism in dogs: 21,583 cases (1981–1990). J Am Vet Med Assoc 1993;203:547–9.
4. Blagburn BL, Lindsay DS, Vaughn JL, et al. Prevalence of canine parasites based on fecal flotation. Compend Contin Educ Pract Vet 1996;18:483–509.
5. Rembiesa C, Richardson DJ. Helminth parasites of the house cat, *Felis catus*, in Connecticut, USA. Comp Parasitol 2003;70:115–9.
6. Flick SC. Endoparasites in cats: current practice and opinions. Feline Practice 1973;3(4):21–34.
7. Dryden MW, Payne PA, Ridley R, et al. Comparison of common fecal flotation techniques for the recovery of parasite eggs and oocysts. Vet Ther 2005;6: 15–28.
8. Levine ND. Capillariins and related nematodes. In: Nematodes parasites of domestic animals and of man. 2nd Edition. Minneapolis: Burgess; 1980. p. 428–44.
9. Campbell B, Little MD. Identification of the eggs of a nematode (*Eucoleus boehmi*) from the nasal mucosa of North American dogs. J Am Vet Med Assoc 1991;198:1520–3.
10. Moravec F. Review of capillarid and trchosomoidid nematodes from mammals in the Czech Republic and the Slovak Republic. Acta Soc Zool Bohem 2000;64: 271–304.
11. Schoning P, Dryden MW, Gabbert NH. Identification of a nasal nematode (*Eucoleus boehmi*) in greyhounds. Vet Res Commun 1993;17:277–81.
12. Zajac AM, Conboy GA. Chapter 1. In: Veterinary clinical parasitology. 7th Edition. Ames (IA): Blackwell; 2006. p. 3–148.
13. Campbell B. *Trichuris* and other Trichinelloid nematodes of dogs and cats in the United States. Compendium on Continuing Education for the Practicing Veterinarian 1991;13:769–78, 801.
14. Evinger JV, Kazacos KR, Cantwell HD. Ivermectin for treatment of nasal capillariasis in a dog. J Am Vet Med Assoc 1985;186:174–5.
15. Conboy GA, Stewart T, O'Brien S. *Eucoleus boehmi* infection in a boxer-Shar pei cross: treatment using milbemycin oxime [abstract 62] In: Proceedings of the 53rd Annual Meeting of the American Association of Veterinary Parasitologists. New Orleans; 2008. p. 69.
16. King RR, Greiner EC, Ackeran N, et al. Nasal capillariasis in a dog. J Am Anim Hosp Assoc 1990;26:381–5.

17. Payne PA, Dryden MW, Smith V, et al. Chronic *Eucoleus boehmi* infection in mixed breed dog [abstract 92]. In: Proceedings of the 52nd Annual Meeting of the American Association of Veterinary Parasitologists. Washington (DC); 2007. p. 93.

18. Barrs VR, Martin P, Nicoll RG, et al. Pulmonary cryptococcosis and *Capillaria aerophila* infection in an FIV-positive cat. Aust Vet J 2000;78:154–8.

19. Burgess H, Ruotsalo K, Peregrine AS, et al. *Eucoleus aerophilus* respiratory infection in a dog with Addison's disease. Can Vet J 2008;49:389–92.

20. Greenlee PG, Noone KE. Pulmonary capillariasis in a dog. J Am Anim Hosp Assoc 1984;20:983–4.

21. Brannian RE. Treatment of bronchial capillariasis in arctic foxes with fenbendazole. Journal of Zoo Animal Medicine 1985;16:66–8.

22. Levine ND. Lungworms and related nematodes. In: Nematodes parasites of domestic animals and of man. 2nd Edition. Minneapolis: Burgess; 1980. p. 222–55.

23. Bihr T, Conboy GA. Lungworm (*Crenosoma vulpis*) infection in dogs on Prince Edward Island. Can Vet J 1999;40:555–9.

24. Unterer S, Deplazes P, Arnold P, et al. Spontaneous *Crenosoma vulpis* infection in 10 dogs: laboratory, radiographic and endoscopic findings. Schweiz Arch Tierheilkd 2002;144:174–9.

25. Conboy G. Natural infections of *Crenosoma vulpis* and *Angiostrongylus vasorum* in dogs in Atlantic Canada and their treatment with milbemycin oxime. Vet Rec 2004;155:16–8.

26. Nelson TA, Gregory DG, Burroughs C, et al. Prevalence of lungworms in Illinois coyotes. Trans Ill State Acad Sci 2007;100:89–95.

27. Hoff B. Lungworm (*Crenosoma vulpis*) infection in dogs. Can Vet J 1993;34:123–4.

28. Lalonde R, Carioto L, Villeneuve A. Infestation pulmonaire par *Crenosoma vulpis* chez le chein. Med Vet Que 2005;35:11.

29. Petersen EN, Barr SC, Gould WJ, et al. Use of fenbendazole for treatment of *Crenosoma vulpis* infection in a dog. J Am Vet Med Assoc 1993;202:1483–4.

30. Shaw DH, Conboy GA, Hogan PM, et al. Eosinophilic bronchitis caused by *Crenosoma vulpis* infection in dogs. Can Vet J 1996;37:361–3.

31. Rinaldi L, Calabria G, Carbone S, et al. *Crenosoma vulpis* in dog: first case report in Italy and use of FLOTAC technique for copromicroscopic diagnosis. Parasitol Res 2007;101:1681–4 [erratum: Parasitol Res 2008;102:569].

32. Conboy GA, Markham RJF. Effects of multiple exposures of *Crenosoma vulpis* infection in dogs on larval fecal shedding patterns [abstract 56] In: Proceedings of the 53rd Annual Meeting of the American Association of Veterinary Parasitologists. New Orleans; 2008. p. 65.

33. Cobb MA, Fisher MA. *Crenosoma vulpis* infection in a dog. Vet Rec 1992;130:452.

34. Conboy G, Bourque A, Miller L, et al. Efficacy of milbemycin oxime in the treatment of dogs experimentally infected with *Crenosoma vulpis*. [abstract 63] In: Proceedings of the 52nd Annual Meeting of the American Association of Veterinary Parasitologists. Washington (DC); 2007. p. 74.

35. Foreyt WJ, Foreyt KM. Attempted transmission of *Oslerus (Oslerus) osleri* = *Filaroides osleri* from coyotes to domestic dogs and coyotes. J Parasitol 1981;67:284–6.

36. Becklund WW. Revised checklist of internal and external parasites of domestic animals in the Unites States and possessions and in Canada. Am J Vet Res 1964;25:1380–416.

37. Urquhart GM, Jarrett FH, O'Sullivan JG. Canine tracheo-bronchitis due to infection with *Filaroides osleri*. Vet Rec 1954;66:143–5.
38. Mills JHL, Nielsen SW. Canine *Filaroides osleri* and *Filaroides milksi* infection. J Am Vet Med Assoc 1966;149:56–63.
39. Dorrington JE. Studies on *Filaroides osleri* infestation in dogs. Onderstepoort J Vet Res 1968;35:225–86.
40. Polley L. Quantitative observations on populations of the lungworm *Oslerus osleri* (Cobbold, 1889) in coyotes (*Canis latrans* Say). Can J Zool 1986;64: 2384–6.
41. Dunsmore JD, Spratt DM. The life history of *Filaroides osleri* in wild and domestic canids in Australia. Vet Parasitol 1979;5:275–86.
42. Polley L, Creighton SR. Experimental direct transmission of the lungworm *Filaroides osleri* in dogs. Vet Rec 1977;100:136–7.
43. Brownlie SE. A retrospective study of diagnosis in 109 cases of canine lower respiratory disease. J Small Anim Pract 1990;31:371–6.
44. Georgi JR. Parasites of the respiratory tract. Vet Clin North Am Small Anim Pract 1987;17(6):1421–42.
45. Clayton HM, Lindsay FE. *Filaroides osleri* infection in a dog. J Small Anim Pract 1979;20:773–82.
46. Burrows CF, O'Brien JA, Biery DN. Pneumothorax due to *Filaroides osleri* infestation in the dog. J Small Anim Pract 1972;3:613–8.
47. Outerbridge CA, Taylor SM. *Oslerus osleri* tracheobronchitis: treatment with ivermectin in 4 dogs. Can Vet J 1998;39:238–40.
48. Whitlock JH. A description of a new dog lungworm, *Filaroides milksi* n sp (Nematoda, Metastrongyloidea). Wien Tierarztl Monatsschr 1956;43:730–8.
49. Hirth RS, Hottendorf GH. Lesions produced by a new lungworm in beagle dogs. Vet Pathol 1973;10:385–407.
50. Georgi JR, Anderson RC. *Filaroides hirthi* sp. n. (Nematoda: Metastrongyloidea) from the lung of the dog. J Parasitol 1975;61:337–9.
51. Georgi JR. Differential characters of *Filaroides milksi* Whitlock, 1956 and *Filaroides hirthi* Georgi and Anderson, 1975. Proc Helminth Soc Wash 1979; 46:142–5.
52. Pence DB. Notes on two species of *Filaroides* (Nematoda: Metastrongyloidea) from carnivores in Texas. Proc Helminthol Soc Wash 1978;45:103–10.
53. Webster WA. *Andersonstrongylus milksi* (Whitlock, 1956) n. comb. (Metastrongyloidea: Angiostrongylidae) with a discussion of related species in North American canids and mustelids. Proc Helminthol Soc Wash 1981;48:154–8.
54. Erb HN, Georgi JR. Control of *Filaroides hirthi* in commercially reared beagle dogs. Lab Anim Sci 1982;32:394–6.
55. Craig TM, Brown TW, Shefstad DK, et al. Fatal *Filaroides hirthi* infection in a dog. J Am Vet Med Assoc 1978;172:1096–8.
56. August JR, Powers RD, Bailey WS, et al. *Filaroides hirthi* in a dog: fatal hyperinfection suggestive of autoinfection. J Am Vet Med Assoc 1980;176: 331–4.
57. Rubash JM. *Filaroides hirthi* infection in a dog. J Am Vet Med Assoc 1986;189:213.
58. Andreasen CB, Carmichael P. What is your diagnosis? Vet Clin Pathol 1992;21: 77–8.
59. Valentine BA, Georgi ME. *Filaroides hirthi* hyperinfection associated with adrenal cortical carcinoma in a dog. J Comp Pathol 1987;97:221–5.
60. Pinckney RD, Studer AD, Genta RM. *Filaroides hirthi* infection in two related dogs. J Am Vet Med Assoc 1988;193:1287–8.

61. Corwin RM, Legendre AM, Dade AW. Lungworm (*Filaroides milksi*) infection in a dog. J Am Vet Med Assoc 1974;165:180–1.
62. Georgi JR, Georgi ME, Fahnestock GR, et al. Transmission and control of *Filaroides hirthi* lungworm infection in dogs. Am J Vet Res 1979;40:829–31.
63. Georgi JR, Georgi ME, Cleveland DJ. Patency and transmission of *Filaroides hirthi* infection. Parasitology 1977;75:251–7.
64. Genta RM, Schad GA. *Filaroides hirthi*: hyperinfective lungworm infection in immunosuppressed dogs. Vet Pathol 1984;21:349–54.
65. Carrasco L, Hervais J, Gomez-Villamandos JC, et al. Massive *Filaroides hirthi* infestation associated with canine distemper in a puppy. Vet Rec 1997;140: 72–3.
66. Georgi JR, Fahnestock GR, Bohm MFK, et al. The migration and development of *Filaroides hirthi* larvae in dogs. Parasitology 1979;79:39–47.
67. Rendano VT, Georgi JR, Fahnestock GR, et al. *Filaroides hirthi* lungworm infection in dogs: its radiographic appearance. J Am Vet Radiol Soc 1979;20:2–9.
68. Bauer C, Bahnemann R. Control of *Filaroides hirthi* infections in beagle dogs by ivermectin. Vet Parasitol 1996;65:269–73.
69. Crawford P. What is your diagnosis? J Small Anim Pract 2000;41:95, 133–4.
70. Caro-Vadillo A, Martinez-Merlo E, Garcia-Real I, et al. Verminous pneumonia due to *Filaroides hirthi* in a Scottish terrier in Spain. Vet Rec 2005;157:586–9.
71. Scott DW. Current knowledge of aelurostrongylosis in the cat. Cornell Vet 1973; 63:483–500.
72. Kennedy MJ. Superfamily metastrongyloidea. In: Synopsis of the parasites of domesticated mammals of Canada. Edmonton (AB): Alberta Agriculture Animal Health; 1986. p. 17–8.
73. Willard MD, Roberts RE, Allison N, et al. Diagnosis of *Aelurostrongylus abstrusus* and *Dirofilaria immitis* infections in cats from a humane shelter. J Am Vet Med Assoc 1988;192:913–6.
74. Hobmaier M, Hobmaier A. Mammalian phase of the lungworm *Aelurostrongylus abstrusus* in the cat. J Am Vet Med Assoc 1935;87:191–8.
75. Hamilton JM. Studies on re-infestation of the cat with *Aelurostrongylus abstrusus*. J Comp Pathol 1968;78:69–72.
76. Ribeiro VM, Lima WS. Larval production in cats infected and re-infected with *Aelurostrongylus abstrusus* (Nematoda: Protostrongylidae). Rev Med Vet 2001;152:815–29.
77. Hamilton JM. *Aelurostrongylus abstrusus* infestation of the cat. Vet Rec 1963;75: 417–22.
78. Hamilton JM. The number of *Aelurostrongylus abstrusus* larvae required to produce pulmonary disease in the cat. J Comp Pathol 1967;77:343–6.
79. Grandi G, Calvi LE, Venco L, et al. *Aelurostrongylus abstrusus* (cat lungworm) infection in five cats from Italy. Vet Parasitol 2005;134:177–82.
80. Traversa D, Lia RP, Ioria R, et al. Diagnosis and risk factors of *Aelurostrongylus abstrusus* (Nematoda, Strongylida) infection in cats in Italy. Vet Parasitol 2008; 153:182–6.
81. Barrs VR, Swinney GR, Martin P, et al. Concurrent *Aelurostrongylus abstrusus* infection and salmonellosis in a kitten. Aust Vet J 1999;77:229–32.
82. Gaglio G, Cringoli G, Rinaldi L, et al. Use of the FLOTAC technique for the diagnosis of *Aelurostrongylus abstrusus* in the cat. Parasitol Res 2008;103:1055–7.
83. Traversa D, Guglielmini C. Feline aelurostrongylosis and canine angiostrongylosis: a challenging diagnosis for two emerging verminous pneumonia infections. Vet Parasitol 2008;157:163–74.

84. Payo-Puente P, Diez A, Gonzalo-Orden, et al. Computed tomography in cats infected by *Aelurostrongylus abstrusus*: 2 clinic cases. Intern J Appl Res Vet Med 2005;3:339–43.
85. Kirkpatrick CE, Megella C. Use of ivermectin in treatment of *Aelurostrongylus abstrusus* and *Toxocara cati* infections in a cat. J Am Vet Med Assoc 1987; 190:1309–10.
86. Freeman AS, Alger K, Guerro J. Feline lungworm: in the absence of clinical signs. Vet Forum 2003;20:20–3.
87. Burgu A, Sarimehmetoglu O. *Aelurostrongylus abstrusus* infection in two cats. Vet Rec 2004;154:602–4.
88. Hamilton JM, Weatherley A, Chapman AJ. Treatment of lungworm disease in the cat with fenbendazole. Vet Rec 1984;114:40–1.
89. Brianti E, Pennisi MG, Risitano AL, et al. Feline aelurostrongylosis sporadic or underestimated disease: prevalence study and therapeutic trial in cats in southern Italy [abstract 54]. In: Proceedings of the 53rd Annual Meeting of the American Association of Veterinary Parasitologists. New Orleans; 2008. p. 64.
90. Foster SF, Martin P, Allan GS, et al. Lower respiratory tract infections in cats: 21 cases (1995–2000). J Feline Med Surg 2004;6:167–80.
91. Bolt G, Monrad J, Koch J, et al. Canine angiostrongylosis: a review. Vet Rec 1994;135:447–52.
92. Morgan ER, Shaw SE, Brennan SF, et al. Angiostrongylus vasorum: a real heartbreaker. Trends Parasitol 2005;21:49–51.
93. Koch J, Willesen JL. Canine pulmonary angiostrongylosis: an update. The Veterinary Journal 2009;179:348–59.
94. Rosen L, Ash I R, Wallace GD. Life history of the canine lungworm *Angiostrongylus vasorum* (Baillet). Am J Vet Res 1970;31:131–43.
95. Verzberger-Epshtein I, Markham RJF, Sheppard JA, et al. Serologic detection of *Angiostrongylus vasorum* infection in dogs. Vet Parasitol 2008;151:53–60.
96. Conboy G, Schenker R, Strehlau G. Efficacy of Milbemax (milbemycin/praziquantel) for the treatment and prevention of *Angiostrongylus vasorum* infection in dogs [abstract 122]. In: Proceedings of the Joint 49th Annual Meeting of the American Association of Veterinary Parasitologists/79th Meeting of the American Society of Parasitologists. Philadelphia; 2004. p. 92.
97. Willesen JL, Kristensen AT, Jensen AL, et al. Efficacy and safety of imidacloprid/moxidectin spot-on solution and fenbendazole in the treatment of dogs naturally infected with *Angiostrongylus vasorum* (Baillet, 1866). Vet Parasitol 2007;147: 258–64.
98. Bowmann DD. Helminths. In: Georgi's parasitology for veterinarians. 9th edition. St. Louis (MO): Saunders Elsevier; 2009. p. 115–239.
99. Rochat MC, Cowell RL, Tyler RD, et al. Paragonimiasis in dogs and cats. Compend Contin Educ Pract Vet 1990;12:1093–100.
100. Bech-Nielsen S, Fulton RW, Cox HU, et al. Feline respiratory tract disease in Louisiana. Am J Vet Res 1980;41:1293–8.
101. Ah H-S, Chapman WL. Extrapulmonary granulomatous lesions in canine paragonimiasis. Vet Parasitol 1976;2:251–8.
102. Pechman RD. Pulmonary paragonimiasis in dogs and cats: a review. J Am Anim Hosp Assoc 1980;21:87–95.
103. Basch PF. Two new molluscan intermediate hosts for *Paragonimus kellicotti*. J Parasitol 1959;45:273.
104. Stromberg PC, Toussant MJ, Dubey JP. Population biology of *Paragonimus kellicotti* metacercariae in central Ohio. Parasitology 1978;77:13–8.

105. Madden A, Pinckney RD, Forrest LJ. Canine paragonimosis. Vet Med 1999;94: 783–91.
106. Lumsden RD, Sogandares-Bernal F. Ultrastructural manifestations of pulmonary paragonimiasis. J Parasitol 1970;56:1095–109.
107. Harrus S, Nyska A, Colorni A, et al. Sudden death due to *Paragonimus kellicotti* infection in a dog. Vet Parasitol 1997;71:59–63.
108. Dubey JP, Stromberg PC, Toussant MJ, et al. Induced paragonimiasis in cats; clinical signs and diagnosis. Am J Vet Res 1978;39:1027–31.
109. Dubey JP, Toussant MJ, Hoover EA, et al. Experimental *Paragonimus kellicotti* infection in dogs. Vet Parasitol 1979;5:325–37.

Heartworm Biology, Treatment, and Control

Dwight D. Bowman, MS, PhD[a],*, Clarke E. Atkins, DVM[b]

KEYWORDS

- *Dirofilaria* • Microfilariae • Right heart failure
- Caval syndrome • Heartworm development units

Dirofilaria immitis, the "inexorable dreaded threadworm," remains the most serious parasitic disease of the dog in North America. These worms are white and approximately a foot in length; males are 12 to 20 cm long and females are 25 to 31 cm long. The worms cause severe lung pathology and morbidity in the dog, shorten the animal's life expectancy, and can cause acute disease and death. Due to the spread of heartworm disease throughout the nation, there are more dogs at risk now than there were 100 years ago. An excellent array of products is available that prevent infection when used on a regular basis. Also, treatment of infected dogs has improved markedly with the introduction of the intramuscularly delivered melarsomine dihydrochloride, but there still can be numerous difficulties and complications, especially in dogs that present after developing severe heartworm associated disease. In most parts of the United States, dogs that are not on preventive therapy are at risk of infection. There is little doubt that cats also get infected with larvae from mosquitoes, though the disease manifestations are different and more subtle than in the dog. Moreover, there have been several reports of these worms causing lesions and clinical signs in the lungs of people throughout the United States. In the United States, coyotes and the unprotected canine population provide reservoir hosts that continue to place dogs, cats, and people at risk of obtaining heartworm infections from the bites of infected mosquitoes.

BIOLOGY
Affinities

The canine heartworm, *Dirofilaria immitis*, is in the phylum Nematoda, class Secernentea, order Spirurida, suborder Spirurina, superfamily Filarioidea, family Onchocercidae, and subfamily Dirofilariinae.[1] This organization of the Nematoda that defines the affinities of the genus *Dirofilaria* based on biologic and morphologic criteria is

[a] Department of Microbiology and Immunology, College of Veterinary Medicine, Cornell University, C4-119 VMC, Tower Road, Ithaca, NY 14853-6401, USA
[b] Department of Clinical Sciences, College of Veterinary Medicine, North Carolina State University, 4700 Hillsborough Street, Raleigh, NC 27606, USA
* Corresponding author.
E-mail address: ddb3@cornell.edu (D.D. Bowman).

Vet Clin Small Anim 39 (2009) 1127–1158
doi:10.1016/j.cvsm.2009.06.003
vetsmall.theclinics.com
0195-5616/09/$ – see front matter © 2009 Elsevier Inc. All rights reserved.

supported by recent ssu RNA gene phylogenies.[2] The Onchocercidae contains some 75 or so genera that have microfilariae found in the blood or skin. By making use of biting vectors that feed on blood or skin and ingest microfilariae, the adult worms can live in tissues of the body that have no direct connections to the external environment, for example, the meninges, lymphatics, and blood vessels, rather than the intestinal tract or tracheal system.[1]

Vertebrate Final Hosts

Although known earlier in Europe, the dog heartworm was first described as a new species in the United States.[3] The worm was first reported in the United States in 1847 in a dog from Erie, Alabama that was described as having a massive number of white worms in its heart and large vessels.[4] The domestic dog, *Canis familiaris*, is the typical host of the heartworm. *Dirofilaria immitis* originated in Asia, had a long history in countries bordering the Mediterranean, and was brought to the Americas in dogs by early explorers and immigrants. At the time of the European arrival in the Americas, there were few representatives of *Canis lupus familiaris* among the Native American population, but there was an indigenous canid population represented by wolves, coyotes, and foxes.

Within the canine hosts of the Americas, heartworms have been recovered from the domestic dog, gray wolf, coyote, red fox, gray fox, maned wolf, and crab-eating fox. Around the world, other wild canids reported to be infected with heartworms include the jackal (*Canis aureus*), the raccoon dog (*Nyctereutes procyonoides*), the dhole (*Cuon alpinus*), and the African wild dog (*Lycaon pictus*).[5,6] A tabular summary of the occurrence of heartworms in the United States by state in coyotes, wolves, and gray and red foxes is presented by Anderson.[7,8] It seems that all members of the genus *Canis* can support the development of patent *D immitis* infections and serve as wildlife reservoirs.[6] The raccoon dog and the African wild dog have also been found to support patent infections with heartworms.[6] Foxes of the *Vulpes* and *Urocyon* genera are not as likely to support long-standing patent infections, and are therefore unlikely to be of major importance as reservoir hosts.[6,9] The other genera of canines have not been examined sufficiently to determine their potential role as reservoirs.[6]

Infections have been reported from hosts other than canines. Felids, both the domestic cat and several other species, can develop infections with heartworms; however, like foxes, felids tend not to serve as biologic reservoirs of the infection.[6] A recent list of hosts included feline hosts: the ocelot (*Leopardus pardalis*), mountain lion (*Felis concolor*), clouded leopard (*Neofelis neburosa*), snow leopard (*Uncia uncia*), Bengal tiger (*Panthera tigris*), and lion (*Panthera leo*).[6] Other hosts occasionally have nonpatent heartworm infections with one to several worms, and such hosts include primates, deer, beavers, muskrats, horses, wolverines, coatimundis, red pandas, raccoons, bears, seals, and sea lions; domestic ferrets can develop heartworm.[5,6,10]

Intermediate Hosts/Vectors

Members of the genus *Dirofilaria* are most commonly transmitted by mosquitoes that ingest blood containing the relatively long unsheathed microfilariae with tapered tails. However, unlike human malarias, in which only the genus *Anopheles* can serve as a vector of the important *Plasmodium* species, *Dirofilaria immitis* is capable of developing in mosquitoes from several different families. More than 60 species of mosquitoes around the world have been shown to be susceptible to infection, and 13 species collected in the field in the United States were infected with *D immitis* larvae.[9] In 1998 Scoles summarized the mosquitoes found to be naturally infected with *D immitis* (**Table 1**).[11]

Table 1
Mosquito species collected naturally infected with filariids presumed to be *Dirofilaria immitis* in the United States

Species	Locations (State)	Total Reports[a]	Number of Reports with L_3[b]
Aedes albopictus	FL, LA	3	1
Aedes canadensis	CT, FL, MA, NJ	4	4
Aedes cantator	NJ	1	1
Aedes excrucians	CT, MA	3	2
Aedes infirmatus	FL	1	1
Aedes sirrensis	CA	1	1
Aedes sollicitans	CT, NC, NJ	4	2
Aedes sticticus	AL, MA	3	3
Aedes stimulans	CT, MA	2	1
Aedes taeniorhynchus	FL, NC	3	3
Aedes triseriatus	IN	1	1
Aedes trivittatus	AL, IA, IN, OK, TN	6	6
Aedes vexans	AL, CA, CT, FL, IN, LA, MD, MI, MN, NH, NY, OK	16	10
Anopheles bradleyi	NC	2	1
Anopheles crucians	AL, FL	2	1
Anopheles freeborni	CA	1	1
Anopheles punctipennis	AL, IA, KY, MA, MD	7	3
Anopheles quadrimaculatus	LA, MA, MI, NY	5	4
Culex nigripalpus	FL	1	1
Culex pipiens	MI	1	1
Culex quinquefasctiatus	AL, FL, LA	3	2
Culex salinarius	MD, NC, NJ	3	2
Psorophora columbae	LA	1	1
Psorophora ferox	CT, FL	2	2

[a] Number of studies that report the collection of suspected *Dirofilaria immitis* in the mosquito species listed.
[b] Number of studies listed in the previous column in which third-stage larvae were present.
    Data from Refs.[2,6,11]

Endosymbionts

Since 1975, bacterialike organisms were observed with the electron microscope in the cells of *D immitis* and other filarioids.[12] Research with molecular methods has shown that the organisms in *D immitis* are *Rickettsia*-like *Wolbachia* endosymbionts of arthropods.[13] In 1999, it was shown that tetracycline had negative effects on the embryogenesis of *D immitis*.[14] The effects of treatments targeting the *Wolbachia* organisms within *D immitis* will be discussed later in this article.

Life Cycle

The summary by Anderson in 2000 remains an excellent presentation of the generalities of the heartworm life cycle.[1] Following a single infection from mosquitoes, a dog that develops adult worms can maintain a patent infection for up to 7.5 years.[10] The adult worms live in the pulmonary arteries of the canine host, and if the pulmonary artery is clamped just before euthanasia, worms are only found in the pulmonary arteries with none in the right ventricle.[15] However, when worms are present in a dog in massive numbers or in large numbers in small dogs, the worms may be regurgitated back into the heart, perhaps from a lack of space for the adult worms or blood pressure changes. In those instances in which adult worms back into the right ventricle and atrium to enter the vena cava, there can be massive hemolysis with associated clinical signs, leading to caval syndrome, a medical emergency.

Fertilized eggs undergo various developmental stages within the uterus: prelarva, developing embryo, pretzel, and stretched microfilaria.[16] Stretched microfilariae are free of the egg membrane, so that microfilariae exiting the vulval opening and entering the blood are not sheathed. Microfilariae transfused into dogs are capable of surviving for up to 2.5 years, and are capable of developing to the infective stage in mosquitoes for at least 3 months after transfusion.[10]

There are dynamics of the microfilarial interactions with dogs and mosquitoes that are very important for the parasite's transmission. There is no demonstrated correlation between circulating microfilarial numbers per cm^3 of blood and the number of adults present in pulmonary arteries.[10] Some homeostatic control is in place on the total number of microfilariae present within the peripheral blood, because microfilariae do not increase uncontrollably during chronic infection even though microfilariae probably live 2.5 years.[10] There is also a daily and seasonal variation in the number of microfilariae found in the blood of dogs.[10] On a daily basis, the circulating levels of *D immitis* microfilariae are defined as subperiodic, that is, the maximum number of microfilariae in circulation seems, in most geographic locations, to occur from late afternoon through late evening, but even at low levels, the peripheral blood contains 5% to 20% of the total microfilariae. Also, somewhat higher numbers of microfilariae are present in the blood of infected dogs in spring and summer compared with fall and winter. The daily and seasonal fluctuations in microfilariae numbers likely correlate with the presence of the vector, and it seems that the temporal availability of vectors within a geographic region can select for the local periodicity of the microfilariae.[17] Furthermore, the ingestion of too many microfilariae by a mosquito is fatal.[10] Mosquitoes can protect themselves somewhat against overwhelming infections by some minimal control of the number of microfilariae ingested in a blood meal from a microfilaremic dog, but they do not prevent ingestion of all microfilariae.[10]

In the mosquito, the microfilaria develops into a first-stage larva and after 2 molts becomes an infective third-stage larva. At 26±1°C in *Aedes aegypti* or *Aedes trivittatus*, the worms undergo a first molt in 7 to 8 days and the second molt a few days later (10 to 11 days after microfilarial ingestion).[18] Similar rates of development were noted for larvae in *Aedes albopictus* held at 28°C.[19] Thus, under constant temperatures of around 26°C (79°F) it takes 10 to 14 days for the larvae to reach the infective stage.[20] In North America where many geographic areas do not maintain steady temperatures near 26°C for much of the year, larval development within the mosquito is affected. These effects on larval development have been used to define expected periods of maps heartworm transmission in Canada and the United States.[21,22] These seasonality/transmission maps are based on Heartworm Development Units (HDUs). HDUs represent the number of Degree Days (°D) that the larval heartworm is above the threshold temperature for development, which has been determined to be 14°C (57°F). Thus, if the temperature is 15°C for 24 hours, this is 1°C above 14°C, so the larva gains 1 HDU; if the temperature is 26°C for 24 hours, this is 12°C above 14°C, so the larva accumulates 12 HDUs. A larva in a mosquito requires around 130 accumulated HDUs to become infective (10 days at 27°C; 20 days at 20.5°C).[21,23] To generate the HDU isolines on the maps for the beginning of the transmission season, a proposed "first date of transmission" is chosen, and then for each weather station's data, the temperatures reported for a day are converted to HDUs [daily °D value = (maximum daily temperature in °C – minimum daily temperature in °C/2] – 14°C; daily values less than 0°D are set to 0 because the larvae do not regress in their development). For the end of the transmission season, the last date of the year is chosen on which 130 HDUs could be accumulated in 30 days, the estimated life span of the mosquito at that time of year. In the map of the United States, it is theorized that transmission would only occur for all 12 months of the year in southern Florida and the extreme southern portion of Texas.[24]

Field studies have supported the HDU-based transmission models; one looked at sentinel dogs, one at collected mosquitoes, and one at yearling coyotes. A total of 96 heartworm-naïve adult beagles were placed in each of three sites in the southeastern United States (32 dogs per site): Tattnall County, Georgia, Orange and Lake Counties, Florida (different site in years 2 and 3), and Pointe-Coupee Parish, Louisiana.[25] The dogs were held in outdoor kennels or runs to allow mosquito access. Between April 1988 and April 1989, 20 dogs were placed at each site: 5 for a full year, and 5 for each of 3 4-month blocks (April to August, August to December, and December to April). Heartworms were found in 93% of the dogs held for a year, 86% of April to August dogs, 73% of August to December dogs, and 0% of December to April dogs. Due to the lack of infection in the latter group, additional dogs were placed at the sites from December through April in the next 2 years, and again, none of these dogs developed infections. HDU-based transmission start dates for these sites were the end of April for Louisiana and Georgia, and February or March for Florida; the stop dates were late October to early November in Louisiana and Georgia, and the first weeks of December in Florida. Molecular probes and polymerase chain reaction technology was used to examine the heads of nearly 110,000 mosquitoes (representing 17 different species) for the DNA of third-stage larvae of D immitis, in Florida and Louisiana.[26] The results supported the conclusion that heartworm transmission in the temperate Gulf coast region of the United States is seasonal rather than continuous. Seasonal heartworm transmission in coyotes in California was examined using coyote carcasses from three counties in north-coastal California (Mendocino, Sonoma, and Napa).[27] For 88 first-year coyotes killed from September through March (1994 to 2002), heartworms were not found in the pulmonary vasculature until the end of October. The HDU transmission season was calculated for the different years as starting from late May through early July and ending in varying weeks of October. Thus, these two studies seem to add good support for the suggested HDU transmission isolines.

There is no doubt that the majority of heartworm transmission occurs during the seasons predicted by the isoline numbers; however, there are reasons to suspect that transmission can be completed "off season." In 1983, Ernst and Slocombe pointed out that "temperatures below 14°C and above 37°C have been reported to be detrimental to mosquito survival. However, when these extremes of temperatures occur, individual mosquitoes may rest and survive where they are protected from temperature extremes."[28] It has also been shown that larvae in mosquitoes that cease development when cooled can resume and complete maturation when the mosquitoes are warmed,[21,28] that is, HDUs do not have to be consecutive. Heartworm larvae have been recovered from overwintering mosquitoes.[29] Furthermore, chilling mosquitoes to 12°C did not affect the viability of third-stage larvae after they were returned to normal conditions.[28] The canine sentinel study from 1988 to 1991 in the southeastern

United States occurred during a major drought, and lack of rainfall one year can have significant effects on mosquito disease transmission the next.[30] The research examining more than 100,000 mosquito heads was designed to examine seasonal prevalence, not to identify the potential transmission of heartworms by low numbers of mosquitoes in winter months, and the investigators state that "winter transmission of heartworms in Gainesville and Baton Rouge cannot be ruled out with absolute certainty."[26] Global climate change also needs to be built into the transmission model, as was suggested when the maps were first drawn.[31]

After the larvae leave the mosquito and enter the dog through the bite wound, they begin their development to the adult stage.[22,32–34] These third-stage larvae are not known to undergo any developmental arrest, that is, there is no apparent ability of the worm to halt the maturation process once it begins. Also, the timing of development is quite consistent, that is, larvae go through their two molts at a fairly defined time points after entry into the dog. The third-stage larvae that enter the dog are a millimeter or so in length.[18,22] Most of these larvae remain in the muscles at the site of inoculation, at least for the first 3 days (**Fig. 1**).[32] It would also seem that most larvae molt to the fourth stage probably before day 3 of the infection and before they begin to move any distance from the initial entry site.[22,32] Newly molted fourth-stage larvae are almost the same length as the infective third-stage larvae. Significant growth of the larvae begins at about 2 to 3 weeks after the infection is initiated, so that by 1 month post infection the worms are around 4 mm long, and by 2 months they are around 1 cm long (**Fig. 2**).

The molt to the adult stage occurs at about this time, between 50 and 58 days post infection.[22] The worms that first appear in the pulmonary arteries are 2 to 3 cm long. At this point, there is a rapid increase in size, and the worms can be 10 cm long by 4 months post infection, and 20 to 30 cm by the time they are 6.5 months old. Adult

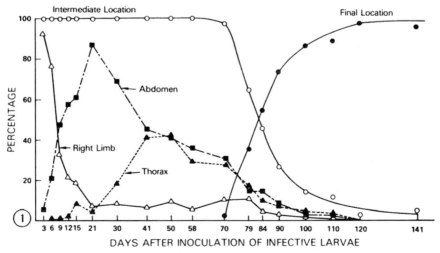

Fig. 1. Distribution and migration patterns of *D immitis* recovered from inoculated dogs, ○, total percentage of larvae recovered from the intermediate locations (subcutaneous and muscle tissues combined) throughout the body. Also included are worms from the abdominal and thoracic cavities, ρ, percentage recovered from the right hindlimb, ■, percentage recovered from the abdomen, π, percentage recovered in the thorax, ●, percentage recovered from final location (right side of the heart, pulmonary arteries, and vena cavae). (*From* Kotani T, Powers KG. Developmental stages of *Dirofilaria immitis* in the dog. Am J Vet Res 1982;43(12):2199–206; with permission.)

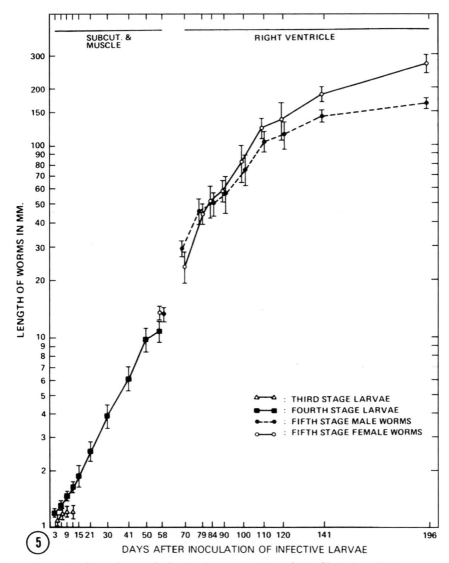

Fig. 2. Stages and larval growth during the maturation of *Dirofilaria immitis* in an experimentally infected dog. (*From* Kotani T, Powers KG. Developmental stages of *Dirofilaria immitis* in the dog. Am J Vet Res 1982;43(12):2199–206; with permission.)

males (12–20 cm long) are shorter and more slender than the females (25–31 cm long), and have a corkscrew-shaped tail that aids in copulation. Fertilization takes place in the pulmonary arteries when the females are approximately 4 months old and reach a length of 7 to 10 cm. Microfilariae first appear after 6 months to as late as 9 months after the induction of an experimental infection,[1] and patency may last up to 7.5 years according to one report.[10]

The route taken by the fourth-stage larvae to get from the abdominal and thoracic muscles to the pulmonary arteries has still not been fully elucidated. Worms entering the pulmonary arteries are typically just a few centimeters long. However, even large adult worms are capable of extensive migration through the tissues.[35]

Life Cycle in the Domestic Cat

In cats, most of the inoculated worms do not mature, and the infections are typically not patent. Worms that survive apparently take longer to reach full maturity, because the prepatent period is 7 to 8 months in cats versus 6 months in dogs.[36] In natural infections, cats have one to eight worms, with two to four being most common.[36] It seems that worms in cats can live for up to 3 to 4 years, although approximately half of infected cats clear their infections without treatment within 3 years.[37]

Geographic Distribution

In recent years, there have been numerous surveys regularly reporting heartworm infections in animals in all of the United States with the exception of Alaska. Also, it is now accepted that most of the lower 48 states and Hawaii support the autochthonous transmission of D immitis, and that the disease can be considered enzootic within the canine population. Surveys have all revealed similar levels of prevalence: nationally, it is somewhat more than 1% in the pet population that visits veterinarians. The overall prevalence based on data from IDEXX reference laboratories and patient-side SNAP tests was around 1.4% (**Fig. 3**).[38] The highest level of infection was in the Southeast at 3.9%, with levels of 0.6% in the Northeast, 0.8% in the Midwest, and 1.2% in the West. This distribution is very similar to other surveys within the pet canine population.[39,40] In most of these studies, a fairly high prevalence was also observed along the Mississippi River (Arkansas 6.8%, Missouri 2.0%, Tennessee 3.6%).

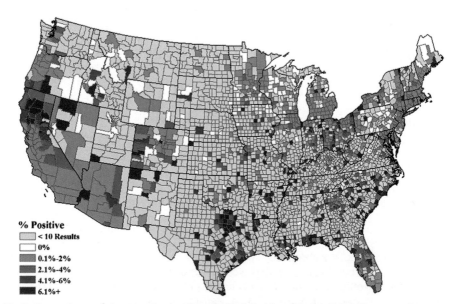

% Positive
- < 10 Results
- 0%
- 0.1%-2%
- 2.1%-4%
- 4.1%-6%
- 6.1%+

Fig. 3. Percentage of dogs testing positive for *D immitis* using the IDEXX Snap test by county throughout the United States. (*From* Bowman DD, Susan EL, Lorentzen L, et al. Prevalence and geographic distribution of *Dirofilaria immitis*, *Borrelia burgdorferi*, *Ehrlichia canis*, and *Anaplasma phagocytophilum* in dogs in the United States: Results of a national clinic-based serologic survey. Vet Parasitol 2009;160(1/2):138–48; with permission.)

Initially concentrated in the southeast and along the Mississippi River, heartworm over the last 50 years has become endemic in much of the United States due to movement of pets and hunting and show dogs.[41] The spread of heartworms has been fairly well documented. In Minnesota, heartworm was first recognized in 1937, but it rapidly spread after 1970.[41] In Canada, the spread has been monitored through a series of triannual surveys.[42] Heartworm is now present over a wide geographic area, is regularly documented in the western states, and endemic transmission is known to occur in California.[43]

The reason for the amazing spread of heartworms over the past few years is probably a combination of several factors. First, mosquito control in the United States was scaled back after the great success of mosquito abatement programs led to a reduction of mosquito-borne disease in humans and the public's fears about the overuse of pesticides. Second, as Dr Roncalli pointed out, pets have been moving rapidly in and out of heartworm-endemic areas, and this has probably exacerbated its spread.[41] Finally, the United States, unlike Europe, has an excellent reservoir host for heartworms: the American coyote, *Canis latrans*. The range of the coyote has expanded eastwardly in the last 50 years, and at the same time heartworms have spread in the coyote reservoir host, a trend that has been carefully detailed in California.[27] In the Sierra Nevada foothills, the prevalence of heartworm-positive coyotes in 1975 to 1985 was 35%, compared with 42% in 2000 to 2002; whereas in the Coastal Range foothills, prevalence increased from 10% to 44%, and in the San Francisco Bay foothills from 8% to 32%.

Cats also serve to give an indication of the distribution of canine heartworm. Cats are for the most part refractory to the development of patent heartworm infection, but adult worms can be found in the hearts of cats.[44] Throughout the United States, antibodies against *D immitis* have been detected in many cats, suggesting that they are being infected by larvae, even if the larvae do not grow into adults. Several national serologic studies of cats using a commercial feline heartworm antibody test found an antibody prevalence in 4.2% to 15.9%, with local prevalences reaching up to 33% in Auburn, California and 21% in Miami, Florida.[45–47]

The prevalence levels detected using antigen or microfilaria tests in dogs, necropsies in coyotes, and antibody tests in cats seem to correlate with the prevalence of the few human cases of *D immitis* reported in the United States. When the reported human cases are mapped on the 2001 American Heartworm Society survey map, it is obvious that human cases occur proportionally to the background prevalence in the dog population.[48]

Diagnosis of Infection

Any control program is based on the ability to diagnose an infection. For heartworm in dogs, the antigen detection assays are excellent diagnostic tests. These tests can be used to ascertain the heartworm status of a dog that has female worms that are greater than 6 months old. These tests should be used annually to verify that preventive programs in individual dogs are successful. The macrolide preventives, ivermectin, milbemycin oxime, moxidectin, and selamectin, result in a significant clearance of microfilariae from the blood of most dogs with circulating microfilariae in 6 to 8 months.[49–53] Therefore the only effective testing modality in the ever-increasing number of dogs receiving monthly preventative is an antigen detection assay.

Prevention

Since the introduction of Heartgard-30 (Merial) in 1987, prevention is achieved almost solely through the administration of one of the many macrocyclic lactones formulated for monthly administration (or as a slow-release injectable formulation [ProHeart-6, Fort Dodge] that provides protection for 6 months; ProHeart-12, effective for 12 months, is available in other countries). The stage killed by the macrocyclic lactones during routine drug testing for monthly preventives is a larva that is 30 days old. In this process, dogs are infected with larvae from a mosquito, and then 30 days later (in a few cases, at 45 days) are given a single dose of the preventive. In most cases, the macrocyclic lactone is present in the body of the host for only a few days. This outcome is not true for moxidectin in the sustained-release formulation ProHeart-6 (Fort Dodge) and for the moxidectin in Advantage Multi [Bayer] that will reach a constant level in the body after several treatments.[50] After treatment, the worms are allowed to mature for 5 to 6 months, and necropsies are performed to assess the number of worms present in the pulmonary arteries of treated versus untreated control dogs. If any dogs develop a single heartworm during the initial trials, the product is likely not to receive approval by the Food and Drug Administration (FDA). In the case of the injectable product, Proheart-6, the dogs are given the injection, then 6 months later they are infected, and about 5 months afterward they are necropsied; here it is slightly more difficult to tell exactly what stage is being killed. It has also been shown that dogs infected with third-stage larvae and then treated 1 day later with the preventive dose of ivermectin are protected from developing adult heartworms.[51] Thus, it seems that ivermectin, and most likely the entire family of macrocyclic lactones, has efficacy against larvae between 1 and 30 days post infection in the dog. These drugs are highly efficacious against larvae up to 2 months of age, but after 2 months the efficacy of the macrocyclic lactones at preventive doses declines.[52]

Current prevention strategies are designed to start dogs on a monthly preventive product as early as possible in their life and continue administration for the life of the pet. There are advocates for year-round preventive therapy, and then others who recommend heartworm prevention only during the predicted seasons of transmission. A good treatment regimen should provide dogs with sufficient protection to allow them to remain heartworm-free even in areas with high infection pressure, where many mosquitoes are actively feeding on infected wildlife or unprotected pets. Adult heartworms are not affected by a single treatment of these macrocyclic lactone formulations, and these products are approved as safe for dogs with circulating microfilariae (selamectin [Revolution, Pfizer] and moxidectin [Advantage Multi, Bayer]) or without any significant effects, that is, only mild hypersensitivity reactions (milbemycin oxime [Sentinel Flavor Tabs, Novartis] and ivermectin [Heartgard Chewables for Dogs, Merial]).

In canine heartworm, the preventive products are not given at dosages designed to be completely microfilaricidal. Some 10% to 20% of dogs with patent infections that are placed on preventatives will continue to have circulating microfilariae for many months after beginning product administration (**Figs. 4** and **5**).[49,53] In a study examining the adulticidal activity of prophylactic doses of Heartgard Plus or Interceptor administered monthly for 16 months to dogs given heartworms by transplantation, some of the five dogs in each of the groups still had microfilariae in the blood after the eleventh (ivermectin) and sixth (milbemycin) treatments.[54] Similar results have been found in studies with selamectin and sustained-release moxidectin.[55,56] In a clinical field trial, seven dogs were given Heartgard and seven Heartgard Plus monthly for 2 years with blood being sampled for microfilariae every 3 to 5 months; two Heartgard dogs and one Heartgard Plus dog were positive 4 months after treatment.[57]

All current heartworm preventives belong to the same class of molecule, the macrocyclic lactones, and thus, one needs to be very prudent in our long-term stewardship of these drugs. Although resistance to macrolides in heartworms has been considered unlikely to develop, this was based on the assumption that preventives were being

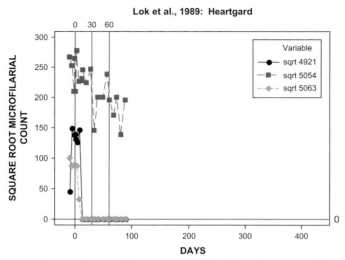

Fig. 4. Microfilarial counts (presented as square roots) in three dogs treated three times with ivermectin (Heartgard). The vertical lines represent the treatment event. Two of the dogs were negative soon after treatment, but one dog remained positive for circulating microfilariae with about 40,000 microfilariae per milliliter of blood. (*Data from* Lok JB, Knight DH, Ramadan EI. Effects of ivermectin on embryogenesis in *Dirofilaria immitis*: age structure and spatial distribution of intrauterine forms as a function of dosage and time posttreatment. In: Proceedings of the Heartworm Symposium. Charleston (SC); 1989. p. 85–94.)

used as per label instructions, and not as adulticides and microfilarial suppressants.[58] To minimize the opportunity for resistance to develop, the products should be used as approved by the FDA: as preventives that should be given to microfilarial negative dogs or to dogs that have been cleared of their heartworm infections.

The hope has been that the *Wolbachia* present in heartworms might prove to be an obligatory mutualistic relationship so that removal of the bacteria with antibiotics would lead to the death of its host, *D immitis*. However, the dog heartworm is not sufficiently dependent on its bacterial symbiont to be killed with simple prolonged antibiotic (doxycycline) therapy.[59] Nonetheless, the killing of *Wolbachia* may prevent the transmission of heartworms. Microfilariae from dogs treated with doxycycline were able to develop to the third larval stage in mosquitoes.[60] However, these larvae did not develop in dogs when they were inoculated subcutaneously. These studies are very difficult to perform, because of the need to grow infective-stage larvae from dogs with suppressed microfilarial counts. The four dogs used in the transmission trials received 40, 40, 6, and a non-disclosed number of infective-stage larvae. Although the controls given approximately 40 larvae were successfully infected while these worms from doxycycline treated dogs did not mature, the number of larvae tested remains small. The potential importance of this work suggests that it should be repeated with larger numbers of larvae and animals.

TREATMENT OF THE COMPANION ANIMAL
Treating the Canine Host

Pathophysiology

In the dog, the primary insult is damage to the pulmonary arteries and lung from the adult *D immitis* living in the pulmonary arteries. The severity of the lesions is related

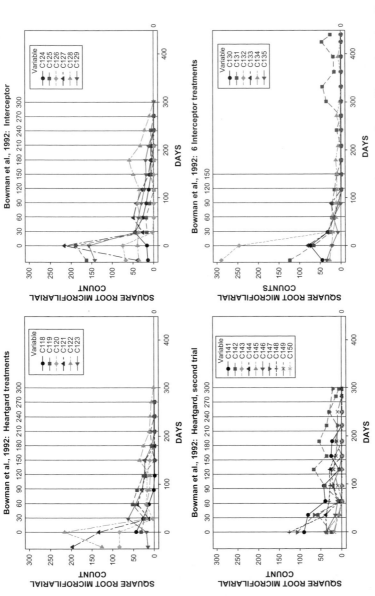

Fig. 5. Microfilarial counts in naturally infected dogs with patent infections treated with ivermectin (Heartgard) or milbemycin oxime (Interceptor) for extended periods. Counts were converted to square roots, and vertical lines on the graphs represent the days on which the dogs were treated. (*Top left*) Dogs treated with Heartgard experienced a precipitous drop in MF, but some dogs were still patent at 300 days post first treatment. (*Top right*) Dogs treated with Interceptor experienced a precipitous drop in MF, but four dogs were still positive at 270 days post first treatment. (*Bottom left*) Of the 10 dogs treated with Heartgard in the second trial, 2 dogs still had patent infections at 300 days. (*Bottom right*) After 6 monthly treatments of Interceptor, 2 dogs remained positive and 1 dog's MF counts appeared to be increasing in number after the termination of treatment. (*Data from* Bowman DD, Johnson RC, Ulrich ME, et al. Effects of long-term administration of ivermectin and milbemycin oxime on circulating microfilariae and parasite antigenemia in dogs with patent heartworm infections. In: Proceedings of the Heartworm Symposium '92. Austin (TX); 1992. p. 151–8.)

to the number of worms present (ranging from 1 to more than 250), amount of exercise, and the duration of infection. In most infections, the worms remain within the caudal pulmonary vascular tree, but they can on occasion migrate into the main pulmonary arteries, the right heart, and even into the great veins in heavy infections. When worms enter these atypical sites, the disease varies from the norm.

Many pathophysiological changes are associated with heartworm disease. The most marked and consistent anatomic pathologic change is a villous proliferation of the intima of the arteries containing worms. Other observed effects are vascular and pulmonary inflammation, pulmonary hypertension, disruption of vascular integrity, and fibrosis. Lesions in the pulmonary arteries appear soon after the arrival of the worms in the lungs. The first changes are endothelial damage and sloughing, villous proliferation, and the activation and attraction of leukocytes and platelets, which release factors that induce smooth muscle cell proliferation with collagen accumulation and fibrosis. The developing proliferative lesions may eventually encroach upon and occlude vascular lumina. Also, the induced endothelial swelling and altered intercellular junctions increase pulmonary vascular permeability. Fortunately, pulmonary infarction is uncommon because the gradual development of vascular occlusion allows extensive collateral circulation in the lung to compensate. For the same reason, obstruction of the pulmonary vessels by living worms is of little clinical significance unless there is a very high worm burden. On the other hand, worms that have died naturally or been killed by treatment induce thromboemboli, arterial obstruction, and vasoconstriction. These dead worms cause reactions by inciting thrombosis, granulomatous inflammation, and rugous villous inflammation. As the disease progresses, the pulmonary arteries become enlarged, thick-walled, and tortuous, with roughened endothelial surfaces.

In dogs with heartworm disease, the pulmonary arteries become varyingly thrombosed, thickened, dilated, tortuous, noncompliant, and functionally incompetent, with the vessels to the caudal lung lobes being the most affected. The damaged vessels cannot respond during increased oxygen demand and resulting diminished exercise capacity. The observed pulmonary vasoconstriction is partly secondary to excessive production of vasoactive substances by vascular endothelial cells.[61] Another contributing factor is hypoxia caused by ventilation-perfusion mismatching secondary to pulmonary thromboembolization, eosinophilic pneumonitis, or pulmonary consolidation. The end result of the prolonged vasoconstriction is pulmonary hypertension and compromised cardiac output.

The right heart's response to increased pulmonary pressure is initially an eccentric hypertrophy with chamber dilatation and wall thickening, Periods of increased cardiac output, such as during exercise, exacerbate the stress. In severe infections there may be decompensation (right heart failure). The response of the heart to modified hemodynamic stresses, geometric changes, and cardiac remodeling may contribute to secondary tricuspid insufficiency, thereby complicating or precipitating cardiac decompensation. Perivascular edema may develop due to the increased pulmonary vascular permeability. This fluid accumulation, along with an accompanying inflammatory infiltrate, may be evident radiographically as increased interstitial and even alveolar density. This presentation is seemingly of minimal clinical significance and should not be misinterpreted as an indication of left heart failure, that is, it is not cardiogenic pulmonary edema and furosemide is not indicated. The role of exercise in the development of pulmonary vascular disease and pulmonary hypertension is still not clear. Rawlings was unable to show an effect of 2.5 months of controlled treadmill exercise on pulmonary hypertension in heavily infected dogs,[62] whereas Dillon and colleagues[63] showed more severe pulmonary hypertension in lightly infected, mildly exercised dogs than in more heavily infected but unexercised dogs.

Generalized pulmonary parenchymal lesions sometimes can develop in heartworm infections. Eosinophilic pneumonitis is an inflammatory reaction to the immune-mediated clearance of antibody-coated microfilariae from the pulmonary microcirculation,[64] and it is therefore reported most commonly in naturally occurring occult heartworm disease (as opposed to iatrogenic occult infections induced by microfilaricidal treatment). Eosinophilic granulomatosis is an uncommon form of parenchymal lung disease associated with heartworm infection. This presentation is induced in a similar manner to eosinophilic pneumonitis, but in this case the trapped microfilariae are surrounded by neutrophils and eosinophils, eventually forming granulomas and associated bronchial lymphadenopathy.[65]

Focal pulmonary parenchymal lesions are more common than generalized disease, and are due to spontaneous or post-adulticidal pulmonary thromboemboli of dead or dying worms. Thromboembolization aggravates the development of pulmonary hypertension and right heart failure, and in rare instances may be the cause of a pulmonary infarction. Dead or moribund worms forced by the flow of blood down into the smaller vessels worsen vascular damage and enhance coagulation, which further restricts pulmonary blood flow and may even lead to consolidation of affected lung lobes. With acute and massive worm death, this insult may be profound, particularly if associated with exercise. The exacerbation of the disease that accompanies exercise likely reflects increased pulmonary arterial flow with escape of inflammatory mediators into the lung parenchyma through badly damaged and permeable arteries. It has been suggested that the lung injury induced by these disintegrating worms is similar to that seen in adult respiratory distress syndrome.

Glomerulonephritis caused by antigen-antibody complex deposition in the kidneys is common in heartworm-infected dogs. This condition results in a measurable proteinuria (albuminuria), and heartworm antigen can be detected in the urine of infected dogs. Progression to renal failure, however, is uncommon.

Heartworms may sometimes migrate to sites other than the pulmonary vasculature of the canine host. The signs associated with worms in atypical sites depend on the organ affected; worms have been described in muscles, brain, spinal cord, or anterior chamber of the eye. Worms have also been observed to migrate into the aortic bifurcation or more distally in the digital arteries.[66] Mature heartworms may sometimes move in a retrograde manner in the pulmonary arteries to the right heart and into the venae cavae, producing the life-threatening caval syndrome, described later.[67]

Clinical signs
Most dogs infected with heartworms show no signs. The clinical signs associated with chronic heartworm disease depend on the severity and duration of infection, and typically, reflect the effects of the parasite on the pulmonary arteries, lungs and, secondarily, the heart. The clinical history may elicit findings that weight loss, diminished exercise tolerance, lethargy, poor condition, cough, dyspnea, syncope, and abdominal distension. Physical examination of the affected animal may disclose evidence of weight loss, a split second heart sound (13%), right-sided heart murmur of tricuspid insufficiency (13%), and rarely cardiac gallop. In dogs with right heart failure, jugular venous distension and pulsation typically accompany hepatomegaly, splenomegaly, and ascites. It is atypical for a dog with chronic heartworm disease to have cardiac arrhythmias or conduction disturbances (<10%). Dogs with pulmonary parenchymal manifestations may have a cough and pulmonary crackles, and in the few dogs that develop eosinophilic granulomatosis there may be muffled lung sounds, dyspnea, and cyanosis. In a dog that has recently undergone massive heartworm-associated

pulmonary thromboembolization, fever and hemoptysis may be present; in such dogs the onset of signs is often associated with exercise.

Diagnosis

Microfilarial and antigen testing The presence of *D immitis* microfilariae in the blood or a positive antigen detection test can be used to confirm a clinical diagnosis of heartworm infection. Some enzyme-linked immunoassay (ELISA) antigen tests can quantitatively predict worm burdens, based on antigen concentrations. The semiquantitative ELISA (Snap Canine Heartworm PF) can predict antigen load and give some indication as to the number of worms present in an infection. The semiquantitative test is useful in predicting thromboembolic complications.[68]

Radiography Thoracic radiographs have been replaced by antigen tests as the routine verification method for heartworm infection. However, thoracic radiography offers an excellent method for determining disease severity and for assessing changes after treatment. In dogs with heartworms, radiographic abnormalities are present in approximately 85% of cases. Radiographic examination of 200 heartworm-infected dogs revealed that 70% had increased prominence of the main pulmonary artery segment, 60% had right ventricular enlargement, 50% had increased size and density of the pulmonary arteries, and 50% had pulmonary artery tortuosity and "pruning."[69] For dogs in right heart failure, additional changes might include enlargement of the caudal vena cava, liver, and spleen, pleural effusion, and ascites.

Different radiographic projections are superior for detailing different heartworm-associated changes. The ventrodorsal projection is preferable for cardiac silhouette evaluation and minimizing patient stress (**Fig. 6**A). The dorsoventral projection is superior for the evaluation of the caudal lobar pulmonary vessels, which are considered abnormal if larger than the diameter of the ninth rib where the rib and artery intersect. The lateral projection is best for the evaluation of the cranial pulmonary artery, which should normally not be larger than its accompanying vein or the proximal one-third of the fourth rib (**Fig. 6**B).

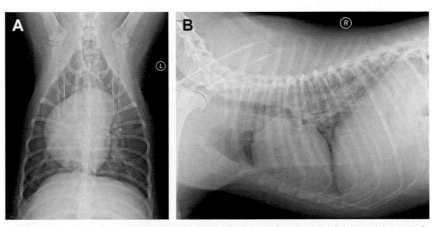

Fig. 6. Radiographs of a 3.5-year-old castrated male dog that had been adopted from a shelter in Georgia 10 months before presentation. (*A*) Ventrodorsal thoracic view showing the classic "reverse D" shape of the cardiac silhouette indicates right heart enlargement. The caudal lobar arteries are markedly enlarged and tortuous. (*B*) Lateral thoracic radiograph in which increased sternal contact is evident. The caudal lobar arteries are enlarged and tortuous in appearance. (*Courtesy of* Amie Knieper, Ithaca, NY.)

Damage to the pulmonary parenchyma is best evaluated radiographically. In pneumonitis, there is a mixed interstitial to alveolar density that typically is most severe in the caudal lung lobes. In eosinophilic granulomatosis, the inflammatory process appears as interstitial nodules associated with bronchial lymphadenopathy and, occasionally, pleural effusion. In pulmonary thromboembolism, there are coalescing interstitial and alveolar infiltrates, occurring particularly in the caudal lung lobes, reflecting the increased pulmonary vascular permeability and inflammation. With massive embolization or pulmonary infarction there may be the appearance of consolidation.

Echocardiography This method is insensitive as a diagnostic tool except in dogs with caval syndrome or heavy worm burdens, because heartworms are only rarely demonstrated in the right ventricle.[70] Two-dimensional echocardiography can sometimes demonstrate worms in the pulmonary artery. Echocardiography is a useful to assess right heart enlargement; with enlargement, the right ventricular end-diastolic dimension and septal and right ventricular free wall thickness will all be increased. It has been reported that 4 of 10 dogs with heartworm disease had abnormal (paradoxic) septal motion. In dogs with heartworm disease, the ratio of left to right ventricular internal dimension is often reduced from a normal value of 3 to 4 to a mean value of 0.7.

Electrocardiography Electrocardiography is useful in detecting arrhythmias, but a less useful method for detecting heartworm-induced chamber enlargement. Arrhythmias are rare in dogs with heartworm disease (2%–4%),[71] except in cases of caval syndrome and heart failure. A right ventricular enlargement pattern is supportive of heartworm disease.

Clinical pathology Hematological and serum chemical abnormalities are useful in providing a framework for evaluating concurrent disease in a dog that is going to undergo adulticide treatment. Dogs with heartworm disease may have a low-grade, nonregenerative anemia (10% of mildly to moderately affected dogs and up to 60% of severely affected dogs), neutrophilia (20%–80% of cases), eosinophilia ($\sim$85% of cases), and basophilia ($\sim$60% of cases).[45] Thrombocytopenia typically occurs 1 to 2 weeks after adulticidal therapy. In severe heartworm disease with heart failure, liver enzyme activities may be increased (10% of cases) and, occasionally, hyperbilirubinemia is noted. Azotemia is present in only about 5% of cases, and may be prerenal in origin if dehydration or heart failure is present, or may be secondary to glomerulonephritis. Albuminuria is present in 10% to 30% of cases, but if glomerular disease is severe, hypoalbuminemia may complicate the clinical picture.

Tracheobronchial cytology can be useful, particularly in the coughing dog with eosinophilic pneumonitis, occult heartworm disease, and cases with minimal supporting radiographic evidence; the examination is likely to reveal evidence of an eosinophilic infiltrate, and occasionally microfilariae. In cases of congestive heart failure, abdominal fluid analysis reveals a modified transudate. Dogs with right heart failure secondary to heartworm disease have a central venous pressure that range from 12 to more than 20 cm H_2O, but ascites can develop at lower pressures if hypoalbuminemia is present.

Microfilaricidal and Preventive Therapy in Heartworm-Positive Dogs

When considering adulticide treatment, a minimum clinical database usually consists of an antigen test, a microfilarial test, chemistry panel, complete blood count (CBC), urinalysis, thoracic radiographic evaluation and, if liver disease is suspected, a serum bile acid evaluation. At this time, monthly macrolide preventive is prescribed. This approach, currently recommended by the American Heartworm Society,[72] is to prevent further infection, reduce circulating microfilariae, and kill larval stages not yet susceptible to adulticide therapy. Dogs with circulating microfilariae should be kept under observation after the first macrolide dose so an adverse reaction might be recognized and promptly treated. Corticosteroids with or without antihistamines (dexamethasone at 0.25 mg/kg intravenously and diphenhydramine at 2 mg/kg intramuscularly, or 1 mg/kg of prednisolone orally 1 hour before and 6 hours after administration of the first dose of preventive) may be given to reduce the potential for adverse reaction in the highly microfilaremic patient. Adverse reactions are unusual with macrolides at preventive doses, but caution should be exercised. Some allow up to 2 to 3 months to lapse after the end of the heartworm transmission season to allow any larvae to mature to adults before commencing adulticide therapy, whereas if the diagnosis is made in the spring or late winter, when infective larvae have matured, adulticidal therapy may be immediately administered.

Adulticidal therapy

Melarsomine dihydrochloride In heartworm disease, the goal of therapy is usually to kill the worms to prevent additional damage to the pulmonary vasculature. The only drug approved currently for this purpose is the organoarsenic compound melarsomine dihydrochloride (Immiticide). With two doses (2.5 mg/kg intramuscularly every 24 hours for two treatments), the efficacy is greater than 96%. The efficacy increases to 99% efficacy with a repeat of the two-dose therapy in 4 months or with a split dosing regimen whereby a single dose is followed by a 2-dose regimen in 1 to 3 months. This product is much safer than the previously prescribed thiacetarsamide, but adverse reactions do occur.

Melarsomine kills the large adults that are carried deeper into the lungs by the vascular flow in the pulmonary arteries. Thromboembolic events are expected following successful adulticide therapy, and the severity of the sequelae can be decreased through strict exercise restriction after melarsomine administration. Cage rest is most easily assured and verified in the veterinary clinic. If financial constraints preclude hospitalization, the owner should be advised that this is an important part of the therapy, and it may be necessary to provide tranquilizers to keep the pet calm at home. The owner needs to be made to understand that failure to restrict the exercise of the pet can increase the opportunity for thromboembolic events that can prove fatal. Patients treated with the split-dosing regimen have a higher seroconversion rate to a negative antigen status than patients treated with the standard dosing regimen.[73] Also, the split-dose method kills only a portion of the worms following the initial intramuscular injection, which lessens the chance of thromboembolic complications. The first dose is then followed in 1 to 3 months with the two-dose regimen. The disadvantages of this method are the additional expense, an increased total arsenic dose, and the need for 2 months of exercise restriction. In 55 dogs with severe heartworm disease treated with the split-dosing method, 96% had a good to very good outcome, with more than 98% testing negative for circulating antigen 90 days post therapy.[74] Of these 55 dogs, 31% had "mild or moderate pulmonary thromboembolization," and there were no fatalities. After treatment, the most common signs were fever, cough, and anorexia that occurred 5 to 7 days later. Signs were associated with mild perivascular caudal lobar pulmonary radiographic densities that subsided spontaneously or after corticosteroid therapy.

Surgical removal of the worms Worms can be removed using flexible alligator forceps.[75] A description of this method in 36 dogs with mild and severe heartworm disease was found to be 90% effective; 2 of the 9 severely affected dogs died of heart and renal failure within 3 months of surgery. In skilled hands, the technique is apparently safe, and subsequent studies have demonstrated superior results as compared with melarsomine, producing less pulmonary thromboembolization and caval syndrome.[76] Dogs treated surgically still require melarsomine treatment to provide a complete cure. The advantages of surgical removal are the diminished potential of arsenic toxicity and fewer worms to cause thromboembolic disease. Of course, disadvantages include the need for general anesthesia and fluoroscopy, as well as the incomplete abrogation of all arsenical use.

Macrolides The macrolides are now known to have some adulticidal properties when administered at the dosages used for preventive therapy.[54] Ivermectin administered monthly at the preventive dose for 31 consecutive months was nearly 100% efficacious in clearing dogs of their heartworm infections.[52] Selamectin, when administered for 18 months at the preventive dose, killed approximately 40% of transplanted worms.[55] Milbemycin and sustained-release moxidectin also seem to have minimal adulticidal efficacy when administered at the preventive dose.[54,55] For different reasons, including the length of treatment required, the lack of control over the thromboembolic events that will occur in the patient, and the potential for induction of resistance as discussed earlier, the current recommendation is that macrolides not be adopted for adulticide therapy.

Post-Adulticide Antigen Testing
Antigen detection is now used to assess the efficacy of adulticide therapy. Circulating antigen will typically become undetectable 8 to 12 weeks after successful therapy; thus, a positive test 12 weeks after completed adulticide therapy suggests a persistent infection.[49] There are cases, however, when the antigen tests may remain positive for longer periods, and one should probably not assume a failure of adulticidal therapy unless antigen is detected ≥ 6 months after therapy has concluded.

Supplemental Therapy
There are several classes of supplemental or ancillary therapy used concurrently with melarsomine therapy; the most common are corticosteroids, aspirin, heparin, and doxycycline. These therapies all have proponents and detractors, and the perceived value of each waxes and wanes every few years. However, it is likely that they all can have value in the hands of certain practitioners in certain cases.

Corticosteroids The agent most often advocated for use in heartworm disease is prednisone, which reduces pulmonary arteritis but worsens the proliferative vascular lesions, diminishes pulmonary arterial flow, and reduces adulticide efficacy. Thus, corticosteroids are indicated only when there are adverse reactions to microfilaricides, pulmonary parenchymal complications, and perhaps to minimize tissue reaction to melarsomine. For allergic pneumonitis, prednisone (1 mg/kg/day) administered for 3 to 5 days and discontinued or tapered as indicated, generally has a favorable outcome.[45] Prednisone at 1 to 2 mg/kg per day with cage rest has been advocated for use in the management of pulmonary thromboembolization, with the treatments being continued until radiographic and clinical improvement are noted.[45] The associated steroid-induced fluid retention is the reason that such therapy should be used with caution when the patient is in borderline heart failure.

Aspirin Antithrombotic agents have been examined numerous times relative to heartworm disease. However, the more recent work has indicated that there are no significant differences in severity of pulmonary vascular lesions between aspirin-treated and control dogs. Thus, the American Heartworm Society no longer endorses aspirin therapy for routine treatment of heartworm disease.[72]

Heparin Heparin therapy has not been studied with respect to melarsomine adulticidal therapy. Low-dose calcium heparin was shown to reduce the adverse reactions associated with thiacetarsemide in dogs with severe clinical signs, including heart failure.[77]

Doxycycline With the realization that *Wolbachia* may contribute to the pathogenesis associated with heartworm infection, efforts to clear *Wolbachia* have been examined in several studies.[60,78] Using surgically transplanted worms, it was shown that a combination of weekly ivermectin (weekly at the monthly preventive dose) and daily doxycycline (10 mg/kg/day) eliminated microfilariae, reduced pulmonary thromboembolization after melarsomine therapy, and reduced heartworm burden compared with control dogs by 78% after 9 months of therapy.[59]

Post-adulticide microfilaricidal therapy
Microfilaricidal therapy has traditionally been instituted 3 to 6 weeks after adulticide administration.[45] Microfilariae are rapidly cleared with ivermectin at 50 μg/kg or milbemycin at 500 μg/kg. Using ivermectin at the 50 μg/kg dose caused adverse reactions (shock, depression, hypothermia, and vomiting) in 8 of 126 dogs receiving ivermectin 3 weeks after adulticide therapy. All dogs recovered within 12 hours after treatment with fluids and corticosteroids; however, one of the 8 dogs died 4 days later. Dogs treated with milbemycin at 500 μg/kg or the elevated ivermectin dose (50 μg/kg) should be hospitalized and observed on the day of treatment. Small dogs (<16 kg) with high microfilarial counts (>10,000/mL) are more apt to suffer adverse reactions.[79] Diphenhydramine (2 mg/kg intramuscularly) and dexamethasone (0.25 mg/kg intravenously) are often administered prophylactically to prevent adverse reactions to microfilaricidal doses of macrolides. Dogs typically are now treated by simply beginning them on a monthly preventive at the time of, or 3 to 6 weeks after the completion of the adulticide therapy.

Complications and specific syndromes
Treating the dog that has no signs from its heartworm infection The typical dog treated for heartworms is an antigen or microfilarial-positive dog with no clinical signs. The dog may have no signs even though it has demonstrable radiographic lesions. Recommended treatment is the split-dose (3) melarsomine regimen. Dogs without signs may develop clinical signs after adulticide therapy due to the induced pulmonary thromboembolization and lung injury following worm kill. The risk of post-adulticide signs can be predicted to some extent using an antigen test to derive a semiquantitative estimate of worm burden and radiographs to assess the existing lung damage.[68] A dog with severe radiographic lesions is not likely to tolerate the treatment as well as one that does not, but radiographic signs do not necessarily correlate directly to worm burden.

Glomerulonephritis Chronic heartworm infection may be associated with glomerulonephritis, which can be severe. The glomerular lesions caused by heartworms are unlikely to produce renal failure, but heartworm infection in a dog with proteinuria and azotemia presents the clinician with a therapeutic dilemma. The worms need to be removed because they contribute to the disease, but doing so carries risks. One approach is to hospitalize the patient and administer intravenous fluids (lactated Ringer solution at 2 to 3 mL/kg/h) for 48 hours (beginning 12 hours before the first melarsomine dose). It is then recommended that the patient return after 48 hours for a blood urea nitrogen and creatinine determination. The second portion of the split-dose treatment is then scheduled for 1 to 3 months later depending on renal function and the response of the patient to the first adulticide administration.

Eosinophilic pneumonitis Eosinophilic pneumonitis affects some 14% of dogs with heartworm disease within the early stages of infection.[45,64] Signs may include cough, dyspnea, weight loss, and exercise intolerance. Radiographs show typical changes associated with heartworm disease with an interstitial infiltrate that is usually worse in the caudal lung lobes. The administration of corticosteroids often results in the rapid attenuation of clinical signs, with radiographic clearing in less than a week. If the signs are ameliorated by the treatment, adulticidal therapy can be started.

Eosinophilic granulomatosis Eosinophilic granulomatosis is a rare presentation in heartworm disease that does not respond as well to treatment as eosinophilic pneumonitis, is characterized by a more organized, nodular inflammatory process associated with bronchial lymphadenopathy, and sometimes accompanying pleural effusion. Cough, wheezes, and pulmonary crackles are often audible; treatment consists of increased levels of prednisone relative to those for eosinophilic pneumonitis, it may take up to 2 weeks for signs to clear, and ultimately, the surgical excision of lobar lesions may be required to control the disease.

Congestive heart failure Right heart failure is caused by increased right ventricular afterload (secondary to chronic pulmonary arterial disease and thromboemboli with resultant pulmonary hypertension). Severe and chronic pulmonary hypertension is often complicated by right heart failure and secondary tricuspid regurgitation. Up to 50% of dogs with severe heartworm-associated pulmonary vascular complications will develop heart failure.[45] Clinical signs may include weight loss, exercise intolerance, ashen mucous membranes with prolonged capillary refill time, ascites, dyspnea, jugular venous distension and pulsation, arrhythmias with pulse deficits, and adventitial lung sounds (crackles and possibly wheezes).

Treatment aims at the reduction of signs of congestion, reducing pulmonary hypertension, and increasing cardiac output. This therapy involves dietary, pharmacologic, and procedural interventions. If congestive heart failure is present before adulticidal therapy, the question arises as to whether melarsomine should be administered. If clinical response to heart failure management is good, adulticidal therapy may be offered in 4 to 12 weeks, as conditions allow, but the adulticide is generally avoided if the heart failure remains refractory to treatment.

Caval syndrome Caval syndrome is an uncommon but severe complication of heartworm disease, characterized by a heavy worm burden (usually >60 worms) and a poor prognosis. Most cases occur in male dogs (75% to 90%). Caval syndrome is due to the retrograde migration of adult heartworms from the pulmonary arteries into the venae cavae and right atrium, which produces partial inflow obstruction to the right heart and, by interfering with the valve apparatus, producing tricuspid insufficiency (with resultant systolic murmur, jugular pulse, and increase in central venous pressure). These dogs have preexisting heartworm-induced pulmonary hypertension, as well as existing or developing cardiac arrhythmias that further compromise cardiac function.

Clinical signs include a sudden onset of anorexia, depression, and weakness, which may occasionally also present with coughing, dyspnea, hemolytic anemia, hemoglobinemia, hemoglobinuria, and hepatic or renal dysfunction. Hemoglobinuria is considered pathognomonic. Hemoglobinemia and microfilaremia have been reported in 85% of dogs suffering from caval syndrome. Physical examination reveals pale mucous membranes, prolonged capillary refill time, weak pulses, jugular distension and pulsation, hepatosplenomegaly, and dyspnea. Thoracic auscultation may disclose a systolic heart murmur of tricuspid insufficiency (87% of cases); loud, split S2 (67%); and cardiac gallop (20%). Other reported signs are ascites (29%), jaundice (19%), and hemoptysis (6%). The body temperature may be subnormal to mildly elevated. Thoracic radiography will reveal signs typical of severe heartworm disease. Sonography reveals heartworm echo shadows.

The hemolytic anemia is caused by the lysis of to red blood cells (RBCs) passing through the sieve of heartworms now in the right atrium and venae cavae. The intravascular hemolysis, along with the induced metabolic acidosis and diminished hepatic function, contributes to an impaired removal of circulating procoagulants. This situation leads to disseminated intravascular coagulation (DIC) with the RBCs being lysed as they are forced past fibrin strands in capillaries, causing further DIC development. The reason for the hepatorenal dysfunction is not clear, but it is likely due to the effects of passive congestion, diminished perfusion, and effects of hemolysis byproducts. Without treatment, death often occurs within 24 to 72 hours.

Hematology and clinical chemistries reveal numerous abnormalities. Hematology will typically show moderate regenerative anemia. The normochromic, macrocytic anemia is associated with the presence of target cells, schistocytes, spur cells, and spherocytes. Leukocytosis with neutrophilia, eosinophilia, and left shift has been described. Dogs with DIC will have thrombocytopenia and hypofibrinogenemia, as well as a prolonged one-stage prothrombin time (PT), partial thromboplastin time (PTT), activated coagulation time (ACT), and high fibrin degradation product concentrations. Serum chemistry analysis typically reveals increases in liver enzymes, bilirubin, and indices of renal function.

Urine analysis reveals high bilirubin and protein concentrations in 50% of cases and more frequently, hemoglobinuria. Central venous pressure is high in some 80% to 90% of cases (mean, 11.4 cm H_2O). Electrocardiographic abnormalities include sinus tachycardia (33% of cases) and atrial and ventricular premature complexes (28% and 6%, respectively). Worms within the right atrium with movement into the right ventricle during diastole are evident echocardiographically; this finding is nearly pathognomonic for caval syndrome when observed with the associated signs. The right ventricular lumen will be enlarged and the left diminished in size; this is probably caused by pulmonary hypertension accompanied by reduced left ventricular preload. Paradoxic septal motion, caused by high right ventricular pressure, is commonly observed.

If the offending heartworms are not removed from the right atrium and venae cavae the prognosis is poor, and even with removal, mortality may occur in almost half of the cases. Fluid therapy is required to improve cardiac output and tissue perfusion, for treating DIC, to prevent hemoglobin nephropathy, and to aid in the correction of metabolic acidosis; however, excessive fluid therapy may precipitate or worsen signs of congestive heart failure. Broad-spectrum antibiotics and aspirin should be administered.

The surgical removal technique for heartworm in dogs with caval syndrome was developed by Jackson and colleagues.[80] This procedure should be undertaken as early as is practical. Sedation is often unnecessary, and the procedure can be accomplished with only local anesthesia. The dog is restrained in left lateral recumbency, the jugular vein is isolated distally and ligated proximally (craniad), and alligator forceps (20 to 40 cm long, preferably of small diameter) are guided gently down the vein past the thoracic inlet Fluoroscopic guidance, when available, can be helpful. A good working goal is the removal of 35 to 50 worms or several consecutive unsuccessful passes, once the worm burden has been reduced. After worm removal has been completed, the jugular vein is ligated distally and the skin incision closed with sutures. Successful worm retrieval is associated with an almost immediate reduction in the intensity of the cardiac murmur and jugular pulsations, rapid clearing of hemoglobinemia and hemoglobinuria, and normalization of serum enzymatic aberrations. Cardiac function should improve immediately with latent improvement during the next 24 hours. The removal of worms does not reduce right ventricular afterload (pulmonary hypertension), and therefore, fluid therapy must be monitored carefully before and after surgery to avoid precipitation or worsening of right heart failure. Cage rest must be enforced for as long as it is deemed necessary. The anemia is likely not to resolve until 2 to 4 weeks after worm removal.

Once the animal has recovered from its crisis, arrangements can be made for the split-dose adulticide therapy to remove whatever worms remain after a month or more. Macrolide preventive therapy is administered just before release from the hospital. Before initiating adulticide therapy, it is important to assess liver and renal function. Often in these cases, aspirin therapy is continued for 3 to 4 weeks after adulticide therapy.

Aberrant migration Young adult worms occasionally appear in locations other than the pulmonary arteries. Worms have been found in the brain, spinal cord, epidural space, anterior chamber of the eye, the vitreous, the subcutis, the peritoneal cavity, and the iliac and femoral arteries. Treatment of heartworms in ectopic locations ranges from no treatment (eg, peritoneal cavity), to surgical excision, adulticidal therapy, or symptomatic treatment (eg, seizure control in the case of brain migration). A method for surgical removal of the worms from the internal iliac and femoral arteries has been described.[66]

Prognosis

When not accompanied by clinical signs, the prognosis for heartworm infection is generally good. The prognosis for severe heartworm disease must be guarded, but most cases can be successfully managed. After the initial crisis and adulticidal therapy, resolution of underlying manifestations of chronic heartworm disease begins, and amazingly many of the changes including the intimal proliferation are partially reversible.[81] The prognosis is poorest when initial presentation is associated with severe DIC, caval syndrome, massive embolization, eosinophilic granulomatosis, severe pulmonary arterial disease, and heart failure. Radiographic and arteriographic lesions usually begin to resolve within 3 to 4 weeks of adulticide therapy, and pulmonary hypertension is reduced within months. Pulmonary parenchymal changes are worsened during the 6 months after adulticidal therapy, but begin to improve and often resolve in the next 2 to 3 months. Persistence of parenchymal lesions suggests that the adulticide therapy may not have been fully successful. Also, signs of heart failure should disappear with the aid of symptomatic therapy, cage rest, and successful removal of all worms.

Treating the Feline Host

The cat can develop disease associated with *D immitis* infection, but infections with mature worms only occur at 5% to 20% of the prevalence that would occur in an unprotected dog population in the same environment.[82] It is more difficult to infect a cat than a dog, and less than 25% of administered third-stage larvae develop to adulthood in cats. Naturally infected cats typically have less than 10 worms and usually only 1 to 4 worms. Cats tend not to support patent infections, thus there is a high percentage of infected cats that have no microfilaremia or very low microfilarial counts. Adult worms also do not live as long in the cat, although a few survive for up to 4 years.[37,83] Heartworm infection has been found in up to 14% of shelter cats.[82] In well-cared-for cats in Texas and North Carolina, heartworm disease with adult worms was diagnosed in 9 of 100 cats with cardiorespiratory signs.[84] Of the 100 Texas and North Carolina cats, 26% had antibodies to *D immitis*, suggesting that they had been host to third-stage larvae that did not fully mature.[84] Aberrant worm migration seems to be a greater problem, or a problem with more severe sequelae, in cats than in dogs.

Pathophysiology

It seems that in cats, more so than in dogs, the immature adult heartworms that enter the lungs cause disease even if they do not mature to adult worms or result in patent infections. This finding has been demonstrated radiographically in experimentally infected cats,[85] and pulmonary vascular lesions have been observed in naturally infected cats with no adult worms.[86] Moreover, pharmacologically abbreviated infections in cats (the worms being killed before becoming adults) has revealed that these infections produce not only proliferative and inflammatory lesions in the pulmonary arteries, but in the bronchioles and lung parenchyma as well. This disease, in which there are respiratory signs due to heartworms but no adult worms, has been termed "heartworm-associated respiratory disease" (HARD) or "pulmonary larval dirofilariasis."[36] Thus, in the cat, pulmonary larval dirofilariasis will produce asthma-like clinical signs even though the worms never fully mature. It is now recognized that 38% to 74% of cats with mature *D immitis* develop clinical signs, as do an estimated 50% of those that never develop mature infections.[36,83]

The worms entering the lungs of cats are around 2 to 3 cm long. The size of the worms relative to the lungs of the cat (versus the dog) along with the presence in cats of pulmonary intravascular macrophages may be reasons why pulmonary inflammation is worse in cats than in dogs.[87] When adult worms were transplanted into heartworm-naïve cats, the significant pulmonary enlargement 1 week after the transplant suggested an intense host-parasite interaction.[88] Cats also exhibit a severe myointimal and eosinophilic response to helminth infections, including to *D immitis*, which produces pulmonary vascular narrowing and tortuosity, thrombosis, and possibly pulmonary hypertension.[89] The feline pulmonary arterial tree is smaller than that of the dog and has less collateral circulation; therefore embolization, even with small numbers of smaller worms, produces disastrous results that can be associated with infarction and even death. Although rare, cor pulmonale and right heart failure can be associated with chronic feline heartworm disease, and the latter is manifested by pleural effusion (hydrothorax or chylothorax), ascites, or both. The lung of the heartworm-infected cat will develop eosinophilic infiltrates in the parenchyma (pneumonitis) and pulmonary arteries. Also, pulmonary vessels may leak plasma, producing pulmonary edema (possibly acute respiratory distress syndrome) and type II cell proliferation, both potentially altering O_2 diffusion.[88] Radiographic findings in cats suggest air trapping, compatible with bronchoconstriction. Overall, cats that have been infected with heartworms can develop multifaceted disease that can vary from virtually no signs to diminished pulmonary function, hypoxemia, dyspnea, cough, and even death.

Clinical signs

Clinical manifestations of heartworm disease in cats can be peracute, acute, or chronic.[84,88,90] Signs in acute or peracute presentations that probably represent cases of worm death, embolization, or aberrant migration variably include: salivation, tachycardia, shock, dyspnea, hemoptysis, vomiting and diarrhea, syncope, dementia, ataxia, circling, head tilt, blindness, seizures, and death. In these acute cases, post-mortem examination often will reveal pulmonary infarction with congestion and edema. Except in the acute or peracute cases, the physical examination of cats with heartworm infection or disease is often unrewarding, although a murmur, gallop, or diminished or adventitial lung sounds (or a combination of these findings) may be noted. In addition, cats may be thin, dyspneic, or both. If heart failure is present, jugular venous distension, dyspnea and, rarely, ascites are detected. In a retrospective study, 28% of cats with mature heartworms seen at a referral center were presented by the owners for signs not referable to the *D immitis* infection.[90] The reported historical findings in cats with chronic heartworm disease include: anorexia, weight loss, lethargy, exercise intolerance, cough, dyspnea, vomiting, and on rare occasions signs of right heart failure. Dyspnea and cough are consistent findings and, when present, should raise suspicion of heartworm disease, especially in endemic areas.[90] Chylothorax, pneumothorax, and caval syndrome have been recognized as rare manifestations of feline heartworm disease.

Diagnosis

Heartworm infection in cats poses a diagnostic problem. Clinical signs are often absent, and if present, are different from those of the dog. The overall prevalence of heartworm in cats is low, so suspicion is lessened. The immunologic tests are often falsely negative in the cat, and microfilariae are usually not present. Electrocardiographic findings are minimal, and radiographic signs are inconsistent and transient.

Microfilarial and antigen testing Because most cats infected with heartworms do not have patent infections, microfilarial testing is not useful. Antigen-positive cats nearly always have more than one mature *D immitis* female, and antibody-positive/antigen-negative cats are not usually be infected with an adult female *D immitis*. However approximately 50% of antibody-positive/antigen-negative cats develop HARD/pulmonary larval dirofilariasis.

Antigen tests are imperfect in cats because of low worm burdens and the fact that only female worms produce detectable antigen.[91] Even in cats that develop detectable numbers of worms, disease can develop before the worms are mature enough to produce antigen.[92]

Screening for antibodies allows a suspicion of pulmonary larval dirofilariasis to be given additional weight, and allows clinicians to alert pet owners of the potential need for further diagnostics. Out of 1962 cats positive for antibodies to heartworms, only 18.6% were antigen positive. About half the cats that are antibody-positive and antigen-negative have postmortem manifestations of heartworm disease. Also, the antibody-positive status of infected cats that clear infection does wane with time.

Radiography Cats without clinical signs rarely have lesions that appear on thoracic radiographs.[83] The most sensitive radiographic criterion (left caudal pulmonary artery greater than 1.6 times the ninth rib at the ninth intercostal space on the ventrodorsal projection) is detected in only about half the cases.[85] Also, the lesions in cats are not specific and are often transient; cats develop lesions when the worms first reach the lungs and these changes can be seen on necropsy even if the worms fail to fully mature.[93] Radiographic findings, when present, include enlarged caudal pulmonary arteries, often with ill-defined margins, pulmonary parenchymal changes that include focal or diffuse infiltrates (interstitial, bronchointerstitial, or even alveolar), perivascular density and, occasionally, atelectasis.

Echocardiography Echocardiography is much more sensitive in cats than in dogs.[84] A double-lined echodensity typically is evident in the main pulmonary artery, one of its branches, the right ventricle, or occasionally at the right atrioventricular junction. Heartworms are found by echocardiography in about three-fourths of cats that have worms in their pulmonary arteries or right ventricle.[84]

Prevention and treatment
There is no reason to screen cats for heartworm infection before beginning them on prophylaxis because there are no microfilariae to speak of, so no risk of a reaction to dying microfilariae. Also, the heartworm preventives have been examined as part of the safety package submitted to the FDA to show that they are not adulticidal. Thus cats, unlike dogs, can be started on a preventive program without prior testing.

Whether preventives should be recommended for cats is a common question by owners and practitioners alike. In the southeastern United States, somewhere between 2.5% to 14% of shelter cats have heartworms at necropsy.[82] A nationwide antibody survey of more than 2000 largely asymptomatic cats revealed that nearly 12% of the cats had been host to third- or later-stage larvae;[46] it has been suggested that the real number is as high as 16%,[46] but other estimates have been lower (1%–8%).[47,94] If one uses a 12% antibody-positive rate as the national prevalence, and assume that 1% to 2% of cats will have mature heartworms in their pulmonary arteries and 5% to 6% of cats will develop signs after exposure consistent with HARD, then a nationwide feline morbidity might be expected to approach 6% to 8%. Also, based on owners' information, nearly one-third of cats diagnosed with heartworm disease at North Carolina State University were housed solely indoors.[90] The consequences of feline heartworm disease can be dire, and there are no standard therapeutic solutions. Therefore, having cats on a heartworm preventive regimen seems the prudent course.

Treatment in cats is currently problematic. Data on efficacy and safety of melarsomine against transplanted *D immitis* in cats are limited and contradictory.[92,95] In addition, the anecdotal clinical experience with melarsomine in naturally infected cats has been generally unfavorable, with an unacceptable mortality. Because of the inherent risk and lack of clear benefit, arsenical treatment is currently not recommended in cats.

Surgical removal of heartworms has been successful and is attractive because it minimizes the risk of thromboembolization.[96,97] The mortality seen in the only published case series was, unfortunately, unacceptable (two of five cats). Overall, the surgical approach still seems impractical for most cases.

Cats that are found to be infected with heartworms or that have heartworm disease should be placed on a monthly preventive and a short-term corticosteroid therapy (prednisone at 1 to 2 mg/kg from every 48 hours, up to two to three times a day) used to manage respiratory signs. If signs resolve initially but then recur, alternate-day steroid therapy (at the lowest dose that controls signs) can be continued indefinitely. Aspirin can be administered to cats with heartworm infections, but should not be prescribed with concurrent corticosteroid therapy.

Prognosis
The verdict is not yet in on heartworm disease in cats. More cats are getting infected than was previously considered; but the majority apparently goes through a period of disease, followed by self cure. However, some cats die unexpectedly and suddenly with heartworm-associated lesions. In cats with heartworm infections without clinical signs in Italy, of 43 infected cats 80% self-cured within 18

to 49 months (23 cats self-cured but had signs, 11 self-cured and never had signs).[36,83] Also, 3 cats died suddenly between 38 and 40 months after diagnosis, and at necropsy, were found to have two to three worms and severe thromboembolic processes.[82] Combining this and another Italian study, of 77 cats without signs seen in general practices in Italy only 58% eventually developed clinical heartworm disease, but of these cats one-third died of heartworm-related sequelae.[36,83] There is still no good and safe treatment for cats, and surgical removal is still in its infancy and may not be developed to any great extent if the outcome does not markedly improve in the cats so treated.

CONTROL RELATIVE TO ERADICATION OR DISEASE SUPPRESSION
Treatment

There are several excellent products to protect the well cared-for pet, but these methods are not suitable or easily applicable to mass treatment or long-term control in wildlife or dogs that are not under an owner's supervision.

Environmental

Mosquito control can have major effects on the transmission of mosquito-borne diseases, and has been shown numerous times with respect to the control of various human diseases such as Yellow fever, Dengue fever, and malaria. Mosquito control and abatement can and does have significant impact on these diseases in the United States and around the world. Dogs have very likely benefited greatly from the control of the mosquitoes that serve as vectors of disease and as major human pests in the United States. Fortunately for dogs, many of the most significant vectors of D immitis are also vectors of human disease. At the same time, due to the source of funding of the mosquito control programs, the targets of mosquito abatement programs are focused mainly on those species known to be important in human disease and comfort, and these might not be the same species affecting dogs. Thus, it is imperative that work be undertaken by different groups to maintain a dialog between the veterinary community and the mosquito control agencies to minimize the impacts of mosquito populations in any given area.

Wildlife

In the United States, the presence of the coyote makes heartworm eradication a difficult proposition. Coyotes are excellent and omnipresent reservoirs of the infection in rural, suburban, and now even urban parts of the country. Also, the existence of a wildlife reservoir raises the risk for heartworm infection of dogs, even if most dogs in a local area are protected and the local prevalence in well cared-for pets is low.

SUMMARY

Heartworm continues to be a parasite that threatens the canine population of the United States. D immitis causes significant morbidity and mortality in dogs, and is now found throughout the United States and in Canada along the United States border. The disease is transmitted by mosquitoes, including rural treehole mosquitoes like Aedes sierrensis and the urban Aedes aegypti and Aedes albopictus. The coyote is a known reservoir of infection and perpetuates heartworms even if all dogs in endemic areas are on preventive therapy. Excellent products to prevent heartworm infections in pets are available, and veterinarians need to be good stewards of their use. Because all the molecules used in the preventive products are from the same class of anthelmintic, veterinarians need to remain vigilant in monitoring heartworm infections in dogs to verify that the emergence of worm populations that are refractory to the preventives does not occur, and if such infections do arise, an active approach needs to be taken to prevent their spread. Dogs that are receiving preventive treatments should be monitored annually to verify that the products are efficacious and that dogs receiving them are being protected. If infected dogs are found, they should be treated with an adulticide, then placed on a monthly preventive. Information on heartworm disease, its prevention and treatment in dogs and cats, new information on the disease, and news and updates can be found by contacting or visiting the websites of the American Heartworm Society (www.heartwormsociety.org) and the Companion Animal Parasite Council (www.capcvet.org).

ACKNOWLEDGMENTS

The authors thank Dr Alice Lee, Department of Microbiology and Immunology, College of Veterinary Medicine, Cornell University, for her careful reading of the manuscript.

REFERENCES

1. Anderson RC. Nematode parasites of vertebrates. Their development and transmission. 2nd edition. Wallingford, Oxon UK: CABI Publishing; 2000. p. 650.
2. Smythe AB, Sanderson MJ, Nadler SA. Nematode small subunit phylogeny correlates with alignment parameters. Syst Biol 2006;55(6):972–92.
3. Osborne TC. Worms found in the heart and blood vessels of a dog; symptoms of hydrophobia. West J Med Surg 1847;8:491–2.
4. Leidy JA. A synopsis of entozoa and some of their ecto-congeners observed by the author. Proc Acad Nat Sci Philadelphia 1856;8:42–58.
5. Trotti GC, Pampiglione S, Rivasi F. The species of the genus *Dirofilaria* Railliet & Henry, 1911. Parassitologia 1997;39(4):369–74.
6. McCall JW, Genchi C, Kramer LH, et al. Heartworm disease in animals and humans. Adv Parasitol 2007;66:193–285.
7. Anderson RC. Filarioid nematodes. In: Samuel WM, Pybus MJ, Kocan AA, editors. Parasitic diseases of wild mammals. 2nd edition. Ames (IA): State University Press; 2001. p. 342–56.
8. Magi M, Calderini P, Gabrielli S, et al. *Vulpes vulpes*: a possible wild reservoir for zoonotic filariae. Vector Borne Zoonotic Dis 2008;8(2):249–52.
9. Lok JB. *Dirofilaria* sp.: taxonomy and distribution. In: Boreham PFL, Atwell RB, editors. Dirofilariasis. London: CRC Press; 1988. p. 1–28.
10. Abraham D. Biology of *Dirofilaria immitis*. In: Boreham PFL, Atwell RB, editors. Dirofilariasis. London: CRC Press; 1988. p. 29–46.
11. Bell LM, Alpert G, Gorton-Slight P. Skin colonization of hospitalized and nonhospitalized infants with lipophilic yeast. In: Programs and abstracts of the 25th Interscience Conference of Antimicrobial Agents and Chemotherapy. Minneapolis (MN); 1985. p. 186–8.
12. McLaren DJ, Worms MJ, Laurence BR, et al. Micro-organisms in filarial larvae (Nematoda). Trans R Soc Trop Med Hyg 1975;69(5/6):509–14.
13. Sironi M, Bandi C, Sacchi L, et al. Molecular evidence for a close relative of the arthropod endosymbiont *Wolbachia* in a filarial worm. Mol Biochem Parasitol 1995;74(2):223–7.
14. Bandi C, McCall JW, Genchi C, et al. Effects of tetracycline on the filarial worms *Brugia pahangi* and *Dirofilaria immitis* and their bacterial endosymbionts *Wolbachia*. Int J Parasitol 1999;29(2):357–64.

15. Wilcox HS. Pulmonary arteriotomy for removal of *Dirofilaria immitis* in the dog. J Am Vet Med Assoc 1960;136(7):328–38.
16. Lok JB, Harpaz T, Knight DH. Abnormal patterns of embryogenesis in *Dirofilaria immitis* treated with ivermectin. J Helminthol 1988;62(3):175–80.
17. Apiwathnasorn C, Samung Y, Prummongkol S, et al. Bionomics studies of *Mansonia* mosquitoes inhabiting the peat swamp forest. Southeast Asian J Trop Med Public Health 2006;37(2):272–8.
18. Christensen BM. Laboratory studies on the development and transmission of *Dirofilaria immitis* by *Aedes trivittatus*. Mosq News 1977;37(3):36772.
19. Zytoon EM, El-Belbasi HI, Konishi E, et al. Susceptibility of *Aedes albopictus* mosquitoes (Oahu strain) to infection with *Dirofilaria immitis*. Kobe J Med Sci 1992;38(5):289–305.
20. Slocombe JOD, Surgeoner GA, Srivastava B. Determination of the heartworm transmission period and its use in diagnosis and control. Proceedings of the Heartworm Symposium. Charleston (SC); 1989. p. 19–26.
21. Lok JB, Knight DH. Laboratory verification of a seasonal heartworm transmission model. In: Recent advances in heartworm disease. Tampa (FL); 1998. p. 15–20.
22. Lichtenfels JR, Pilitt PA, Kotani T, et al. Morphogenesis of developmental stages of *Dirofilaria immitis* (Nematoda) in the dog. Proc Helm Soc Wash 1985;52(1):98–113.
23. Knight DH, Lok JB. Seasonality of heartworm infection and implications for chemoprophylaxis. Clin Tech Small Anim Pract 1998;13(2):77–82.
24. Knight DH, Lok J B. Seasonal timing of heartworm chemoprophylaxis in the United States. In: Proceedings of the Heartworm Symposium '95. Auburn (AL); 1995. p. 37–42.
25. McTier TL, McCall JW, Dzimianski MT, et al. Epidemiology of heartworm infection in beagles naturally exposed to infection in three southeastern states. In: Proceedings of the Heartworm Symposium '92. Austin, Texas; 1992. p. 47–57.
26. Watts KJ, Reddy GR, Holmes RA, et al. Seasonal prevalence of third-stage larvae of *Dirofilaria immitis* in mosquitoes from Florida and Louisiana. J Parasitol 2001;87(2):322–9.
27. Sacks BN, Woodward DL, Colwell AE. A long-term study of non-native-heartworm transmission among coyotes in a Mediterranean ecosystem. Oikos 2003;102(3):478–90.
28. Ernst J, Slocombe JOD. The effect of low temperature on developing *Dirofilaria immitis* larvae in Aedes triseriatus. In: Proceedings of the Heartworm Symposium '83. Orlando (FL); 1983. p. 1–4.
29. Price DL. Microfilariae other than those of *Dirofilaria immitis* in dogs in Florida. In: Proceedings of the Heartworm Symposium '83. Orlando (FL); 1983. p. 8–14.
30. Hulden L, Hulden L, Heliovaara K. Endemic malaria: an 'indoor' disease in northern Europe. Historical data analysed. Malar J 2005;4:19.
31. Slocombe JOD, Srivastava B, Surgeoner GA The transmission period for heartworm in Canada. In: Proceedings of the Heartworm Symposium '95. Auburn (AL); 1995. p. 43–8.
32. Kotani T, Powers KG. Developmental stages of *Dirofilaria immitis* in the dog. Am J Vet Res 1982;43(12):2199–206.
33. Kume S, Itagaki S. On the life-cycle of *Dirofilaria immitis* in the dog as the final host. Br Vet J 1955;111:16–24.
34. Orihel TC. Morphology of the larval stages of *Dirofilaria immitis* in the dog. J Parasitol 1961;47(2):251–62.

35. Hayasaki M. Re-migration of fifth-stage juvenile *Dirofilaria immitis* into pulmonary arteries after subcutaneous transplantation in dogs, cats, and rabbits. J Parasitol 1996;82(5):835–7.
36. Venco L, Genchi C, Grandi G, et al. Clinical evolution and radiographic findings of feline heartworm infection in asymptomatic cats. Vet Parasitol 2008;158:232–7.
37. Genchi C, Venco L, Ferrari N, et al. Feline heartworm infection: a statistical elaboration of the duration of the infection and life expectancy in asymptomatic cats. Vet Parasit 2008;158:177–82.
38. Bowman DD, Susan EL, Lorentzen L, et al. Prevalence and geographic distribution of *Dirofilaria immitis, Borrelia burgdorferi, Ehrlichia canis*, and *Anaplasma phagocytophilum* in dogs in the United States: Results of a national clinic-based serologic survey. Vet Parasitol 2009;160(1/2):138–48.
39. Guerrero J, Nelson CT, Carithers DS. Results and realistic implications of the 2004 AHS-Merial heartworm survey. In: Proceedings AAVP 51st Annual Meeting, Honolulu (HI): 2006. p. 62–3.
40. Apotheker EN, Glickman NW, Lewis HB, et al. Prevalence and risk factors for heartworm infection in dogs in the United States, 2002–2005. Presented at the Proceedings of the 2006 Merck/Merial National Veterinary Scholar Symposium. August 3–6, 2006.
41. Roncalli RA. Tracing the history of heartworms: a 400 year perspective. In: Recent advances in heartworm disease: Symposium '98. Tampa (FL); 1998. p. 1–14.
42. Slocombe JOD. Reflections on heartworm surveys in Canada over 15 years. Presented at the Proceedings of the Heartworm Symposium. Austin, Texas, May 1–3, 1992.
43. Roy BT, Chirurgi VA, Theis JH. Pulmonary dirofilariasis in California. West J Med 1993;158(1):74–6.
44. Nelson CT, Young TS. Incidence of *Dirofilaria immitis* in shelter cats from Southeast Texas. In: Recent advances in heartworm disease: Symposium '98. Tampa (FL); 1998. p. 63–6.
45. Calvert CA, Rawlings CA, McCall JW. Canine heartworm disease. In: Fox PR, Sisson D, Moise SN, editors. Textbook of canine and feline cardiology. Philadelphia: WB Saunders; 1999. p. 702–26.
46. Piche CA, Cavanaugh MT, Donoghue AR, et al. Results of antibody and antigen testing for feline heartworm infection at HeskaR veterinary diagnostic laboratories. In: Recent advances in heartworm disease: Symposium '98. Tampa, Florida: 1998. p. 139–43.
47. Lorentzen L, Caola AE. Incidence of positive heartworm antibody and antigen tests at IDEXX Laboratories: trends and potential impact on feline heartworm awareness. Vet Parasit 2008;158(3):183–90.
48. Theis JH. Public health aspects of dirofilariasis in the United States. Vet Parasitol 2005;133(2/3):157–80.
49. Bowman DD, Johnson RC, Ulrich ME, et al. Effects of long-term administration of ivermectin and milbemycin oxime on circulating microfilariae and parasite antigenemia in dogs with patent heartworm infections. In: Proceedings of the Heartworm Symposium. Austin (TX); 1992. p. 151–8.
50. Cruthers LG, Arther RG, Basel CL, et al. New developments in parasite prevention. Veterinary Forum 2008;25(Suppl):1–3.
51. Blair LS, Williams E, Ewanciw DV. Efficacy of ivermectin against third-stage *Dirofilaria immitis* larvae in ferrets and dogs. Res Vet Sci 1982;33(3):386–7.
52. McCall JW, Guerrero J, Roberts RE, et al. Further evidence of clinical prophylactic, retroactive (reach-back) and adulticidal activity of monthly administrations

of ivermectin (Heartgard Plus™) in dogs experimentally infected with heartworms. In: Recent advances in heartworm disease. San Antonio (TX); 2001. p. 189–200.

53. Lok JB, Knight DH, Ramadan EI. Effects of ivermectin on embryogenesis in *Dirofilaria immitis*: age structure and spatial distribution of intrauterine forms as a function of dosage and time posttreatment. In: Proceedings of the Heartworm Symposium. Charleston (SC); 1989. p. 85–94.

54. McCall JW, Ryan WG, Roberts RE, et al. Heartworm adulticidal activity of prophylactic doses of ivermectin (6 µg/kg) plus pyrantel administered monthly to dogs. In: Recent advances in heartworm disease. Tampa (FL); 1998: p. 209–15.

55. Dzimianski MT, McCall JW, Steffens WL, et al. The safety of selamectin in heartworm infected dogs and its effect on adult worms and microfilariae. In: Recent advances in heartworm disease. San Antonio (TX); 2001. p. 135–40.

56. Blagburn BL, Paul AJ, Newton JC, et al. Safety of moxidectin canine SR (sustained release) injectable in ivermectin-sensitive collies and in naturally infected mongrel dogs. In: Recent advances in heartworm disease. San Antonio (TX); 2001. p. 159–63.

57. Venco L, McCall JW, Guerrero J, et al. Efficacy of long-term monthly administration of ivermectin on the progress of naturally acquired heartworm infections in dogs. Vet Parasitol 2004;124(3/4):259–68.

58. Prichard RK. Is anthelmintic resistance a concern for heartworm control? What can we learn from the human filariasis control programs? Vet Parasitol 2005; 133(2/3):243–53.

59. Bazzocchi C, Mortarino M, Grandi G, et al. Combined ivermectin and doxycycline treatment has microfilaricidal and adulticidal activity against *Dirofilaria immitis* in experimentally infected dogs. Int J Parasitol 2008;38(12):1401–10.

60. McCall JW, Genchi C, Kramer LH, et al. Heartworm and *Wolbachia*: therapeutic implications. Vet Parasit 2008;158(3):204–14.

61. Kramer LH. Treating canine heartworm infection. NAVC Clinician's Brief 2006;4: 19–20.

62. Rawlings CA. Exercise in the dog with *Dirofilaria immitis* infection. Am J Vet Res 1981;42:2057–60.

63. Dillon AR, Brawner WR, Hanrahan L. Influence of number of parasites and exercise on the severity of heartworm disease in dogs. In: Proceedings of the Heartworm Symposium '95. Auburn (AL); 1995. p. 113.

64. Calvert CA, Losonsky JM. Occult heartworm-disease associated allergic pneumonitis. J Am Vet Med Assoc 1985;186(1):1096–8.

65. Confer AW, Qualls CW, MacWilliams PS, et al. Four cases of pulmonary nodular granulomatosis in dogs. Cornell Vet 1983;73(1):41–51.

66. Frank JR, Nutter FB, Kyles AE, et al. Systemic arterial dirofilariasis in five dogs. J Vet Intern Med 1997;11(3):189–94.

67. Atkins CE. Heartworm caval syndrome. Semin Vet Med Surg 1987;2:64–71.

68. Rawlings CA, Tonelli Q, Lewis R, et al. Semiquantitative test for *Dirofilaria Immitis* as a predictor of thromboembolic complications associated with heartworm treatment in dogs. Am J Vet Res 1993;54(6):914–9.

69. Losonsky JM, Thrall DE, Lewis RE. Thoracic radiographic abnormalities in 200 dogs with heartworm infestation. Vet Radiol 1983;24(3):120–3.

70. Lombard CW, Buergelt CD. Echocardiographic and clinical findings in dogs with heartworm-induced cor pulmonale. Compend Cont Educ 1983;5(12):971–9, 982.

71. Lombard CW, Ackerman N. Right heart enlargement in heartworm infected dogs. A radiographic, electrocardiographic, and echocardiographic correlation. Vet Radiol 1984;25(5):210–7.

72. American Heartworm Society. Guidelines for the diagnosis, prevention, and management of heartworm (*Dirofilaria immitis*) in dogs. Available at: http://www.heartwormsociety.org. Accessed August 1, 2009.

73. Miller MW, Keister DM, Tanner PA, et al. Clinical efficacy of melarsomine dihydrochloride (RM340) and thiacetarsemide in dogs with moderate (class 2) heartworm disease. Presented at the Proceedings of the Heartworm Symposium. Auburn, AL, March 31–April 2, 1995.

74. Vezzoni A, Genchi C, Raynaud J-P: Adulticide efficacy of RM 340 in dogs with mild and severe natural infections. In: Proceedings of the Heartworm Symposium '92. Austin (TX); 1992. p. 231–40.

75. Sasaki Y, Kitagawa H, Ishihara K. Clinical and pathological effects of heartworm removal from the pulmonary arteries using flexible alligator forceps. In: Proceedings of the Heartworm Symposium '89. Charleston (SC); 1989, p. 45–51.

76. Morini S, Venco L, Fagioli P, et al. Surgical removal of heartworms versus melarsomine treatment of naturally-infected dogs with risk of thromboembolism. In: Recent advances in heartworm disease: Symposium '98. Tampa (FL); 1998. p. 235–40.

77. Vezzoni A, Genchi C: Reduction in post-adulticide thromboembolic complications with low-dose heparin therapy. In: Proceedings of the Heartworm Symposium '89. Charleston (SC); 1989. p. 73–83.

78. Kramer LH, Tamarozzi F, Morchon R, et al. Immune response and tissue localization of the *Wolbachia* surface protein (WSP) in dogs with natural heartworm (*Dirofilaria immitis*) infection. Vet Immunol Immunopathol 2005;106(3/4):303–8.

79. Atwell RB, Sutton RH, Carlisle CH. The reduction of pulmonary thromboembolic disease (*D immitis*) in the dog associated with aspirin therapy. In: Proceedings of the Heartworm Symposium '83. Orlando, Florida: 1983. p. 115–8.

80. Jackson RF, Seymour WG, Growney RJ, et al. Surgical treatment of caval syndrome of canine heartworm disease. J Am Vet Med Assoc 1966;171: 1065–9.

81. Rawlings CA, Keith JC, Schaub RG. Development and resolution of pulmonary disease in heartworm infection: Illustrated review. J Am Anim Hosp Assoc 1981;17(5):711–20.

82. Ryan WG, Newcomb KM. Prevalence of feline heartworm disease—a global review. In: Proceedings of the Heartworm Symposium '95. Auburn (AL); 1995. p. 79–86.

83. McCall JW, Dzimiansnki MT, McTier TL, et al. Biology of experimental heartworm infection in cats. In: Proceedings of the Heartworm Symposium '92. Austin (TX); 1992. p. 71–9.

84. Atkins CE, DeFrancesco TD, Miller MW, et al. Prevalence of heartworm infection in cats with signs of cardiorespiratory abnormalities. J Am Vet Med Assoc 1997; 212:517–20.

85. Selcer BA, Newell SM, Mansour MS, et al. Radiographic and 2-D echocardiographic findings in eighteen cats experimentally exposed to *D immitis* via mosquito bites. Vet Radiol Ultrasound 1996;37:37–44.

86. Browne LE, Carter TD, Levy JK, et al. Pulmonary arterial lesions in cats seropositive for *Dirofilaria immitis* but lacking adult heartworms in the heart and lungs. Am J Vet Res 2005;66:1544–9.

87. Dillon AR. Activity of pulmonary intravascular macrophages in cats and dogs with and without adult *Dirofilaria immitis*. Vet Parasitol 2008;158:171–6.

88. Dillon R. Feline dirofilariasis. Vet Clin North Am 1984;14(6):1185–99.

89. Holmes RA, Clark JN, Casey HW, et al. Histopathologic and radiographic studies of the development of heartworm pulmonary vascular disease in experimentally infected cats. In: Proceedings of the Heartworm Symposium '92. Austin (TX); 1992. p. 81–9.
90. Atkins CE, DeFrancesco TC, Coats JR, et al. Heartworm infection in cats: 50 cases (1985–1997). J Am Vet Med Assoc 2000;217(3):355–8.
91. McTier, TL, Supakorndej N, McCall JW, et al. Evaluation of ELISA-based adult heartworm antigen test kits using well-defined sera from experimentally and naturally infected cats. In: AAVP 38th Annual Meeting. Minneapolis (MN); 1993. p. 37.
92. Schafer M, Berry CR. Cardiac and pulmonary artery mensuration in feline heartworm disease. Vet Radiol Ultrasound 1995;36(6):499–505.
93. DeFrancesco TD, Atkins CE, Miller MW, et al. Use of echocardiography for the diagnosis of heartworm disease in cats: 43 cases (1985–1997). J Am Vet Med Assoc 2001;218(1):66–9.
94. Goodman DA, McCall JW, Dzimianski MT, et al. Evaluation of a single dose of melarsomine dihydrochloride for adulticidal activity against *Dirofilaria immitis* in cats. In: Proceedings AAVP 41st Annual Meeting. Louisville (KY); 1996. p. 64.
95. McLeroy LW, McCall JW, Dzimianski MT, et al. Evaluation of melarsomine dihydrochloride (Immiticide) for adulticidal activity against *Dirofilaria immitis* in cats. In: Proceedings AAVP 43rd Annual Meeting. Baltimore (MD); 1998. p. 67.
96. Rawlings CA. Pulmonary arteriography and hemodynamics during feline heartworm disease. J Vet Intern Med 1990;4(6):285–91.
97. Small MT, Atkins CE, Gordon SG, et al. Use of a nitinol gooseneck snare catheter for removal of adult *Dirofilaria immitis* in two cats. J Am Vet Med Assoc 2008;233(9):1442–5.

Mites and Lice: Biology and Control

Robert G. Arther, PhD

KEYWORDS

- Mites • Mange • Lice • Pediculosis • Acaricide • Insecticide

External parasite infestations caused by mites and lice frequently present challenges to small animal practitioners from various perspectives, including identification of the parasite, treatment options, and animal husbandry or management practices to prevent transmission. Mites (class Arachnida) are small (usually less than 1 mm in length), without body segmentation. They have a life cycle with development of six-legged larvae to eight-legged nymphs, which may have from one to three nymph instars, to eight-legged adults. Mite life cycles may be completed in 8 days to 4 weeks. Mites are highly adaptable and are capable of living in various habitats. Sarcoptoid mites (including *Sarcoptes scabiei* and *Notoedres cati*) burrow into the skin, producing channels in which eggs are deposited. Nonburrowing mite species pierce the skin, causing inflammation, exudations, pruritus, and scab formation. The word "mange" is used loosely in reference to both types of mite infestations.

Lice (class Insecta) are wingless ectoparasites, have three pairs of stout legs with claws for clinging to hair and fur, and have a dorsoventrally flattened segmented body divided into a head, thorax, and abdomen. They have adapted to spend their entire lives on the host, with a preference for specific anatomic sites. They feed on epidermal tissue debris, sebaceous fluids, and blood. Lice belonging to the order Mallophaga, with chewing/biting mouthparts, frequently infest dogs and cats. Lice of the order Anoplura, with sucking mouthparts, infest dogs but not cats.

SARCOPTES SCABIEI—BIOLOGY

S scabiei, the burrowing mite or itch mite (**Fig. 1**), is the cause of sarcoptic mange or scabies on dogs, foxes, and humans. The mite species is able to infest a range of mammals with different degrees of adaptation. Each subpopulation may be highly adapted to a particular host, so some strains may not easily infest a different species. Different subpopulations may be distinguished by the presence or absence of dorsal and/or ventral spines but differ more physiologically than morphologically. When interspecies transmission occurs, infestations tend to be mild and cure spontaneously.

Animal Health Research and Development, Bayer HealthCare, 12809 Shawnee Mission Parkway, Shawnee, KS 66216, USA
E-mail address: bob.arther.b@bayer.com

Vet Clin Small Anim 39 (2009) 1159–1171
doi:10.1016/j.cvsm.2009.06.009
0195-5616/09/$ – see front matter © 2009 Elsevier Inc. All rights reserved.

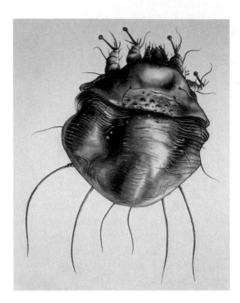

Fig. 1. *S scabiei.*

Although only one species is recognized, the mite found on dogs is often referred to as *S scabiei* var *canis*. This mite is rare in cats.

Adult female mites are 300 to 600 by 250 to 400 μm, whereas males measure 200 to 240 by 140 to 170 μm. The first two pairs of legs in both sexes each terminate in a small suckerlike pulvillus on the long, unsegmented pretarsi, which helps the mite grip the substrate as it moves. The posterior pair of legs in the female and the third pair of legs in the male end in long bristles, whereas the fourth pair of legs in the male also bears suckers on the distal end of the legs. The third and fourth pairs of legs do not project beyond the posterior body margin. The nymphs resemble the female adults.[1,2]

The life cycle of *S scabiei* var *canis* takes place exclusively on dogs, passing from egg to larva and through two nymphal stages, in 2 to 3 weeks. After mating on the skin surface, the females burrow into the epidermis, making tunnels up to 1 cm long that are parallel to the surface. After a maturation phase of 4 to 5 days, the females deposit one to three oval eggs daily into these tunnels for about 2 months. The six-legged larvae hatch 3 to 4 days after oviposition and most of them crawl from the burrows to the skin surface, although some remain in the tunnels where they continue to develop. The larvae molt first to protonymphs, then to tritonymphs, and then to adults. They feed on damaged skin and tissue fluids. After mating, the newly developed males die, whereas the adult females look for a suitable site on the host for burrowing and subsequently depositing their eggs. The total egg-to-adult life cycle typically requires 17 to 21 days, but may be as short as 14 days.[3] Mites can survive off the host for 2 to 3 weeks in sleeping areas and on grooming equipment, which should also be considered as potential sources of contamination.[1]

Sarcoptic mange often begins on relatively hairless areas of skin on the head (**Fig. 2**), with frequent distribution to the lower abdomen, chest, and legs. The ears are almost always affected, particularly the inside of the pinna, as is the lateral aspect of the elbow. Lesions consist of follicular papules, yellow crusts of dried serum, and excoriations from scratching due to intense pruritus. Secondary bacterial infections are frequent complications. The lesions usually spread rapidly, sometimes covering

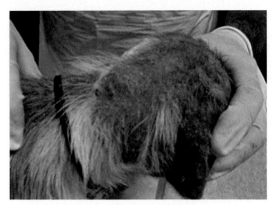

Fig. 2. Clinical lesions resulting from *S scabiei* infestation.

the entire body. The affected sites also display alopecia caused by self-inflicted trauma. Chronic cases result in thickening of the skin with hyperkeratosis, wrinkling, and hyperpigmentation. In the most seriously affected skin areas, histopathologic examination indicates severe chronic inflammation of the epidermis, with variable hyperkeratosis and parakeratosis.[1]

Despite obvious clinical lesions and intense pruritus, a diagnosis is often difficult. Dogs infested with these mites frequently display a pinnal-pedal scratch reflex.[4] Direct parasite detection should be performed with microscopic examination of skin scrapings. Samples should be taken from the edges of the lesions adjacent to intact tissue, that is, not from open wounds or chronically inflamed excoriations. The preferred areas for obtaining skin scrapings are those covered with clearly visible, raised, yellowish crusts and papules. The accuracy of this diagnostic procedure depends on the number of examined skin scrapings. Up to 10 scrapings are advised per dog,[5] although mites are not found in approximately 50% of cases and diagnosis is based on clinical manifestations and response to treatment.[2]

SARCOPTES SCABIEI—CONTROL

The coat should be clipped, and crusty lesions and scale should be removed with an antiseborrheic shampoo.[4] Traditional treatments have included the use of an acaricidal dip, such as lime sulfur, repeated weekly.[6] Fipronil (0.25%) spray treatment (Frontline Spray, Merial) has been used successfully to treat sarcoptic mange.[7,8] The preferred method of treatment includes the use of systemic macrocyclic lactones. Topical selamectin (Revolution, Pfizer) applied at a dose of 6 mg/kg given twice with a 30-day interval is highly effective.[9,10]

Although not labeled for this claim, two treatments have been reported to be efficacious against canine scabies: (1) 10% imidacloprid + 2.5% moxidectin (Advantage Multi for Dogs, Bayer) applied at the rate of 0.1 mL/kg (to provide 10.0 mg/kg imidacloprid + 2.5 mg/kg moxidectin) and administered twice at a 30-day interval; and (2) milbemycin oxime (Interceptor, Novartis) administered orally at a dose of 2 mg/kg for a total of three treatments (days 0, 7, and 14).[11–13]

All dogs having contact with infested dogs should be treated. Because mites are able to survive off the host, potential sources of contamination should be disinfected, including bedding, brushes, and combs.

NOTOEDRES CATI—BIOLOGY

N cati (**Fig. 3**) is the cause of face or head mange in cats and other felines. These mites closely resemble large Sarcoptes species. Females are about 230 to 300 by 200 to 250 μm, whereas males measure 150 to 180 by 120 to 145 μm. Notoedric mange lesions consist principally of alopecia and marked hyperkeratosis around the head and ears, with abundant epidermal scaling. Mites are easily demonstrated from skin scrapings. Advanced lesions may produce thickened skin with hyperkeratosis and hyperpigmentation, which may give cats an "old age" appearance. The mite may also infest dogs and can cause a transient dermatitis in humans.

Mating takes place on the surface of the skin. Males die after mating. Females burrow into the epidermis, making tunnels parallel to the surface, and then begin to deposit eggs. After 3 to 4 days, six-legged larvae hatch from the eggs, most of which migrate to the skin surface where they molt to protonymphs, then to tritonymphs, and eventually to adults. The life cycle is completed in about 2 to 3 weeks. Each stage feeds on damaged skin components and tissue exudates. The mites are highly infectious, and transmission occurs primarily by animal-to-animal contact by larvae or nymphs.[1]

NOTOEDRES CATI—CONTROL

Currently there are no products labeled for the treatment and control of notoedric mange in cats. Traditional treatments have included the use of lime sulfur dip.[14]

Macrocyclic lactones have been used successfully to treat these mite infestations, including two to three treatments of ivermectin (0.3 mg/kg) given subcutaneously at 7-day intervals.[15] Topically applied selamectin, administered once at a dose of 6 mg/kg, has been used successfully to treat infested cats.[16]

OTODECTES CYNOTIS—BIOLOGY

The ear mite, Otodectes cynotis, is the most common mange mite found on cats, dogs, and other carnivores (**Fig. 4**). Female mites are 400 to 500 by 270 to 300 μm,

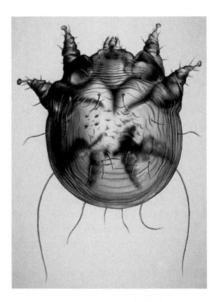

Fig. 3. N cati.

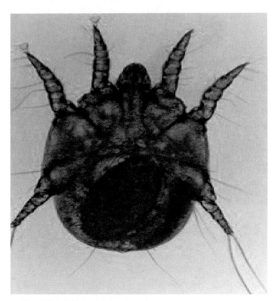

Fig. 4. Female *O cynotis* with visible egg.

whereas the males measure 320 to 400 by 210 to 300 μm. The first two pairs of legs of the adult female terminate in cup-shaped suckers on short, unsegmented pretarsi. The third and fourth pairs of legs each have two long terminal setae. In the male, all four pairs of legs have cup-shaped suckers on short, unsegmented pretarsi. The fourth pair of legs is shorter in both sexes. Sexual dimorphism only occurs in the adult stage. The mites generally live deep in the ear canal but may be found on other areas of the body.

O cynotis develops from egg to adult mite within about 3 weeks, via one larval and two nymphal stages. This mite has a life span of about 2 months.[1] The mites cause irritation and local inflammatory reaction in the external ear canal by piercing the skin surface, feeding, and migrating. The external ear canal of infested animals frequently has an accumulation of dark cerumen, dried blood, and mite excretory products, which resemble coffee grounds (**Fig. 5**). Aural pruritus may cause the animal to rub, scratch, and shake its head violently, resulting in excoriations, erythema, hematomas, and swelling of the ears.

The mite occurs worldwide, and it is often prevalent in animal shelters and breeding establishments. It has been estimated that more than 50% of all cases of otitis externa in dogs and more than 80% of the cases in cats are caused by *O cynotis*, and a considerable proportion of dogs and cats harbor subclinical infestations.[2] Mites are transferred through direct contact and from infested females to pups and kittens.

Mites may be identified (1) by direct examination of the ear canal using an otoscope with an attached magnifying lens or (2) by swabbing the ear canal with a cotton applicator to remove the waxy deposits and observing the mites or eggs in the exudate with a hand lens or microscope.

OTODECTES CYNOTIS—CONTROL

The ear canal of infested animals should be flushed and cleansed with a mild ceruminolytic agent. Traditional treatments have included using preparations of acaricides or mineral oil instilled directly into the ear canal.[4] Frequent reapplications may be

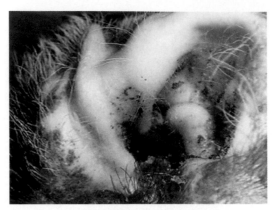

Fig. 5. Debris in ear canal of cat infested with *O cynotis.*

required. An otic suspension containing 0.01% ivermectin controls adult mites and also prevents the hatching of larvae from eggs.[17] Systemic products providing extended residual activity are highly efficacious and convenient to apply. Topically applied imidacloprid + moxidectin solution is efficacious for treatment of otodectic mange in cats,[18–20] and topically applied selamectin solution is efficacious for the treatment of otodectic mange in cats and dogs.[10,21]

When a case of otoacariasis is confirmed, all dogs and cats in the household having direct contact should be treated. In addition, grooming equipment and bedding should be disinfected because mites are able to survive for a period of time off the host.

DEMODEX CANIS —BIOLOGY

Demodex canis is a minute, specialized mite, with a cigar-shaped body measuring 100 to 300 μm in length and four pairs of stout legs ending in small blunt claws (**Fig. 6**). The opisthosomal region (behind the legs) is at least one-half of the body length and has a transversely striated cuticle.

Demodex mites live in the hair follicles and sebaceous glands of a wide range of wild and domestic animals, including humans. Feline demodicosis (caused by *Demodex cati* or *Demodex gatoi*) is a rare parasitic disease. Most dogs naturally carry a small number of *D canis* without displaying clinical infestation. Under certain conditions, however, the mites can cause demodectic mange or demodicosis (red mange), regarded as one of the most important skin diseases in dogs. Demodicosis is more common in purebred dogs.[4]

The mites live embedded head-down in hair follicles as well as sebaceous and meibomian glands, where they spend their entire lives. Demodex mites are unable to survive without their host. Female mites lay 20 to 24 eggs in the hair follicle, which develop via two six-legged larval stages followed by two nymphal stages. Mites in the immature stages are moved to the edge of the follicle by sebaceous flow, where they mature. All stages of the life cycle may exist concurrently in one follicle. The life cycle is completed in 18 to 24 days. Transmission of *D canis* from bitch to puppies occurs during the first 3 days of life through close physical contact while nursing.

Demodectic mange has been classified in various ways depending on the clinical manifestations. These categories include juvenile demodicosis, adult-onset demodicosis, localized demodicosis, and generalized demodicosis.

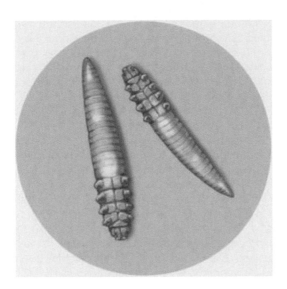

Fig. 6. *Demodex.*

Juvenile demodicosis, which occurs in young dogs between 3 and 15 months of age, results in nonpruritic areas of focal alopecia on the head and forelimbs. The hind limbs and torso are rarely affected. The first lesions are frequently observed just above the eye, with small patches of depilation around the eye resulting in a "spectacled" appearance. This form of the disease is self-limiting, and recurrences are rare. Immunosuppressive therapy with glucocorticoids, however, may cause deterioration leading to generalized and pustular manifestations.[2]

Adult-onset demodicosis is often associated with concurrent staphylococcal pyoderma and is a pustular form of the disease. It can be localized or generalized. Clinical signs include erythema, pustules, crusts, and pruritus. The localized form is often confined in an area of 1 or 2 feet. Generalized conditions include six or more localized lesions or more than two affected limbs. The skin often becomes hyperpigmented in chronic cases. The generalized form commonly develops as a consequence of an underlying debilitating disease, such as hypothyroidism, hyperadrenocorticism, diabetes mellitus, prolonged immunosuppressive therapy, or neoplasia, or various infectious diseases, such as leishmaniasis, which reduce the host's immune defense mechanisms and are followed by a massive multiplication of mites.[1,2,4]

The diagnosis of demodicosis is based on the demonstration of large numbers of adult mites or significantly increased numbers in the immature stage as a proportion of adults. Deep skin scrapings taken from the edge of the lesions increase the chances of detecting the mites. Skin folds should be squeezed firmly to expel the mites from the depths of the hair follicles. Skin scrapings revealing low mite numbers should be considered normal hair fauna. Mites may also be detected by plucking hair samples for microscopic examination of the follicles.

DEMODEX CANIS—CONTROL

Localized demodicosis usually resolves spontaneously within 6 to 8 weeks, with or without the use of an acaricidal treatment.[1]

Treatment of generalized demodicosis is challenging, difficult, and frequently requires extended and intensive therapeutic intervention. Amitraz, a formamidine derivative, is approved for the treatment of canine generalized demodicosis, applied as a dip at the rate of 250 ppm (0.025%) of active drug. About three to six applications that are 14 days apart may be necessary. Treatments should be preceded with a benzoyl peroxide shampoo to remove crusts and debris and to flush the follicles, allowing for better penetration of the acaricide. Not all dogs respond to amitraz treatments, and relapses of dogs previously thought to be cured are common.[22] Single spot application of 14.24% metaflumizone + 14.34% amitraz (ProMeris, Fort Dodge) is labeled for the control of demodectic mange mites on dogs.

Macrocyclic lactones have also been used successfully for treatment of generalized demodicosis. The spot-on formulation containing 10% imidacloprid + 2.5% moxidectin, applied topically at the recommended rate of 0.1 mL/kg, 2 to 4 times at 4-week intervals, provided clinical improvement, and no mites were detected after treatment in 26 of 30 dogs.[23] Milbemycin oxime administered orally with dosages ranging from 0.5 to 2.2 mg/kg/d and treatment durations ranging from 9 to 26 weeks have been reported to be effective. Oral doses of ivermectin at 300 to 600 μg/kg/d with treatment duration extending 1 month beyond negative skin scrapings have also been effective.[22] The extralabel use of avermectins or milbemycins for the treatment of canine demodicosis should be approached with caution, especially for breeds with known sensitivity to these compounds.

While a dog is being treated for demodicosis, skin scrapings should be collected every 2 to 4 weeks, preferably from the same locations at each sampling site (at least one sample from the head and foreleg, respectively), undergoing microscopic examination for mites to monitor treatment progress. The total number of detectable mites, the ratio of live to dead mites, and the ratio of adult *Demodex* mites to those in immature stages should be determined. These ratios can then be used to determine the success of the initial treatment. A quantitative reduction in the numbers of adult and immature mites or an abundance of dead mites are indications of a successful healing process. A continued presence of numerous mites and a comparatively large number in the immature stages relative to adult mites may indicate further progression of the disease.[1,4]

Female dogs with generalized demodectic mange or a history of demodectic mange should be spayed because the condition may worsen or relapse during estrus or pregnancy and because of the inheritable predisposition of the disease.[22]

CHEYLETIELLA SPP—BIOLOGY

Three similar *Cheyletiella* species are of importance to small animal practitioners, including *C yasguri* in dogs, *C blakei* in cats, and *C parasitivorax* in rabbits. Adult mites are rather large with an ovoid shape, measuring about 400 μm in length, with curved palpal claws. They move rapidly and induce branlike exfoliative debris on the rump and backs of animals, resulting in a "walking dandruff" appearance. Adult mites can live up to 1 month off their host without feeding.

The mites spend their entire lives on the host, living in the skin debris at the base of the hair. They do not burrow, but pierce the skin with styletlike chelicerae to feed on lymph. Eggs are attached to the hair above the skin. The prelarva and larva develop within the egg. Fully developed nymphs emerge from eggs, developing through two nymphal stages before becoming adults. Young animals, especially when housed in cages or kennels, and debilitated ones are particularly susceptible to infestation.

Heavily infested dogs may have excessive shedding of hair, inflammation, and hyperesthesia of the dorsal skin. Cats are primarily affected around the head and trunk. The mites are readily transferred to humans causing papular lesions.[2]

CHEYLETIELLA SPP—CONTROL

Currently there are no products labeled for the treatment of cheyletiellosis in either cats or dogs. Spray, shampoo, or spot-on formulations containing pyrethrins or pyrethroids are effective for treatment of cheyletiellosis on dogs; pyrethroids should not be applied to cats.[6,24] Fipronil spot-on or spray formulations have been used for treatment of cheyletiellosis in dogs and cats.[25,26]

Spot-on treatment with 10% imidacloprid + 2.5% moxidectin solution has been shown to be effective for the treatment of canine cheyletiellosis,[27] whereas spot-on selamectin solution provided efficacy for the treatment of feline cheyletiellosis.[28]

The bedding and grooming equipment of infested animals should be disinfected.

TROMBICULA SPP—BIOLOGY

Cats and dogs are frequently infested with mite larvae of the family Trombiculidae, more commonly known as "chiggers" or "harvest mites." The six-legged larvae are orange-red or yellow and measure 200 to 300 μm. The nymphs and adults are free-living. These mites are strongly seasonal and generally encountered in late summer or fall. Mites in larval stages develop on the ground. They climb on vegetation, where they wait for passing hosts. They are likely to be found on the ears, eyes, nose, or other areas of thin skin, including the abdomen and regions between the toes. They usually occur in large clusters.

The larvae attach to the host and pierce the superficial epidermal layers with blade-like chelicerae to inject salivary gland enzymes into the skin. They then feed on liquefied tissues, body secretions, and blood. After feeding, the engorged larvae drop to the ground to continue their development. Infestations may cause intense pruritus, erythema, excoriations, and alopecia. Different responses to the infestations may be due to individual hypersensitivity reactions to the mites.[1]

TROMBICULA SPP—CONTROL

Infested animals generally have a history of roaming through woods or fields. Topically applied fipronil and selamectin have been used successfully to treat trombiculosis in cats and dogs,[29,30] and topical pyrethroid + pyriproxyfen formulations have been used to control these mite infestations on dogs.[31]

LICE INFESTATIONS

Dogs may be infested with two different lice species, *Trichodectes canis* (biting lice) and *Linognathus setosus* (sucking lice), whereas cats are infested with only one lice species, *Felicola subrostratus* (sucking lice). The term "pediculosis" is used in reference to infestation with lice.

Lice species can be distinguished by the characteristic shape of their heads. Females lay white operculated eggs (nits) on the animal's fur, gluing each egg firmly to a hair shaft. Nymphs hatch from the eggs, and undergo three molts before becoming adults. The life cycle can be completed in 14 to 21 days. Lice infestations may be diagnosed by examination of adhesive tape impressions or skin scrapings from affected sites. Lice are able to survive for more than 1 to 2 days off their host but usually remain with a single host animal throughout their lives. Transfer of lice between hosts is through close physical contact between animals.

TRICHODECTES CANIS—BIOLOGY

T canis, the biting or chewing louse species of dogs (**Fig. 7**), are 1 to 2 mm in length, yellowish, and dorsoventrally flattened and have a clearly recognizable head, thorax, and abdomen. They attach to hair shafts typically around the head, neck, back, and tail area, where they feed on dermal debris and exudates from skin lesions. Mature females lay several eggs per day. Nymphs, which resemble the adults, hatch from the eggs within 1 or 2 weeks of oviposition. Adults live for about 1 month. The lice are active and produce intense irritation, pruritus, and scratching. They often congregate around body openings or wounds.

LINOGNATHUS SETOSUS—BIOLOGY

L setosus, the sucking louse species of dogs, are brownish-yellow, measuring 1.5 to 1.7 mm. The head is long, narrow, and pointed, whereas the abdomen is slender and elongated. The lice feed on blood. Females lay one egg per day. Sucking lice infestations are most commonly found on long-hair breeds, such as spaniels, basset hounds, and Afghan hounds. Preferred sites for these lice include the ears, neck, and back. The infestations may result in pruritus, alopecia, and excoriations. Severely infested dogs may become anemic.

FELICOLA SUBROSTRATUS—BIOLOGY

F subrostratus, the biting louse species of cats, are yellow to beige and measure 1 to 1.5 mm. This is the only louse species that is commonly found on cats. The lice have a distinctive triangular-shaped head and mouthparts with a median longitudinal groove to grasp an individual hair. Infestations most commonly occur on the face, back, and pinnae. Long-haired breeds are more prone to severe infestations, especially under matted or neglected fur. Lice infestations in cats may result in dull and ruffled hair, scaling, crusts, and alopecia. Severe infestations are rare and usually confined to elderly or debilitated cats.

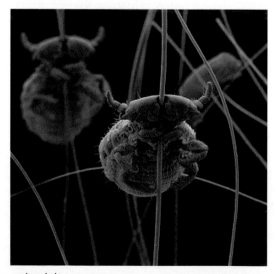

Fig. 7. *Trichodectes canis* adult.

PEDICULOSIS—CONTROL

Lice infestations are frequently encountered in neglected animals subjected to overcrowding and poor sanitation.

Lice are easily killed, and traditional treatments have included the use of conventional insecticidal shampoos, sprays, and powders. Biting and sucking lice infestations on dogs have been successfully treated, following a single topical spot-on application with 9.1% wt/wt imidacloprid (Advantage, Bayer).[32] Biting lice infestations on dogs have been successfully treated following a single topical spot-on application with 10% imidacloprid + 2.5% moxidectin,[33] 10% fipronil,[34] or 65% permethrin.[35] Biting lice on cats and dogs have been successfully treated with a single topical spot-on application of selamectin.[36] All pets in the household should be treated. Bedding and grooming equipment from infested animals should be cleaned and disinfected.

SUMMARY

Dogs and cats frequently encounter a diverse variety of mite and lice species, which may result in mild to severe consequences depending on husbandry conditions, the severity of the infestation, and the nature of the localized or systemic defense mechanisms mobilized by the host in response to the parasite. Some of these external parasites are obvious to detect, identify, and control, although others may offer a significant challenge to the practitioner. Traditional acaricide and insecticide formulations, including dips, sprays, powders, and shampoos, have been used to treat and control these infestations. Some of the more recently developed, low-volume, topically applied insecticides and systemically acting macrolide formulations, although not always labeled for specific claims, may offer safe, efficacious, and convenient alternatives. The practitioner may wish to consider these products when implementing treatment and control programs involving these pests.

REFERENCES

1. Schneider T, editor. Veterinary parasitology, special excerpt. 6th edition. Stuttgart: Parey; 2006. p. 13–39.
2. Wall R, Shearer D. Veterinary ectoparasites, biology, pathology & control. 2nd edition. Oxford: Blackwell Science; 1997. p. 23–54.
3. Arlian LG, Vyszewski-Moher DL. Life cycle of *Sarcoptes scabiei* var *canis*. J Parasitol 1988;74(3):427–30.
4. Scott DW, Miller WH, Griffin CE, editors. Muller & Kirk's small animal dermatology. 6th edition. Philadelphia: W.B. Saunders; 2001. p. 423–516.
5. Grant DI. Notes on parasitic skin diseases in the dog and cat. Br Vet J 1985;141: 447–62.
6. Curtis CF. Current trends in the treatment of *Sarcoptes*, *Cheyletiella*, and *Otodectes* mite infestations in dogs and cats. Vet Dermatol 2004;15:108–14.
7. Curtis C. Use of 0.25% fipronil spray to treat sarcoptic mange in a litter of 5-week old puppies. Vet Res 1996;139:43–4.
8. Koutinas A, Saridomichelakis M, Soubasis N, et al. Treatment of canine sarcoptic mange with fipronil spray. Aust Vet Pract 2001;31(3):115–9.
9. Shanks D, McTier T, Behan S, et al. The efficacy of selamectin in the treatment of naturally acquired infestations of *Sarcoptes scabiei* on dogs. Vet Parasitol 2000; 91:269–81.

10. Six RH, Clemence RG, Thomas CA, et al. Efficacy and safety of selamectin against *Sarcoptes scabiei* on dogs and *Otodectes cynotis* on dogs and cats presented as veterinary patients. Vet Parasitol 2000;91:291–309.

11. Fourie L, DuRand C, Hein J. Evaluation of the efficacy of an imidacloprid 10% moxidectin/2.5% spot-on against *Sarcoptes scabiei var canis* on dogs. Parasitol Res 2003;90(3):135–6.

12. Krieger K, Heine J, DuMont P, et al. Efficacy and safety of imidacloprid 10% plus moxidectin 2.5% spot-on in the treatment of sarcoptic mange and otoacariosis in dogs: results of a European field study. Parasitol Res 2005;97(1):81–8.

13. Bergvall K. Clinical efficacy of milbemycin oxime in the treatment of canine scabies: a study of 56 cases. Vet Dermatol 1998;9:231–3.

14. Bowman DD. Georgis' parasitology for veterinarians. 7th edition. Philadelphia: W.B. Saunders Co.; 1999. p. 1–78.

15. Foley RH. A notoedric mange epizootic in an island's cat population. Feline Practice 1991;19:8–10.

16. Itoh N, Muraoka N, Aoki M, et al. Treatment of *Notoedres cati* infestation in cats with selamectin. Vet Rec 2004;154:409.

17. Bowman D, Kato S, Fogarty E. Effects of an ivermectin otic suspension on egg hatching of the cat ear mite, *Otodectes cynotis*, in vitro. Vet Ther 2001;2(4):311–6.

18. Davis W, Arther R, Settje T. Clinical evaluation of the efficacy and safety of typically applied imidacloprid plus moxidectin against ear mites (*Otodectes cynotis*) in client-owned cats. Parasitol Res 2007;101(1):19–24.

19. Farkas R, Germann T, Szeidemann Z. Assessment of the ear mite (*Otodectes cynotis*) infestation and the efficacy of an imidacloprid plus moxidectin combination in the treatment of otoacariosis in a Hungarian cat shelter. Parasitol Res 2007; 101(1):35–44.

20. Fourie L, Kok D, Heine J. Evaluation of the efficacy of an imidacloprid 10%/moxidectin 1% spot-on against *Otodectes cynotis* in cats. Parasitol Res 2003;90(3):112–3.

21. Shanks D, McTier T, Rowan T, et al. The efficacy of selamectin in the treatment of naturally acquired aural infestations of *Otodectes cynotis* on dogs and cats. Vet Parasitol 2000;91:283–90.

22. Paradis M. New approaches to the treatment of canine demodicosis. Vet Clin North Am Small Anim Pract 1999;29(6):1425–37.

23. Heine J, Krieger K, DuMont P, et al. Evaluation of the efficacy and safety of imidacloprid 10% plus moxidectin 2.5% spot-on in the treatment of generalized demodicosis in dogs: results of a European field study. Parasitol Res 2005;97(1):89–96.

24. Endris R, Rueter V, Nelson J, et al. Efficacy of 65% permethrin applied as a topical spot-on against walking dandruff caused by the mite, *Cheyletiella yasguri*, in dogs. Vet Ther 2000;1(4):273–9.

25. Chadwick AJ. Use of 0.25 percent fipronil pump spray formulation to treat canine cheyletiellosis. J Small Anim Pract 1997;38:261.

26. Scarampella F, Pollmeier M, Romano D. et al. Efficacy of frontline spot-on in the treatment of feline chyletiellosis. Proc. 77th International Symposium on Ectoparasites of Pets. League City, TX, April 13–16, 2003.

27. Loft KE, Willesen JL. Efficacy of imidacloprid 10 percent/moxidectin 2.5 percent spot-on in the treatment of cheyletiellosis in dogs. Vet Rec 2007;160:528–9.

28. Chailleux N, Paradis M. Efficacy of selamectin in the treatment of naturally acquired cheyletiellosis in cats. Can Vet J 2004;43:767–70.

29. Nuttall TJ, French AT, Cheetham HC. Treatment of *Trombicula autumnalis* infestations in dogs and cats with a 0.25% fipronil pump spray. J Small Anim Pract 1998; 39:237–9.

30. Leone F, Albanese F. Efficacy of selamectin spot-on formulation against *Neotrombicula autumnalis* in eight cats [abstract]. Vet Dermatol 2004;15(1):49.
31. Small D, Jasmin P, Mercier P. Treatment of *Neotrombicula autumnalis* dermatitis in dogs using two topical permethrin-pyriproxyfen combinations. J Small Anim Pract 2004;45:98–103.
32. Hanssen I, Mencke N, Asskildt, et al. Field study on the insecticidal efficacy of advantage against natural infestations of dogs with lice. Parasitol Res 1999;85: 347–8.
33. Stanneck D, Doyle J, Ketzis J, et al. Efficacy of imidacloprid 10% plus moxidectin 2.5% against natural lice (*Trichodectes canis*) infestations in dogs. Parasitol Res 2007;101(1):13–9.
34. Pollmeier M, Pengo G, Jeannin, et al. Evaluation of the efficacy of fipronil formulations in the treatment and control of biting lice *Trichodectes canis* (DeGeer, 1778) on dogs. Vet Parasitol 2002;107:127–36.
35. Endris R, Rueter V, Nelson J, et al. Efficacy of a topical spot-on containing 65% permethrin against dog louse, *Trichodectes canis*, (Mallophaga: Trichodectidae). Vet Ther 2000;2(2):135–9.
36. Shanks DJ, Gautier P, McTier TL, et al. Efficacy of selamectin against biting lice on dogs and cats. Vet Rec 2003;154(8):234–7.

Biology, Treatment, and Control of Flea and Tick Infestations

Byron L. Blagburn, BS, MS, PhD[a],*, Michael W. Dryden, DVM, PhD[b]

KEYWORDS

• Flea • Tick • Biology • Treatment • Control • Disease

Flea and tick infestations of pets and the home environment are a common occurrence and their elimination can be an expensive and time-consuming problem. Many problems in control can be related to a lack of understanding of parasite biology and ecology. In fact many advances in control of fleas can be directly linked to advances in our knowledge of the intricacies of flea host associations, reproduction, and survival in the premises. Understanding tick biology and ecology is far more difficult than with fleas, because North America can have up to nine different tick species infesting cats and dogs compared to one primary flea species. The range and local density of certain tick species has increased in many areas because of changes in climate, vegetation, agricultural practices, wildlife host abundance, acaricide usage, and probably several other factors. Whatever the reason, tick infestation pressure may be much higher and associated tick-transmitted diseases may be more prevalent in some locations today than in the past.

FLEA OVERVIEW

Flea infestations are probably the most common ectoparasitic affliction of dogs and cats in North America. Although more than 2200 species and subspecies of fleas are known throughout the world, only *Ctenocephalides felis felis* (cat flea), *Ctenocephalides canis* (dog flea), *Pulex simulans,* and *Echidnophaga gallinacea* (poultry sticktight flea) occur in large numbers on dogs and cats with enough regularity to be of importance as nuisance pests.[1,2] In North America, the most commonly encountered flea species on dogs and cats is *C f felis* (**Fig. 1**).[1,2]

The term "cat flea," which is the approved common name for *C f felis*, can occasionally cause confusion. When it appears in print, it refers to the specific flea genus and

[a] Department of Pathobiology, 166 Greene Hall, College of Veterinary Medicine, Auburn University, Auburn AL 36849-5519, USA
[b] Department of Diagnostic Medicine/Pathology, College of Veterinary Medicine, Kansas State University, Manhattan, KS 66506, USA
* Corresponding author.
E-mail address: blagbbl@auburn.edu (B.L. Blagburn).

Vet Clin Small Anim 39 (2009) 1173–1200
doi:10.1016/j.cvsm.2009.07.001   vetsmall.theclinics.com

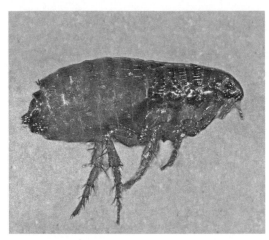

Fig. 1. Adult female cat flea (*C felis*).

species and not to fleas recovered from cats. There are four recognized subspecies of *C felis* throughout the world: *Ctenocephalides felis damarensis* and *C felis strongylus* occur primarily in East Africa, *C felis orientis* occurs in India and Australia, and the widespread *C f felis* occurs in all continents except Antarctica and is the only subspecies that occurs in North America.[2] Therefore, most of the North American literature refers to the cat flea as *C felis*. Because the cat flea is the most common flea on domestic dogs and cats in North America and has been extensively investigated, the following discussions on flea biology will be confined to the cat flea.

The cat flea, *C felis,* is a clinically important parasite of domestic pets, being responsible for the production of allergic dermatitis, serving as the vector of various bacterial pathogens, and being the intermediate host for filarid and cestode parasites.

Flea allergy dermatitis (see later discussion for detail) is the most common dermatologic disease of dogs and a major cause of feline miliary dermatitis.[1,2] It is an immunologic disease in which a hypersensitive state is produced in a host, resulting from the injection of antigenic material from the salivary glands of fleas. Blood consumption by fleas can produce iron deficiency anemia and even death in heavy infestations.[1,2] *Ctenocephalides felis* has also been recently implicated in the transmission of *Rickettsia typhi*, *Rickettsia felis*, *Bartonella henselae* and other *Bartonella spp*, *Mycoplasma haemofelis,* and in rare cases, even *Yersinia pestis*.[3–6] *Ctenocephalides felis* also serves as an intermediate host of the nonpathogenic subcutaneous filarid nematode of dogs, *Acanthocheilonema* (*Dipetalonema*) *reconditum*. Several species of cestodes can also be carried by *C felis*, including *Dipylidium caninum* and *Hymenolepis nana*.[1,2]

FLEA BIOLOGY

Flea eggs are pearly white and oval, with rounded ends, and are 0.5 mm in length. Eggs will usually hatch in 1 to 10 days, depending on temperature and humidity.[7,8] Newly hatched flea larvae are slender, white, segmented, sparsely covered with short hairs, and 2 to 5 mm in length; they possess a pair of anal struts (**Fig. 2**). Larvae are free living, feeding on adult flea feces (which are essential for successful development), on organic debris that is found in their environment, and on flea eggs.[1,2] Once the larvae have ingested adult flea feces or other material, they become darker. Flea larvae avoid

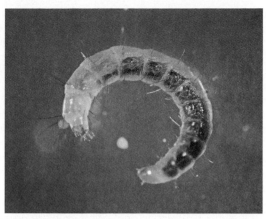

Fig. 2. Third instar larva of *C felis*.

direct sunlight in their microhabitat, actively moving deep into carpet fibers or under organic debris (grass, branches, leaves, or soil).[2] Flea larvae undergo two molts, usually over 5 to 11 days, before developing into the pupal stage.[7,8]

Flea larvae are extremely susceptible to heat and desiccation.[8,9] Moisture in the larval environment is essential for development, with relative humidity lower than 50% causing desiccation, and larvae that are maintained in soil with low moisture levels fail to develop.[8] Because larvae are susceptible to heat and desiccation, development outdoors probably occurs only where the ground is shaded and moist. The flea-infested host also needs to spend a significant amount of time in these areas, so that adult flea feces will be deposited into the larval environment.

The mature third instar larva produces a 0.5-cm–long, whitish, loosely spun silklike cocoon in which it undergoes pupation. The cocoon is sticky and becomes coated with debris from the environment. Cocoons are found in soil, in carpets, under furniture, and on animal bedding. At 27°C (80.6°F) and 80% relative humidity, fleas begin to emerge approximately 5 days after pupation, and they reach peak emergence in 8 to 9 days.[10,11] Once the pupa has fully developed, the pre-emerged adult flea within the cocoon can be stimulated to emerge from the cocoon by physical pressure, carbon dioxide, and heat.[12] If the pre-emerged adult does not receive an emergence stimulus, it may remain quiescent in the cocoon for several weeks or months until a suitable host arrives.[12]

The entire life cycle of *C felis* can be completed in 12 to 14 days, or it can be prolonged up to 174 days, depending on temperature and humidity within the microenvironment.[12] However, under most household conditions, nearly all cat fleas will complete their life cycle within 3 to 8 weeks.

The adult *C felis* depends primarily on visual cues to locate hosts.[13] Factors such as flea age, CO_2, and temperature modify their responsiveness.[13] It has been determined that *C felis* adults are most sensitive to green light with wavelengths between 510 and 550 nm.[13,14] *Ctenocephalides felis* adults that have emerged in dark areas, such as under porches, in crawl spaces, or under beds or sofas, will orient and move toward a light source. They then jump when the light source is suddenly and temporarily interrupted (host-shadow).

If the newly emerged *C felis* adults do not immediately acquire a host, they can survive several days before requiring a blood meal. As with immature life stages, survival of adult fleas is highly dependent on temperature and humidity. In moisture-saturated air, 62% of adult C felis survived for 62 days, whereas only 5% survived for 12 days when maintained at 22.5°C and 60% RH (relative humidity).[10,15] It is unlikely that adult or immature fleas in the premises can survive during winter in northern temperate regions. It has been shown that no life cycle stage (egg, larva, pupa, or adult) can survive for 10 days at 3°C (37.4°F) or 5 days at 1°C (33.8°F).[10]

Numerous warm blooded animals play host to C felis. In North America, various nondomesticated hosts that harbor cat fleas have been reported, including coyotes, red and gray fox, bobcats, skunks, several rodent species, raccoons, opossums, Florida panthers, poultry, calves, and ferrets.[1,2] With such a large number of alternative hosts, several of which often live in close proximity to humans and their pets, it is likely that flea-infested wild animals or feral dogs and cats are serving as continual sources of reinfestation. Newly emerged fleas, in carpets or outdoors, often bite humans before colonizing their preferred host. Because C felis is not highly cold-tolerant, it has been postulated that it is surviving in cold climates in the urban environment, as adults on untreated dogs and cats or on small wild mammals, such as opossums and raccoons.[1,2] Because these animals pass through yards in the spring, or establish nesting sites in crawl spaces or attics, eggs drop off and develop into adults. Cat fleas may also survive the winter, as pre-emerged adults in microenvironments that are protected from the cold.[1,2]

Once on a host, C felis initiates feeding within seconds to minutes.[16] In one study, approximately 25% of fleas were blood-fed within 5 minutes, and in another, the volume of blood consumed by fleas was quantifiable within 5 minutes.[17,18] Mating occurs on the host after feeding and can occur within 8 to 24 hours.[16] Female cat fleas begin egg production within 24 to 36 hours of their first blood meal.[19] They lay eggs within the pelage of the host, but because the eggs are not sticky, they drop out of the hair into the surrounding premises. Ctenocephalides felis is a highly fecund organism, with the female reaching peak egg production at 40 to 50 eggs per day and producing approximately 1300 eggs during the first 50 days on a host. Ctenocephalides felis can continue to produce eggs at a gradually declining rate for more than 100 days.[19] To produce such a large quantity of eggs, female cat fleas consume an average of 13.6 μL of blood per day, which is equivalent to 15.15 times their body weight.[16] While feeding, female cat fleas excrete large quantities of incompletely digested blood, which dries within minutes into reddish-black fecal pellets or tubular coils that are often called "flea dirt" or "frass." Flea feces can often be found matted into the pelage.

Actively feeding and reproducing C felis adults are fairly permanent ectoparasites. When normal grooming activity of cats was restricted, an average of 85% of female and 58% of male fleas were still present on cats after 50 days.[19] When fleas that have been on a host for several days are removed, they die within 1 to 4 days.[15] Although cat fleas rarely leave their host voluntarily, the host's grooming activity plays a significant role in their survival and longevity on that host. When cats are allowed to groom freely, they will ingest or groom off a substantial number of fleas in a few days.[10,20] When cat fleas were allowed to feed for only 12 hours and then removed from their host, 5% were still alive at 14 days.[15] This is of particular importance, because one study showed that when cats were housed adjacent to each other but physically separated, 3% to 8% of the fleas moved from one cat to another. However, when cats were housed in the same cage, 2% to 15% of the fleas transferred. Therefore, it is possible for a few adult fleas to transfer from one host to another.[21] However, it is far more likely that most flea infestations originate from previously unfed fleas emerging from environments that have supported development of immature life stages.

TICK OVERVIEW

There are two primary tick families, Argasidae (soft ticks) and Ixodidae (hard ticks). In North America, the ticks of most importance to dogs, cats, and their owners are the Ixodidae or hard ticks. Hard ticks are characterized by a hardened dorsal shield (scutum) and a head (capitulum) that extend in front of the body. Many species also have eye spots on the scutum and posterior indentations called festoons that can be used to aid in identification. Additionally, the Ixodidae commonly found on dogs and cats in North America are all three-host ticks, feeding once on a different host after molting in each motile stage (larva, nymph, and adult).[22,23]

Most ticks in motile life stages that infest dogs and cats use an ambush technique called questing, although *Ixodes spp* may use ambush and hunter tactics.[23] Ticks do not jump onto hosts or drop out of trees. Ticks that use the ambush strategy climb onto weeds, grasses, bushes, or other leafy vegetation, extend their forelegs that contain a sensory apparatus called the Haller organ, and wait for passing hosts to brush against the vegetation. When the host brushes against the plant, the tick immediately releases the vegetation and crawls onto the host.

Mating by ticks in the genera *Amblyomma, Dermacentor,* and *Rhipicephalus* occurs on the host after feeding. Certain species of *Ixodes* often mate off the host before feeding, but may mate while on the host.[24] During the first 24 to 36 hours following attachment to the host, little or no ingestion of blood takes place.[25] During this period, ticks use their chelicerae to cut the epidermis and insert their hypostome, which contains backward directed spines. Following insertion of the hypostome, many ticks reinforce their attachment by secreting a cementlike substance from their salivary glands.[23,26] Once the feeding site is established, the tick begins the second slow feeding phase, which lasts for several days. The slow feeding phase is followed by a rapid feeding phase. During the rapid feeding phase, which occurs 12 to 36 hours before detachment, the mated female tick may increase dramatically in size, often reaching 100 times her unfed body weight.[25,26]

TICKS SPECIES INFESTING DOGS AND CATS

The tick species that most commonly infest dogs and cats in North America are *Amblyomma americanum* (Lone Star tick), *Amblyomma maculatum* (Gulf Coast tick), *Dermacentor occidentalis* (Pacific Coast tick), *Dermacentor variabilis* (American dog tick), *Dermacentor andersoni* (Rocky Mountain wood tick) *Ixodes pacificus* (western black-legged tick), *Ixodes scapularis* (black-legged tick), *Otobius megnini* (spinose ear tick) and *Rhipicephalus sanguineus* (brown dog tick).[22,23]

Amblyomma *spp*

Amblyomma americanum (Lone Star tick) is named for the characteristic and easily recognizable single white spot that occurs on the dorsal shield of the female (**Fig. 3**). The males are also ornate but have several white to yellow lines on the edge of their scutum instead of the single white spot (see **Fig. 3**). *Amblyomma americanum* have long palpi, a long hypostome, eye spots, and festoons.

The range of *A americanum* seems to be increasing across the southern plains and Midwestern and eastern states. It was once considered to occur primarily in the south, with southern New Jersey being its northernmost range; its geographic range has since expanded.[27] Focal populations now occur in many northern states, including Connecticut, Maine, Massachusetts, Michigan, New Jersey, and New York.[27,28] The range of distribution extends south into Florida, west to Texas, and north through eastern Oklahoma and Kansas to Michigan.[27]

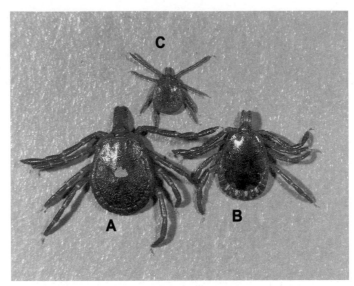

Fig. 3. Female (A), male (B), and nymph (C) of *A americanum* ("Lone Star tick").

Several factors have contributed to the increased range of *A americanum*, including increased habitat and wide host range that includes deer, small mammals, birds, and humans.[27,29] This tick occurs most commonly in woodland habitats with dense underbrush. Substantial reforestation over the last century, in urban and rural habitats, has provided increased areas of habitat for white-tailed deer and for survival and expansion of *A americanum*.[27,29] The white-tailed deer is considered a preferred host for *A americanum*, and all life stages will feed on white-tailed deer.[27,29]

It is well recognized that before and in the early-to-middle part of the nineteenth century, white-tailed deer were numerous and widespread throughout North America. Throughout the nineteenth century, unregulated hunting, loss of natural predators, and extensive loss of habitat decimated deer populations.[27,29] By the beginning of the twentieth century, only an estimated 300,000 to 500,000 deer remained in North America.[31] During the early and middle part of the twentieth century, restrictions were placed on deer hunting, numerous states began restocking efforts, and combined with an increase in natural habitat, there was a marked resurgence in deer populations to an estimated 18 million by 1992.[29] As deer expanded their range and increased their numbers, there was a corresponding increase in the tick species that are closely associated with deer.

White-tailed deer populations are so important to the long-term survival of *A americanum* that exclusion of deer has a profound effect on its populations. In one study, exclusion of deer from a 71-ha forest over a 4-year period resulted in reductions of 88%, 53%, and 51% of the larvae, nymphs, and adults, respectively, as compared with control plots.[30]

Another excellent host for larvae and nymphs that uses similar habitats is the wild turkey.[27,31] Areas with a deciduous forest canopy and high populations of white-tailed deer and wild turkey can have remarkably large populations of *A americanum*. Many other animals can be parasitized by this aggressive tick. Immature stages can be found on various ground-dwelling birds and numerous mammals such as red fox, rabbits, squirrels, raccoons, dogs, cats, coyotes, deer, and humans.[22,27] Adult

A americanum also feeds on various hosts, including cats, cattle, coyotes, deer, dogs, horses, sheep, raccoons, and humans.[22,27]

As *A americanum* populations expand into new areas, seasonality of ticks found on dogs and cats can change. Nymphs are found from March to September, larvae are frequently encountered in the late summer into the fall, and adults are often encountered from late February to early June.[27,31] Because all life stages can parasitize dogs and cats, *A americanum* could be encountered on pets, 8 to 9 months out of the year. Once hosts are acquired, larvae and nymphs engorge over a period of 3 to 9 days, and adults typically engorge within 9 days, but may take up to 2 weeks to do so.[27,31] As with most ticks, peak seasonal activity can vary widely by geographic region.

Similar to other ixodid ticks, unfed adults may survive for prolonged periods (>400 days) if hosts are not available. In temperate climates, the life cycle often takes 2 years to complete, whereas in warmer coastal climates, it can be completed within 1 year.[32]

A americanum is considered a major vector of animal and human pathogens, including *Ehrlichia chaffeensis* (causing human monocytic ehrlichiosis) and *Ehrlichia ewingii*.[27] The Lone Star tick can also transmit *Borrelia lonestari*.[33] It has also been implicated in the transmission of *Francisella tularensis* (causing tularemia).[34] The Lone Star tick has also recently been demonstrated to be a competent vector of *Cytauxzoon felis*, the highly pathogenic and usually fatal protozoan parasite of cats.[35]

Another *Amblyomma* species that parasitizes dogs is the Gulf Coast tick, *A maculatum* (**Fig. 4**). *Amblyomma maculatum* is a three-host tick with larvae and nymphs feeding on small rodents and ground dwelling birds, such as quail, meadow larks, and cattle egrets. Adults primarily parasitize the ears of large mammals, such as cattle, but they will also feed on horses, pig, goats, dogs, bear, birds, bobcats, coyotes, rabbits, raccoons, deer, and humans.[36] Once considered to be restricted within a 100-mile strip along the Gulf and Atlantic Coasts, *A maculatum* is now recognized to extend further inland, particularly in the Central United States, with expansion into Oklahoma and eastern Kansas.[37–39] *A maculatum* transmits *Hepatozoon americanum*, the etiologic agent of American canine hepatozoonosis. The transmission of this disease is unique, in that dogs must ingest the tick to become infected.[40] *Amblyomma maculatum* also has been documented to cause tick paralysis.[22]

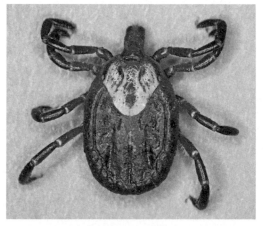

Fig. 4. Adult female *A maculatum* ("Gulf Coast tick").

Dermacentor *spp*

Dermacentor variabilis is an ornate Ixodidae. The scutum, which covers the entire dorsal surface of the male and the anterior one-third of the unengorged female, is covered with white markings. It also has festoons on the posterior abdomen, eye spots, and short palpi (**Fig. 5**).

Dermacentor sp ticks are one of the most widespread and common ticks, infesting dogs and cats in North America. *Dermacentor variabilis* (American dog tick) occurs in the eastern United States from Florida to southern New England and from the Atlantic Coast to the eastern sections of the Plains States.[41] Populations also occur along the Pacific Coast. This tick commonly occurs in grassy meadows, young forests, and along roadways and trails.[41]

The seasonal tick activity of *D variabilis* is similar across its wide geographic range, but variations in peak activity do occur. In the northern areas of the United States and Canada, adults are active from April to August, with a single period of peak activity in May to June.[41] In Kentucky, adults became active in early-to-mid–April followed by two periods of peak activity, one from mid-to-late–May and another in July.[42]

Larvae of *D variabilis* feed on small rodents, such as voles and mice. In the southern United States, larvae, hatching from eggs that are laid during the early summer, can undergo two distinct periods of host seeking. Some larvae may seek hosts in late summer, but others will enter diapause in the fall. These larvae will not seek hosts until early February and will continue this activity for 2 to 3 months.[41] Once attached, larvae can take from 3 to 12 days to engorge, averaging 4 days typically.[41]

Questing activity of nymphs quickly follows larval activity during the spring and early summer, as soil temperatures warm.[41] Common hosts for nymphs include cats, dogs, opossums, rabbits, raccoons, and other medium-to-small sized mammals. Similar to larvae, nymphs feed for only a few days and require from 3 to 11 days to engorge.[41]

Adults may seek hosts that same summer after molting but often overwinter and begin questing the following spring.[41] Common hosts for adult *D variabilis* include cats, dogs, cattle, horses, and other large mammals, including humans. Similar to males in the genera *Amblyomma* and *Rhipicephalus*, males in the genus *Dermacentor* feed sparingly and do not engorge. Female *D variabilis* are typical of many ixodid ticks,

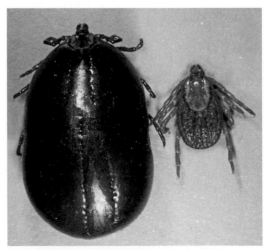

Fig. 5. Engorged (*left*) and nonengorged females of *D variabilis* ("American dog tick").

in that they engorge markedly on blood and often increase more than 100 times in size. Fully engorged *D variabilis* females drop from their hosts within 4 to 10 days and deposit between 4000 to 6500 eggs.[42] The life cycle can be completed in 3 months in the southern United States, but it may take up to 2 years in more northern climates. Similar to other ixodid ticks, unfed adults can survive for protracted periods without feeding. Adult *D variabilis* can live more than 2 years without feeding if hosts are not available.[41] An adult tick found on a dog may have originated from eggs laid 2 to 4 years previously, because it can survive the various stages for prolonged periods, awaiting appropriate hosts on which to feed, and because it often takes 2 years to complete development from egg to adult.

Dermacentor andersoni is found in at least 14 western US states and in south-western Canada.[43,44] In the United States, populations extend from western Nebraska and the Dakotas to Washington and Oregon, south through the eastern counties of California, then east through northern Arizona and New Mexico.[43] The life cycle of this three-host tick often takes 2 to 3 years. Similar to *D variabilis,* the larvae and nymphs of *D andersoni* feed on small mammals for 3 to 5 days. Adult *D andersoni* parasitize large mammals including horses, cattle, dogs, sheep, deer, bears, coyotes, and humans.[43] Adults usually occur from March to June, but are most numerous in April.[43,44] This tick can also survive for prolonged periods without feeding, with larvae and nymphs surviving for more than a year without a host, and adults, for more than 2 years.[43] It is similar in appearance to *D variabilis*, but adults of *D andersoni* have larger goblets on the spiracular plates than *D variabilis*.

Another *Dermacentor* species that is also regionally important is *D occidentalis* (Pacific Coast tick). It is widely distributed in the state of California, except for the very dry regions of the central valley and the southeast. The only other areas from which it has been collected are southwest Oregon and Baja, Mexico.[45,46] It is a three-host tick, commonly feeding on rodents, rabbits, and squirrels in the immature stages, and on cattle, dogs, horses, deer, and humans as adults.[46]

Dermacentor sp ticks are important vectors of disease. *Dermacentor variabilis* has been implicated in the transmission of cytauxzoonosis (*Cytauxzoon felis*).[47] *Dermacentor variabilis* and *D andersoni* are the primary vectors of Rocky Mountain spotted fever (etiologic agent, *Rickettsia rickettsii*) to dogs and humans.[23] In North America, both species are most commonly associated with tick paralysis. They can also transmit *Francisella tularensis*.[35]

Ixodes *sp*

Ixodes scapularis, the black-legged tick, (deer tick or Lyme disease tick) is an inornate tick without eyes or festoons. Larvae are small and often difficult to see. They are about 0.5 mm long, flat, six-legged, and nearly translucent.[48] Nymphs are approximately 1 mm long and darker. Unfed males are approximately 2 mm long and unfed females, about 2.5 mm.[48] There are considerable morphologic differences between male and female *Ixodes* (**Fig. 6**). Males are dark brown, almost black, with shorter palps than females. Females have longer mouthparts and appear two-toned. In the unengorged female, the inornate dorsal shield covers the anterior one-third of the body, leaving the orange-brown posterior portion of the body exposed.

Ixodes scapularis is widely distributed in the eastern and central United States in at least 35 states.[48,49] Its distribution is from Florida to Maine, west into far eastern South Dakota, and south through eastern Kansas into central Texas.[48,49] *Ixodes scapularis is* also located in central and eastern Canada.[50]

Similar to *A americanum,* the distribution of *I scapularis* correlates to the distribution and abundance of white-tailed deer.[48,51] Exclusion of deer dramatically decreases

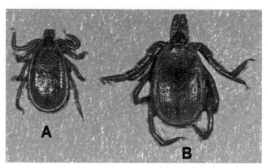

Fig. 6. Male (A) and female (B) of *I scapularis* ("eastern black-legged tick"; "deer tick").

I scapularis populations.[52] On Mohegan island, off the coast of Maine, annual fall flagging for ticks produced an average of 6 to 17 adult *I scapularis* per hectare, and up to 18 larvae per rat.[52] During an approximate 2.5-year period, all the deer were removed from the island. Within 4 years of deer removal, no immature ticks were found on rats and only 0.67 adult ticks per hectare were found during flagging of vegetation.[52]

Although white-tailed deer are widely distributed across the central and eastern United States, the abundance of *I scapularis* is not always directly related to the abundance of deer populations. Tick populations can vary markedly across a region due to soil type, moisture, and forest cover.[53,54] In the north central United States, *I scapularis* was found to be more numerous in areas with a deciduous forest canopy and where soil textures were classified as sandy or loam-sand.[53]

Seasonal activity varies by geographic region, but larval activity is generally highest in August and September. Larvae attach to and feed on various small mammals, including mice, chipmunks, and shrews. Larvae also feed on birds and lizards.[50] The white-footed mouse (*Peromyscus leucopus*) is of particular importance in tick life cycle and disease transmission, because it serves as a good host for larval *I scapularis* and it is a major reservoir of *Borrelia burgdorferi*.[50,55]

Immature ticks engorge typically for 2 to 4 days before dropping off to molt in moist protected areas, such as under leaf litter in forested habitats.[56] Larvae overwinter and then molt to nymphs in the spring. Nymphs will feed for 3 to 4 days on various hosts, including mice, squirrels, chipmunks, raccoons, opossums, skunks, shrews, cats, birds, and humans.[48,49,51] Nymphs occur primarily from May through July in the north and January through September in the south.[48,56] Adults occur most commonly from October to December. Adults that do not find a host will quest again, typically from March to May.[51] Adults feed for 5 to 7 days, primarily on white-tailed deer, but also on bobcats, cattle, coyotes, dogs, foxes, horses, humans, opossums, raccoons, and other mammals.[48,55]

Ixodes scapularis is the vector of *B burgdorferi* (causing Lyme disease) in the central, upper Midwestern, and northeastern United States; it is also the vector of *Anaplasma phagocytophilum* (causing human granulocytic ehrlichiosis), and *Babesia microti* (causing human babesiosis).[23] *Ixodes scapularis* may also cause tick paralysis.

The western black-legged tick, *I pacificus,* is morphologically similar to *I scapularis.* It is the vector for *B burgdorferi* and *A phagocytophilum* in the western United States.[55] Populations of *I pacificus* are distributed from Mexico to British Columbia, with localized populations in Utah and Arizona.[46,49,57,58] It is found primarily in leaf litter, under deciduous trees, and it favors cooler, moister coastal climatic conditions. Larvae and nymphs feed on various animals, including lizards, small rodents, squirrels, rabbits, cougars, black-tailed deer, ground nesting birds, and humans.[59,60] The primary hosts for larvae and nymphs are the western fence lizard *(Sceloporus occidentalis)* and the southern alligator lizard *(Elgaria multicarinata)*. Adults are also found on a various hosts, including deer, elk, black bear, bobcats, dogs, cats, coyotes, cougars, horses, cattle, and humans.[60]

Nymphs, typically, are present and active by mid-March, peak by early May, and are absent by late July to mid-August.[59] Adult ticks are found most often, from October to June (winter/spring), during the period of the year when humidity is usually high.

Rhipicephalus *sp*

Rhipicephalus sanguineus (brown dog tick) is reddish brown and inornate (**Fig. 7**). The basis capitulum is hexagonal and eyes and festoons are present. Tick species are often restricted in their distribution because of evolutionary adaptation to specific hosts and ecological factors. However, because dogs are the primary host for *R sanguineus,* they are widely distributed in tropical and temperate regions, wherever dogs are found. *Rhipicephalus sanguineus* seems to be well adapted to dogs as their natural host. Consequently, dogs do not develop resistance to *R sanguineus* infestations.[61] Although dogs are the primary host, immature life stages can be found on rodents and other small mammals. Rarely, adults can be found on other mammals, such as cats and humans.[61]

Most ixodid ticks develop outdoors. *Rhipicephalus sanguineus*, an exception, is commonly found in indoor environments. It is the only tick that infests human dwellings and kennels in North America. Although it seems to be cold-intolerant, *R sanguineus* can withstand areas of low humidity, and it persists in temperate regions by inhabiting kennels and homes.[61] These ticks often crawl up walls and can be found above artificial ceilings.[1,60]

Adult ticks can be found throughout the hair coat, but they are most commonly located in the ears or between the toes of dogs. Adults ticks feed for 5 to 21 days.[61] After engorgement, adult females drop off and deposit up to 4000 eggs. The eggs are often deposited in cracks and crevices along floors, behind dog cages, or even in ceilings.[61] Eggs can hatch within 20 to 30 days. Although preferring dogs, immature ticks will also feed on rodents and rabbits.[23] Larvae and nymphs feed over a period of 3 to 11 days, and they are commonly distributed along the back and neck of dogs.[61] As with many hard ticks, ticks in unfed stages can survive for prolonged

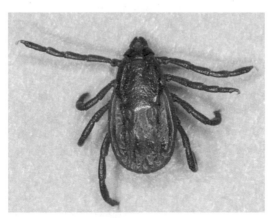

Fig. 7. Male *R sanguineus* ("brown dog tick").

periods in the environment. Unfed larvae, nymphs, and adults can survive for up to 8, 6 and 19 months, respectively.[61] The life cycle may be completed in as little as 63 to 91 days. This results in a rapid increase in tick populations, and it can make infestations of homes or kennels extremely difficult to eradicate.[61]

Previously attached *R sanguineus* has been shown to transfer from one dog to another.[62] In cohoused dogs, ticks, previously attached to one dog, emigrated to other dogs. This was particularly evident in males, when female ticks were no longer present.[62] This movement of ticks between hosts has major potential implications for intrastadial (within life cycle stage) disease transmission. *Rhipicephalus sanguineus* is the vector of numerous important pathogens, including *Ehrlichia canis* (causing canine monocytic ehrlichiosis) and *Babesia canis* (causing canine babesiosis).[23] It may also transmit *Anaplasma* (formerly *Ehrlichia*) *platys* and *Babesia gibsoni*.[63,64] Recently, in the southwestern United States, *R sanguineus* was identified as a vector for *R rickettsii*, the etiologic agent of Rocky Mountain spotted fever.[65]

Otobius *sp*

Otobius megnini (spinose ear tick) is the only soft tick (Argasidae) that is an important ectoparasite of dogs and cats in North America. It has no dorsal shield and the capitulum is positioned under the body (**Fig. 8**). *O megnini* is unusual, with only the larvae and nymphs being parasites. Larvae, which resemble small shriveled grapes, infest the ears of livestock and occasionally, dogs and cats.[66,67] Larvae feed for 6 to 9 days before molting to the first stage nymph on the host.[66,67] First stage nymphs stay in the ear and feed for 8 to 9 days. They molt to second stage nymphs and feed for an additional 10 to 12 days.[67] Both nymphal stages have a spiny cuticle from which the tick derives its name. Engorged nymphs drop from the host and crawl into cracks and crevices, under stones, or under tree bark, where they develop to adults. Development from larva to adult requires 62 to 107 days.[67] Adults do not feed, and mating occurs in the environment. Several hundred to more than 1000

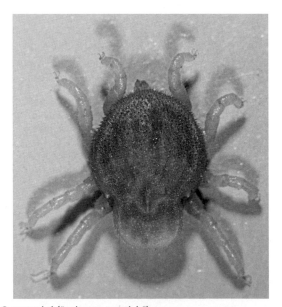

Fig. 8. Nymph of *O megnini* ("spinose ear tick").

eggs are deposited into the environment over a few weeks.[67] Larvae and nymphs feed on numerous mammals, including cats, cattle, coyotes, deer, dogs, goats, horses, humans, mules, rabbits, and sheep (including bighorn sheep).[67] In North America, the spinose ear tick is generally found in drier areas of the western and southwestern United States, but it also occurs in Hawaii and British Columbia.[67,68] It can easily be transported to other areas, while in the ear canals of dogs, cats, and livestock. *O megnini* has been implicated in the transmission of *Coxiella burnetii* (causing Q fever).[69]

CONTROL OF FLEAS AND TICKS

Control of fleas and ticks on companion animals and in the environment can be challenging.[1,2,70–72] Strategies for successful elimination of fleas from pets and their environments will differ in some respects from measures used for successful tick control. Each will be addressed separately and will be followed by a discussion of the available agents commonly used for flea or tick control. These agents are summarized in **Table 1**.

Flea Control

Successful control of pet flea infestations usually involves a combination of strategies.[70,73,74] These include host-targeted and environmental insecticides and mechanical means of reducing or eliminating environmental flea stages. Mechanical means of environmental control include washing of pet bedding or bed cloths frequented by pets. Vacuuming of carpets, furniture cushions, rugs, or other substrata, with a vacuum machine containing a "beater bar," will remove many of the flea eggs and larvae. In addition, cocooned pupae at the upper levels of the carpet can also be affected. The vibration also stimulates adult fleas to emerge from their cocoons so that they can be collected in the vacuum machine. Therefore frequent vacuuming, during a flea infestation, can reduce the overall flea burden in the home. It should be ensured that vacuum bags are disposed of properly, to prevent recolonization of the home with flea stages previously removed by vacuuming. Because outdoor development of immature flea life stages is limited to shaded areas, altering outdoor environments to eliminate such habitats can effectively reduce flea populations. Because urban wildlife, such as opossums, raccoons, and foxes, are good hosts for cat fleas, pet owners should avoid encouraging visitations by wildlife, which will affect flea and tick control (see later discussion). Treatment of indoor and outdoor environments with insecticides requires knowledge of what to use and where to use it. For this reason, it is suggested that pet owners consult with a licensed pest control specialist for such applications.

Numerous safe and effective host-targeted flea-control agents are available. Available agents include topical (imidacloprid, dinotefuran, fipronil, metaflumizone, selamectin) and oral (spinosad, nitenpyram) adulticides (see **Table 1**). Some single entity or combination flea products are also effective against ticks. Because topical products reside in the superficial layers of the skin, their residual efficacy can be affected by excessive water immersion and shampooing.[74] However, available research suggests that topical products have substantial residual activity, if wetting or bathing is not practiced in excess. Certain descaling and follicle-flushing shampoos are more likely to affect residual flea control than are simple detergent (grooming) shampoos. Orally administered flea-control products remain unaffected by wetting and bathing; however, these products have activity against fleas only (see **Table 1**). Some flea-control formulations also combine adulticides with insect growth regulators

Table 1
Summary of selected flea and tick control products

Active Ingredients (Product Name)	Target Animal (Minimum Age)	Formulations[a]	Parasite Claims														
			C Felis Adult	C Felis Eggs	Ticks Unspecified	A Americanum	A Maculatum	D Variabilis	I Scapularis	R Sanguineus	Cheyletiella Yasguri	Otodectes Cynotis	Sarcoptes Scabiei	Chewing Lice	Biting Flies	Mosquitoes	Gnats
Amitraz (Preventic Tick Collar)	Dog (12 Wk)	9% amitraz collar			■												
Dinotefuran, pyriproxyfen, permethrin (Vectra 3D)	Dog (7 Wk)	4.95% Dinotefuran, 36.8% permethrin, 0.44% pyriproxyfen topical spot-on	■	■[b]		■	■	■	■	■				■[b]	■[b]	■	
Dinotefuran, pyriproxyfen (Vectra for Cats)	Cat (8 Wk)	22% dinotefuran, 0.44% pyriproxyfen topical spot-on	■	■[b]													
Fipronil, (S)-methoprene (Frontline Plus)	Dog, cat (8 Wk)	9.8% fipronil, 11.8% (C) or 8.8% (D) (S)-methoprene topical spot-on	■	■	■	■		■	■	■			■D	■			
Fipronil (Frontline Top Spot, Frontline Spray)	Dog, cat (8 Wk)	9.7% fipronil topical spot-on; 0.29% fipronil spray	■	■	■	■		■	■	■			■D	■			
Imidacloprid (Advantage)	Dog, cat (7 Wk [D]; 8 Wk [C])	9.1% imidacloprid topical spot-on	■											■D			

Drug	Species (Min. Age)	Formulation								
Imidacloprid, permethrin	Dog (7 Wk)	8.8% imidacloprid, 44.0% permethrin topical spot-on	■		■	■	■		■	■
Imidacloprid, moxidectin (Advantage Multi)	Dog, cat (7 Wk, 3 lbs [D]; 9 Wk, 2 lbs [C])	10% Imidacloprid, 2.5% moxidectin [dog], 1% moxidectin [cat] topical spot-on (w/v)	■		■	■	■	■C		
Lufenuron (Program, Sentinel)	Dog, cat (4 Wk, 6 Wk [injectable])	46, 115, 230, or 460 mg per tablet (dog), 90, 204 mg per tablet (cat), 135, 270 mg suspension (cat), 0.4 mL, 0.8 mL injectable syringes (cat)	■							
Metaflumizone, amitraz (Promeris for dogs)c	Dog (8 Wk)	14.34% metaflumizone, 14.34% amitraz topical spot-on	■		■	■	■			■
Metaflumizone (Promeris for cats)	Cat (8 Wk)	18.53% metaflumizone topical spot-on	■							

(continued on next page)

Table 1
(continued)

Active Ingredients (Product Name)	Target Animal (Minimum Age)	Formulations[a]	C Felis Adult	C Felis Eggs	Ticks Unspecified	A Americanum	A Maculatum	D Variabilis	I Scapularis	R Sanguineus	Cheyletiella Yasguri	Otodectes Cynotis	Sarcoptes Scabiei	Chewing Lice	Biting Flies	Mosquitoes	Gnats
Nitenpyram (Capstar)	Dog, cat (4 Wk, 2 lbs)	11.4 and 57 mg tablets	■														
Permethrin (Proticall)	Dog (4 Wk)	65% permethrin topical spot-on	■			■		■	■	■	■			■		■	
Permethrin, pyriproxyfen (Virbac Long Acting Knockout Spray)	Dog (6 months)	2% permethrin, 0.05% pyriproxyfen spray	■	■	■												
Pyrethrins (Virbac Pyrethrin Dip)	Dog, cat (12 Wk)	1% pyrethrin dip	■		■									■	■	■	■
Selamectin (Revolution)	Dog, cat (6 Wk [D], 8 Wk [C])	6% (C) or 12% (D) spot-on; tubes contain 15, 30, 45, 60, 12 or 240 mg of selamectin (w/v)	■	■				D				■	D				
Spinosad (Comfortis)	Dog (14 Wk)	140, 270, 560, 810, 1620 mg per tablet	■														

See specific product inserts for dosage regimens and other details of product use. Certain products also prevent heartworm infection and treat or control certain gastrointestinal parasites in dogs or cats.

Abbreviations: C, cat; D, dog; w/v, weight/volume; w/w, weight/weight.

[a] All percentage concentrations are w/w unless specified as w/v.
[b] Also labeled for control of flea larvae and pupae and sand flies, sucking lice, and mites that cause dandruff and scale.
[c] Also labeled for control of *Demodex* spp.

(IGRs) (eg, methoprene, pyriproxyfen) or insect development inhibitors (IDIs) (eg, lufenuron).

Several product properties should be considered when designing a flea-control program and selecting flea-control agents. Among them are speed of action, duration and spectrum of activity, route of administration, and systemic versus topical action of the product.[73] These properties may be important if the pet suffers from flea allergy dermatitis (FAD), if owner compliance (including capability to administer the product) is inconsistent, if pet wetting or bathing is excessive, or if treatment or control of other parasites is necessary or desirable. Speed of action can be important if limited flea feeding is desirable, as in severely flea-allergic pets, or if fleas are biting pet owners. Once flea control is initiated, even if aggressive environmental flea control is a component, immature flea life stages will continue to develop, and fleas are still likely to emerge at some level. Therefore, a continuing flea problem should be expected for several weeks after treatment has begun. This necessitates an understanding of the cause of the problem and the persistence to see it through.

As mentioned previously, FAD is probably the most common allergic canine skin disease in certain regions of the United States.[75] It is caused by an atypical and exaggerated immune response to antigens present in flea saliva. At present, at least 15 potentially immunogenic (allergenic) components have been described. These are complete antigens and not haptens. Dogs with FAD can present with several types of hypersensitivity: Type I (immediate) hypersensitivity; Type IV delayed hypersensitivity; and cutaneous basophil hypersensitivity (CBH). Type I hypersensitivity is a humoral response that occurs in a few minutes. It is triggered by immunoglobulin E (reaginic antibody) binding to mast cells, resulting in the release of inflammatory mediators, such as histamine, serotonin, and leukotrienes. Type IV reactions are cell-mediated and involve interactions of T lymphocytes. Release of numerous lymphokines results in the release of pruritogenic inflammatory mediators. CBH is a transient delayed-type reaction in which basophils comprise the principal cell population. Type I and Type IV reactions (particularly Type I) are the reaction basics sought in intradermal skin tests for flea allergy.

Flea bite dermatitis (FBD), the typical reactions to irritation caused by flea bites, and FAD are two distinctly different conditions. Some think that all cases of FBD involve some degree of allergy. In the experience of the authors, nonallergic dogs usually present with fleas and demonstrate few signs of typical FAD. Normally, they have mild skin irritation, acute moist dermatitis ("hot spots"), or acral lick granulomas. Often between 3 and 5 years of age, allergic dogs present with crusted papules with erythema and/or alopecia, lichenification, or hyperpigmentation, usually on the dorsal lumbosacral area, caudomedial thighs, or ventral abdomen. In many cases, atopic dogs also suffer concurrently from FAD. In true cases of FAD, the ears, feet, and face are usually devoid of lesions. Dogs with FBD and FAD are frequently infected with *Dipylidium* tapeworms. FAD in dogs must be differentiated from food and atopic allergies; other parasitic dermatoses, such as lice and *Cheyletiella*; dermatophytosis; demodicosis; and superficial pyoderma. Dogs that are intermittently exposed to fleas are more likely to develop FAD than dogs that are chronically exposed to fleas. Consequently, if a dog is treated irregularly or flea control is discontinued until fleas reappear, the intermittent nature of this flea challenge is more likely to result in the development of FAD. The authors have observed this in their colonies of cats that are used as propagation subjects for fleas. The cats are infested weekly with fleas. Because cats tend to remove many fleas from the hair coat during grooming, the authors are, in essence, pulsing them with fleas at weekly intervals. This has lead to the frequent development of FAD in their colonies. When severe FAD exists, persistent or fast-acting host-directed agents, combined with aggressive environmental control measures, are usually necessary to control fleas and maintain pets below their responsive allergic threshold

Tick Control

Control of ticks also involves targeting pet animals and addressing the pet's environment. The former is more difficult for ticks than for fleas, because most ticks of veterinary importance use many hosts other than dogs or cats to complete their life cycle (the exception is *R sanguineus*). Reducing exposure to ticks by being informed about predominant species in the local area and avoiding periods when most ticks are active may also reduce the pet and pet owner's risks of exposure.

Numerous studies support the efficacy of host-targeted tick control products.[76–81] Year-round use of these products is justified because of the various tick species that may infest companion animals, and because ticks are more likely than fleas to be active in colder months or to emerge and quest for hosts during warm-weather breaks. The authors are often asked about proper mechanical methods of removing attached ticks from dogs or cats. Although several tick detachment devices are available, the authors recommend the slow deliberate removal of ticks, with a single slow-motion application of steady pressure, while grasping the ticks as close to the skin at the attachment site as possible.[82] Twisting or crushing the tick should be avoided, because this may result in either failure to remove the intact mouthparts or expulsion of tick gut contents into the host. Leaving mouth parts in the host can result in inflammatory swellings at the site of attachment. Inflammation, due to residual tick mouthparts in the host, is more severe for species that have longer mouthparts, such as *Amblyomma* and *Ixodes*. Expulsion of tick gut contents may further increase the potential for introducing infectious agents. Topical application of fingernail polish, alcohol, petroleum jelly, or any other moiety to attached ticks is ineffective and imprudent. Likewise the use of direct heat (ie, cigarettes or lighters) should be avoided for obvious reasons.

In cases where more aggressive tick control strategies are needed, host-targeted tick control products can be administered in combination, or the frequency of application can be increased. Another option is to move pets to the next product weight range, if the pet's weight is within 10% of the higher weight range. Any or all of these recommendations may be a violation of product label claims.

Environmental control of fleas and ticks usually involves destroying refuge areas of animals that may serve as alternative hosts.[70] It is important to eliminate piles of yard waste such as grass, weeds, and brush, particularly if they are near buildings or kennels that house pets. Although controlled burning of tick habitats, such as grasslands or forest canopies, can provide brief respites from tick infestation, these procedures can be dangerous and unpopular with environmentalists. Brown dog ticks require aggressive kennel- and domicile-control because all stages can use dogs as a suitable hosts. Successful strategies for brown dog tick control include appropriate use of environmental acaricides (ie, synthetic pyrethroids) behind, under, and around cages and in cracks and crevices in floors, walls, and ceiling. Including the ceilings is particularly important because brown dog ticks are inclined to climb upwards in indoor environments. As discussed for fleas earlier, application of environmental tick control products should be performed by professional pest control specialists. It is also prudent to limit access to crawl spaces under homes, decks, and outbuildings, to discourage visits by wildlife. Product properties or issues to be considered when designing regimens for successful tick control include numbers and species of ticks in the pet's environment, expected level of exposure to ticks, prevalence and spectrum of tick-borne diseases, and severity of reactions to tick bites. Several published studies suggest that available tick control products can aid in the prevention of transmission of vector-borne diseases.[83–89]

FLEA AND TICK CONTROL AGENTS
Carbamates, Organophosphates, Organochlorines, Pyrethrins, Pyrethroids, and Others

These traditional flea and tick control agents have largely given way to newer agents that are discussed in the following sections. Although they remain as active ingredients in some ethical and over-the-counter target animal products and also in many environmental products, they are no longer used for flea and tick control with the frequency that they once were. One exception is permethrin, which remains a component of several newer products. Permethrin will be discussed later with tick control strategies.

Imidacloprid

Imidacloprid is a member of the nitroguanidine subclass of neonicotinoid insecticides[90] (see **Table 1**). These agents were so named because they are related to nicotine in structure and function. Imidacloprid and other neonicotinoids act specifically on insect nicotinic acetylcholine receptors, resulting in rapid inhibition of insect nervous system function.[91] The neonicotinoids can be used safely in dogs and cats because of unique and important structural differences between mammalian and insect acetylcholine receptors. Imidacloprid targets adult fleas, although skin scales, hair, and debris that are shed from treated animals were shown to be larvicidal, when coming into contact with these stages in the pet's environment.[91]

Another strength of imidacloprid is that it can be administered as frequently as once-weekly.[91] This is particularly helpful for animals with severe flea-associated dermatitis.

Dinotefuran

Dinotefuran is a new third generation member of the neonicotinoid class of insecticides. Other members of this class include imidacloprid and nitenpyram. Imidacloprid and nitenpyram bear some resemblance to the nicotine molecule in being chlorinated compounds that share the aromatic pyridine ring of nicotine. Dinotefuran is a non-chlorinated, nonaromatic compound, more similar in structure to acetylcholine than to nicotine.[92] It binds poorly to the insect acetylcholine receptor, suggesting that it possesses a novel site of action. Dinotefuran is available as the single ingredient for adult flea control in cats and is combined with permethrin for adult flea and tick control in dogs. In dog and cat products, dinotefuran is combined with pyriproxyfen to expand its flea activity to include eggs, larvae, and pupae (see **Table 1**).

Nitenpyram

Nitenpyram is a nitroenamine compound. It is chemically similar to imidacloprid, but it differs in formulation, being administered orally rather than topically at a minimum target dose of 1 mg/kg.[91] Nitenpyram is marketed as a rapid flea removal adulticide.[93] Nitenpyram is rapidly eliminated following oral administration. Peak blood levels are achieved in approximately 1 hour. Nitenpyram is eliminated from dogs, mostly by urinary excretion, within 24 hours. Complete elimination requires a bit more time in the cat, with activity for up to 48 hours (see **Table 1**).

Fipronil

Fipronil is a phenylpyrazole insecticide/acaricide currently marketed as a 0.29% alcohol-based spray, and as a 9.7% solution for spot-on administration to dogs and cats. The more popular spot-on product combines fipronil and methoprene (see later discussion) for additional control of flea egg and larvae stages.[94] The mechanism of action of fipronil probably involves fipronil and its principal metabolite, fipronil sulfone.[91] Both molecules act on gamma-aminobutyric acid (GABA)- and gluta-mate-gated chloride ion channels that are located in the insect nervous system. Gluta-mate-gated channels have only been observed in invertebrates. Binding of fipronil and fipronil sulfone to GABA receptor sites is much reduced in mammals compared with insects. The target dosage for the fipronil spray formulation is 3 mL/lb (one to two pumps of formulated product per pound). The spot-on is administered at a minimum target dosage of approximately 7.5 mg/kg (see **Table 1**).

Selamectin

Selamectin is a semi-synthetic avermectin compound, derived from doramectin.[95] It is marketed as a isopropanol/dipropylene glycol monomethyl ether-based topical liquid (6% or 12% active) for spot-on application to dogs and cats. Selamectin is the first broad spectrum, single entity endectocide (effective against endo- and ectoparasites) available in a topical formulation for small animals. Selamectin is positioned principally as a topical heartworm preventive and flea-control agent for use in dogs and cats at a minimum target dose of 6 mg/kg.[96] Claims in the dog, in addition to controlling heart-worm and fleas (including flea eggs), include controlling *Sarcoptes scabiei*, *Otodectes cynotis*, and *Dermacentor variabilis*. Claims in the cat, again in addition to controlling heartworm and fleas and flea eggs, include controlling *Otodectes cynotis*, intestinal roundworms (*Toxocara cati*) and hookworms (*Ancylostoma tubaeforme*) (see **Table 1**).

Spinosad

The spinosyns are natural products obtained by fermentation from the actinomycete *Saccharopolyspora spinosa*.[97] Several spinosyn products were recovered during the fermentation and purification process. Spinosyns A and D appeared to be the most active and were selected for further development (hence that name spinosad). Spino-sad binds to specific sites on insect nicotinic acetylcholine receptors that are different from sites targeted by other nicotinoids and neonicotinoids. Spinosad induces nervous system hyperexcitation in insects, resulting in paralysis. Spinosad also binds secondarily to GABA sites and, as such, may provide additional potentiation of nervous system dysfunction. Spinosad is absorbed quickly after oral administration and is known to exert its effects quickly.[97] Its action remains persistent for approxi-mately 1 month because of extensive plasma protein binding. Spinosad is adminis-tered orally with food, monthly, to dogs in five dose bands at a minimum target dose of 30 mg/kg (see **Table 1**).

Metaflumizone

Metaflumizone is a semicarbazone compound derived from the dihydropyrazole insecticides.[98] Metaflumizone exerts its effects by binding to voltage-dependent sodium channels in target insects. Metaflumizone is related to indoxacarb, an oxadia-zine sodium channel-blocking insecticide. Pyrazoline insecticides bind to tonic sensory receptors and pacemaker neurons, which are very sensitive, resulting in insect paralysis. Metaflumizone is the first compound with this unique mode of action to be used in the animal health market. Metaflumizone is marketed alone for cats and is combined with amitraz for flea and tick control in dogs. The minimum target dose of metaflumizone in the feline and canine formulations is 40 mg/kg (see **Table 1**).

Permethrin

Permethrin is a third-generation synthetic pyrethroid that exerts its effect, primarily by modulating gating kinetics of sodium channels in nerves.[91,99] This action results in either repetitive discharges or membrane depolarization and subsequent death of the target arthropod. Recent research also indicates that pyrethroid and permethrin insecticides suppress GABA and glutamate receptor-channel complexes and voltage-activated calcium channels.[97] Permethrin and other synthetic pyrethroids possess quick-kill and contact-repellency effects. Permethrin is the active ingredient in several tick control products (see **Table 1**).

Amitraz

Amitraz is a formamidine compound that exerts its lethal effects by inhibiting mixed function oxidases.[91] Although amitraz is known to inhibit monoamine oxidase, this effect seems to be less important than its effect on mixed function oxidases. Affected ticks show interesting behavioral changes, such as hyperactivity, leg waving, and detachment. These effects are thought to be due the effects of amitraz on octopaminergic G-coupled protein. Other amitraz-induced effects are reduced fecundity, inhibition of oviposition, and diminished egg hatchability. Amitraz has a broad spectrum of activity against various ticks and mites, but it possesses no significant activity against insects. Amitraz in an active ingredient in several tick control products for dogs (see **Table 1**).

IGRS OR IDIS

Lufenuron, methoprene, pyriproxyfen, and other IGRs or IDIs exert their effects on flea eggs, larvae, or pharate (early) pupae.[72,100–104] They do so by either interfering with the development of chitin or chitinous structures (lufenuron) or by disrupting the hormonal signals necessary for successful development or molting (methoprene, pyriproxyfen). These agents are either administered orally or by injection (lufenuron) or topically (pyriproxyfen, methoprene) and provide long-term (generally 30 days or more) ovicidal and larvicidal effects. Recent products that combine dinotefuran and pyriproxyfen also carry label claims against pharate (early) pupae. The strength of a combination of adulticide and IGRs or IDIs is that they are likely to decrease the time necessary to control flea infestations. This is particularly important in the case of heavy flea infestations or when pet owners are experiencing flea bites. Secondly, when used in combination with adulticidal compounds, the likelihood of developing resistance is diminished considerably, because the flea life cycle is being disrupted at different points and by entirely different mechanisms.

Vaccination Against Flea or Ticks

Vaccination strategies for control of fleas and ticks are based on the induction of antibodies (or other factors) that attack and destroy "concealed" or "hidden" gut antigens.[105–107] These strategies presume that moieties from the midgut of fleas and ticks are not revealed to the host during feeding and engorgement (thus "hidden" antigens). They are isolated, purified, and introduced into target animals, together with adjuvanting substances, to enhance contact with immune competent cells. Although some success has been achieved using these strategies for ticks of production animals[106] and fleas of companion animals,[107] the achieved levels of efficacy, thus far, are not likely to be satisfactory to veterinarians and pet owners. To the best of the authors' knowledge, the availability of commercial tick vaccines to date has been limited to cattle ticks (*Boophilus microplus*), and they are available only in Australia and Cuba. Continued improvements in molecular methods of identification and isolation, and the delivery of putative immunogens, may eventually lead to the development and marketing of such vaccines in dogs and cats. The authors' opinion is that they are more likely to be useful as agents to prevent accumulations of environmental stages of fleas or ticks, given that their principal effects are to reduce engorgement (hence egg-laying) of the female arthropod. They also may be useful in reducing the transmission of arthropod-borne diseases, if the period of feeding and engorgement can be reduced sufficiently.

SUMMARY

Fleas (*C felis*) are important causes of primary disease (FBD) in dogs and cats. They may also cause allergic skin disease (FAD) and may serve as vectors of bacterial, rickettsial, viral, and parasitic diseases. Adult fleas on animals comprise just 5% of the total flea population. Understanding the life cycle of fleas and the habits of the adult and immature stages are important in successful prevention of flea-associated diseases. Modern host-targeted adulticides or adulticide-IGR combinations are highly effective in treating and preventing on-animal and environmental flea infestations. Ticks are also causes of primary irritation and are effective vectors for important diseases such as Lyme borreliosis, Rocky Mountain spotted fever, ehrlichiosis, anaplasmosis, babesiosis, cytauxzoonosis, and hepatozoonosis. Four genera (eight species) of hard ticks (family Ixodidae) are important ectoparasites in North America. Immature stages of a single soft tick (family Argasidae; *O megnini*) parasitize dogs and cats in North America. Hard ticks that infest dogs and cats are three-host ticks, so named because the different stages (larvae, nymphs, and adults) feed on different individual hosts. Immature ticks usually feed on small mammals (although they will feed on dogs, cats, and humans), birds, or reptiles. Adult ticks are more commonly found on larger mammals, including dogs, cats, and humans. The brown dog tick (*R sanguineus*) is uniquely important because it only requires dogs for completion of its life cycle. Consequently, it can be especially problematic in homes and kennels. Effective tick control is more difficult to achieve than effective flea control, because of the abundance of potential alternative hosts in the tick life cycle. Several effective host-targeted tick control agents are available, also possessing activity against adult or immature fleas and other parasites. Compliant use of host-targeted flea and tick control products, together with a knowledge of flea and tick life cycles, is necessary to control fleas and ticks on the animal, in the home, and in outdoor environments.

REFERENCES

1. Dryden M, Rust M. The cat flea: biology, ecology and control. Vet Parasitol 1994; 52:1–19.
2. Rust M, Dryden M. The biology, ecology and management of the cat flea. Annu Rev Entomol 1997;42:451–73.
3. Breitschwerdt EB. Feline bartonellosis and cat scratch disease. Vet Immunol Immunopathol 2008;123(1–2):167–71.
4. Kamrani A, Parreira VR, Greenwood J, et al. The prevalence of *Bartonella, hemoplasma*, and *Rickettsia felis* infections in domestic cats and in cat fleas in Ontario. Can J Vet Res 2008;72(5):411–9.

5. Woods JE, Brewer MM, Hawley JR, et al. Evaluation of experimental transmission of *Candidatus Mycoplasma haemominutum* and *Mycoplasma haemofelis* by *Ctenocephalides felis* to cats. Am J Vet Res 2005;66(6):1008–12.

6. Eisen RJ, Borchert JN, Holmes JL, et al. Early-phase transmission of *Yersinia pestis* by cat fleas (*Ctenocephalides felis*) and their potential role as vectors in a plague-endemic region of Uganda. Am J Trop Med Hyg 2008;78:949–56.

7. Lyons H. Notes on the Cat Flea, *Ctenocephalides felis* (Bouché). Psyche 1915; 22:124–32.

8. Silverman J, Rust MK, Reierson DA. Influence of temperature and humidity on survival and development of the cat flea, *Ctenocephalides felis* (Siphonaptera: Pulicidae). J Med Entomol 1981;18:78–83.

9. Thiemann T, Fielden LJ, Kelrick MI. Water uptake in the cat flea *Ctenocephalides felis* (Pulicidae: Siphonaptera). J Insect Physiol 2003;49(12):1085–92.

10. Hudson BW, Prince FM. A method for large scale rearing of the cat flea, Ctenocephalides felis felis (Bouché). Bull World Health Organ 1958;19:1126–9.

11. Silverman J, Rust MK. Some abiotic factors affecting the survival of the cat flea, *Ctenocephalides felis* (Siphonaptera: Pulicidae. Environ Entomol 1983;12: 490–5.

12. Silverman J, Rust MK. Extended longevity of the pre-emerged adult cat flea (Siphonaptera: Pulicidae) and factors stimulating emergence from the pupal cocoon. Ann Entomol Soc Am 1985;78:763–8.

13. Dryden M, Broce A. Development of a flea trap for collecting newly emerged *Ctenocephalides felis* (Siphonaptera: Pulicidae) in homes. J Med Entomol 1993;30:901–6.

14. Crum GE, Knapp FW, White GM. Response of the cat flea, *Ctenocephalides felis* (Bouché), and the oriental rat flea, *Xenopsylla cheopis* (Rothschild), to electromagnetic radiation in the 300–700 nanometer range. J Med Entomol 1974;11: 88–94.

15. Dryden MW. Evaluation of certain parameters in the bionomics of Ctenocephalides felis felis (Bouché 1835). M.S. Thesis, Purdue University, W. Lafayette, IN; 1988. p. 115.

16. Dryden M, Gaafar S. Blood consumption by the cat flea, *Ctenocephalides felis* felis (Siphonaptera: Pulicidae). J Med Entomol 1991;28(3):394–400.

17. Cadiergues MC, Hourcq P, Cantaloube B, et al. First bloodmeal of *Ctenocephalides felis felis* (Siphonaptera: Pulicidae) on cats: time to initiation and duration of feeding. J Med Entomol 2000;37(4):634–6.

18. McCoy C, Broce AB, Dryden MW. Flea blood feeding patterns in cats treated with oral nitenpyram and the topical insecticides imidacloprid, fipronil and selamectin. Vet Parasitol 2008;156(3–4):293–301.

19. Dryden MW. Host association, on-host longevity and egg production of *Ctenocephalides felis felis*. Vet Parasitol 1989;34:117–22.

20. Wade SE, Georgi JR. Survival and reproduction of artificially fed cat fleas, *Ctenocephalides felis* Bouché (Siphonaptera: Pulicidae). J Med Entomol 1988;25: 186–90.

21. Rust MK. Interhost movement of adult cat fleas (Siphonaptera: Pulicidae). J Med Entomol 1994;31(3):486–9.

22. Dryden MW, Payne PA. Biology and Control of ticks infesting dogs and cats in North America. Vet Ther 2004;26:2–16.

23. Sonenshine DE, Lane RS, Nicholson WL. Ticks (Ixodida). In: Mullen G, Durden L, editors. Medical and veterinary entomology. Amsterdam: Academic Press Elsevier Science; 2002. p. 517–58.

24. Kiszewski AE, Matuschka FR, Spielman A. Mating strategies and spermiogenesis in ixodid ticks. Annu Rev Entomol 2001;46:167–82.
25. Soneshine DE. The midgut. In: Sonenshine DE, editor, Biology of ticks, vol. 1. New York: Oxford University Press; 1991. p. 159–76.
26. Kaufman WR. Tick-host interaction: a synthesis of current concepts. Parasitol Today 1989;5:47–56.
27. Childs JE, Paddock CD. The ascendancy of *Amblyomma americanum* as a vector of pathogens affecting humans in the United States. Annu Rev Entomol 2003;48:307–37.
28. Merten HA, Durden LA. A state-by-state survey of ticks recorded from humans in the United States. J Vector Ecol 2000;25:102–13.
29. Paddock CD, Yabsley MJ. Ecological havoc, the rise of white-tailed deer, and the emergence of *Amblyomma americanum*-associated zoonoses in the United States. Curr Top Microbiol Immunol 2007;315:289–324.
30. Bloemer SR, Mount GA, Morris TA, et al. Management of lone star ticks (Acari: Ixodidae) in recreational areas with acaricide applications, vegetative management, and exclusion of white-tailed deer. J Med Entomol 1990;27(4):543–50.
31. Kollars TM, Oliver JH, Durden LA, et al. Host associations and seasonal activity of *Amblyomma americanum* (Acari: Ixodidae) in Missouri. J Parasitol 2000;86:1156–9.
32. Teel PD. Ticks. In: Williams RE, Hall RD, Broce AB, editors. Livestock entomology. New York: John Wiley & Sons; 1985. p. 129–50.
33. Bacon RM, Gilmore RD Jr, Quintana M, et al. DNA evidence of *Borrelia lonestari* in *Amblyomma americanum* (Acari: Ixodidae) in southeast Missouri. J Med Entomol 2003;40:590–2.
34. Soneshine DE. Tick-borne bacterial diseases. In: Sonenshine DE, editor, Biology of ticks, vol. 2. New York: Oxford University Press; 1993. p. 255–319.
35. Reichard MV, Meinkoth JH, Edwards AC, et al. Transmission of *Cytauxzoon felis* to a domestic cat by Amblyomma americanum. Vet Parasitol 2009, doi:10.1016/j.vetpar.2008.12.016.
36. Barker RW, Kocan AA, Ewing SA, et al. Occurrence of the Gulf Coast tick (Acari: Ixodidae) on wild and domestic mammals in north-central Oklahoma. J Med Entomol 2004;41(2):170–8.
37. Goddard J, Norment BR. Notes on the geographical distribution of the Gulf Coast tick, *Amblyomma maculatum* (Koch) [Acari: Ixodidae]. Entomol News 1983;94:103–4.
38. Semtner PJ, Hair JA. Distribution, seasonal abundance, and hosts of the Gulf Coast tick in Oklahoma. Ann Entomol Soc Am 1973;66:1264–8.
39. Broce AB, Dryden MW. Gulf Coast ticks make their presence known in Kansas. Vet Q 2005;8(2):2.
40. Ewing SA, Panciera RJ. American canine hepatozoonosis. Clin Microbiol Rev 2003;16:688–97.
41. Soneshine DE. Tick paralysis and other tick-borne toxicosis. In: Sonenshine DE, editor, Biology of ticks, vol. 2. New York: Oxford University Press; 1993. p. 320–30.
42. Burg JG. Seasonal activity and spatial distribution of host-seeking adults of the tick *Dermacentor variabilis*. Med Vet Entomol 2001;15(4):413–21.
43. James AM, Freier JE, Keirans JE, et al. Distribution, seasonality, and hosts of the Rocky Mountain wood tick in the United States. J Med Entomol 2006;43(1):17–24.
44. Eisen L. Seasonal pattern of host-seeking activity by the human-biting adult life stage of *Dermacentor andersoni* (Acari: Ixodidae). J Med Entomol 2007;44(2):359–66.

63. Sanogo YO, Davoust B, Inokuma H, et al. First evidence of *Anaplasma platys* in *Rhipicephalus sanguineus* (Acari: Ixodida) collected from dogs in Africa. Onderstepoort J Vet Res 2003;70(3):205–12.

64. Higuchi S, Kuroda H, Hoshi H, et al. Development of *Babesia gibsoni* in the midgut of the nymphal stage of the tick, *Rhipicephalus sanguineus*. J Vet Med Sci 1999;61(6):697–9.

65. Demma LJ, Eremeeva M, Nicholson WL, et al. An outbreak of Rocky Mountain Spotted Fever associated with a novel tick vector, *Rhipicephalus sanguineus*, in Arizona, 2004: preliminary report. Ann N Y Acad Sci 2006;1078:342–3.

66. Soulsby EJL. Arthropods in helminths, arthropods and protozoa of domestic animals. 7th edition. Philadelphia: Lea & Febiger; 1982. p. 357–504.

67. Jagannath MS, Lokesh YV. The life cycle of Otobius megnini (Acari: Argasidae). In: Progress in Acarology Volume 1: papers presented at the VII International Congress of Acarology held during August 3–9, 1986 at Bangalore. G.P. Channabasavanna, C.A. Viraktamath, Brill Archive; 1989. p. 91–4.

68. Rich GB. The Ear Tick, *Otobius megnini* (Duges). (Acarina: Argasidae), and its record in British Columbia. Can J Comp Med 1957;12:415–8.

69. Jellison WL, Bell EJ, Huebner RJ, et al. Q fever studies in Southern California. IV. Occurrence of *Coxiella burnetii* in the spinose ear tick, *Otobius megnini*. Public Health Rep 1958;63:1483–9.

70. Blagburn BL. Changing trends in ectoparasite control. In: Thoday K, Foil C, Bond R, editors. Advances in veterinary dermatology. Oxford: Blackwell Publishing; 2002. p. 59–68.

71. Blagburn BL, Lindsay DS. Ectoparasiticides. In: Richard Adams H, editor. Veterinary pharmacology and therapeutics. 8th edition. Ames, IA: Iowa State University Press; 2001. p. 1017–39.

72. Rust MK. Advances in the control of *Ctenocephalides felis* (cat flea) on cats and dogs. Trends Parasitol 2005;21(5):232–6.

73. Perrins N, Hendricks A. Recent advances in flea control. In Practice 2007;29:202–7.

74. Marsella R. Advances in flea control. Vet Clin North Am Small Anim Pract 1999; 29:1407–24.

75. Medleau L, Hnilica KA. Small animal dermatology: a color atlas and therapeutic guide. St. Louis (MO): Saunders; 2006. p. 526.

76. Endris RG, Hair JA, Anderson G, et al. Efficacy of two 65% permethrin spot-on formulations against induced infestation of *Ctenocephalides felis* (Insecta: Siphonaptera) and *Amblyomma americanum* (Acari: Ixodidae) on beagles. Vet Ther 2003;4:47–55.

77. Estrada-Pena A, Ascher F. Comparison of an amitraz-impregnated collar with topical administration of fipronil for prevention of experimental and natural infestations by the brown dog tick (*Rhipicephalus sanguineus*). J Am Vet Med Assoc 1999;214(12):1799–803.

78. Jernigan AD, McTier TL, Chieffo C, et al. Efficacy of selamectin against experimentally induced tick (*Rhipicephalus sanguineus* and *Dermacentor variabilis*) infestations on dogs. Vet Parasitol 2000;91:359–75.

79. Dryden MW, Payne P, McBride A, et al. D. Efficacy of fipronil (9.8% w/w)+(*S*)-methoprene (8.8% w/w) and imidacloprid (8.8% w/w)+permethrin (44% w/w) against *Dermacentor variabilis* (American dog tick) on dogs. Vet Ther 2008;9: 15–25.

80. Hellmann K, Adler K, Parker L, et al. Evaluation of the efficacy and safety of a novel formulation of metaflumizone plus amitraz in dogs naturally infested with fleas and ticks in Europe. Vet Parasitol 2007;150:239–45.

81. Hellmann K, Knoppe T, Krieger K, et al. European multicenter field trial on the efficacy and safety of a topical formulation of imidacloprid and permethrin (Advantix) in dogs naturally infested with ticks and/or fleas. Parasitol Res 2003;90(Suppl 3):S125–6.
82. Hendricks A, Perrins N. Recent advances in tick control. In Practice 2007;29: 284–7.
83. Elfassy OJ, Goodman FW, Levy SA, et al. Efficacy of an amitraz-impregnated collar in preventing transmission of Borrelia burgdorferi by adult Ixodes scapularis to dogs. J Am Vet Med Assoc 2001;219:185–9.
84. Hunter JS, McCall JW, Alva R, et al. The use of frontline spray treatment to prevent transmission of borrelia burgdorferi, the causative agent of lyme disease, from infected black-legged ticks, ixodes scapularis, to dogs. Proceedings of the Annual Meeting of the American Association Veterinary Parasitology 2002;42 [abstract].
85. Davoust B, Marie JL, Mercier S, et al. Assay of fipronil efficacy to prevent canine monocytic ehrlichiosis in endemic areas. Vet Parasitol 2003;112:91–100.
86. Spencer JA, Butler JM, Stafford KC, et al. Evaluation of permethrin and imidacloprid for prevention of Borrelia burgdorferi transmission from black-legged ticks (Ixodes scapularis) to Borrelia burgdorferi-free dogs. Parasitol Res 2003;90: S106–7.
87. Blagburn BL, Spencer JA, Billeter SA, et al. Use of imidacloprid-permethrin to prevent transmission of Anaplasma phagocytophilum from naturally infected Ixodes scapularis ticks to dogs. Vet Ther 2004;5:212–7.
88. Jacobsen R, McCall J, Hunter J, et al. The ability of fipronil to prevent transmission of Borrelia burgdorferi, the causative agent of Lyme Disease to dogs. International Journal of Applied Research in Veterinary Medicine 2004;2:39–45.
89. Blagburn BL, Spencer JA, Butler JM, et al. Prevention of transmission of Borrelia burgdorferi and Anaplasma phagocytophilum from ticks to dogs using imidacloprid/permethrin (K9 Advantix) and fipronil/(S)-methoprene (Frontline Plus) applied 25 days before exposure to infected ticks (Ixodes scapularis). Int J Appl Res Vet Med 2005;3:69–75.
90. Everett R, Cunningham J, Arther R et al: Comparative evaluation of the speed of kill of Advantage (Imidacloprid) and Revolution (Selamectin) on dogs. In: International flea control symposium, Compendium of Continuing Education for the Practicing Veterinarian 2000; (Suppl);22:9–14.
91. Page SW. Antiparasitic drugs. In: Maddison JE, Page SW, Church DB, editors. Small animal clinical pharmacology. 2nd edition. New York: Saunders; 2008. p. 198–260.
92. Matsuda K, Buckingham SD, Kleier D, et al. Neonicotinoids. insecticides acting on insect nicotinic acetycholine receptors. Trends Pharmacol Sci 2001;22(11):573–80.
93. Rust MK, Waggoner MM, Hinkle NC, et al. Efficacy and longevity of nitenpyram against adult cat fleas (Siphonaptera: Pulicidae). J Med Entomol 2003;40: 678–81.
94. Franc M, Beugnet M, Vermot S. Efficacy of fipronil-(S)-methoprene on flea, flea egg collection, and flea egg development following transplantation of gravid fleas onto cats. Vet Ther 2008;8:285–92.
95. Bishop BF, Bruce CI, Evans NA, et al. Selamectin: a novel broad-spectrum endectocide for dogs and cats. Vet Parasitol 2000;91:163–76.
96. Boy MG, Six RH, Thomas CA, et al. Efficacy and safety of selamectin against fleas and heartworms in dogs and cats presented as veterinary patients in North America. Vet Parasitol 2000;91:233–50.

97. Synder DE, Meyer J, Zimmerman AG, et al. Preliminary studies on the effectiveness on the novel pulicide, spinosad, for the treatment and control of fleas on dogs. Vet Parasitol 2007;150:345–51.
98. Salgado VL, Hayashi JH. Metaflumizone is a novel sodium channel blocker insecticide. Vet Parasitol 2007;150:182–9.
99. Blagburn BL. Permethrin, A Type I synthetic pyrethroid: history and properties. Comp Cont Ed Pract Vet 2003;25:7–10.
100. Blagburn BL. Advances in ectoparasite control: insect growth regulators and insect development inhibitors. Vet Med 1996;(Suppl):9–14.
101. Cadiergues MC, Steffan J, Tinembart O. Efficacy of an adulticide used alone or in combination with an insect growth regulator for flea infestations of dogs. Am J Vet Res 1999;60:1122–5.
102. Blagburn BL, Vaughan JL, Butler JM, et al. Dose titration of an injectable formulation of lufenuron in cats experimentally infested with fleas. Am J Vet Res 1999; 60:1513–5.
103. Jacobs DE, Hutchinson MJ, Ryan WG. Control of flea populations in a simulated home environment model using lufenuron, imidacloprid, or fipronil. Med Vet Entomol 2001;25:73–7.
104. Maynard L, Houffschmitt P, Lebreux B. Field efficacy of a 10% pyriproxyfen spot-on for the prevention of flea infestations on cats. J Small Anim Pract 2001;42:491–4.
105. Heath AW, Arfsten A, Yamanaki M, et al. Vaccination against the cat flea (*Ctenocephalides felis felis*). Parasite Immunol 1994;16:187–91.
106. Willadsen P, Jongejan F. Immunology of the tick-host interaction and the control of ticks and tick-borne diseases. Parasitol Today 1999;15:258–62.
107. Nisbet AJ, Huntley JF. Progress and opportunities in the development of vaccines against mites, fleas, and myiasis-causing flies of veterinary importance. Parasite Immunol 2006;28:165–72.

Index

Note: Page numbers of article titles are in **boldface** type.

A

Aberrant migration, heartworm and, 1148
Aelurostrongylosis
    canine, 1118–1119
    feline, 1116–1117
Aelurostrongylus spp.
    A. abstrusus, in cats, 1116–1117
    A. vasorum, in dogs, 1118–1119
Amblyomma spp., in dogs and cats, 1177–1179
American canine hepatozoonosis, **1035–1038.** See also *Hepatozoonosis, in dogs.*
American trypanosomiasis, **1055–1064.** See also *Chagas disease.*
Amitraz, in flea and tick control, 1186, 1193
Ancyclostoma spp., biology of, 1093–1094
    A. braziliense, 1094
    A. caninum, 1093–1094
    A. tubaeforme, 1094
Antigen testing, in heartworm diagnosis
    canine host, 1141
    feline host, 1150
Ascaridae, biology of, 1091–1093
Aspirin, for heartworm, 1144–1145

B

Babesia spp. See also *Babesiosis.*
    characteristics of, 1040–1043
        B. canis vogeli, 1042–1043
        B. conradae, 1041–1042
        B. gibsoni, 1040–1041
        North Carolina *B.* sp., 1043
    life cycle of, 1039–1040
    transmission of, 1039–1040
Babesiosis. See also *Babesia spp.*
    in dogs, **1039–1045**
        described, 1039
        diagnosis of, 1043–1044
        treatment of, 1044–1045
Blanchard, R.A.E., 995
Bronchitis, verminous nodular, canine, 1114

Vet Clin Small Anim 39 (2009) 1201–1211
doi:10.1016/S0195-5616(09)00157-0
0195-5616/09/$ – see front matter © 2009 Elsevier Inc. All rights reserved.

vetsmall.theclinics.com

45. Easton ER, Keirans JE, Gresbrink RA, et al. The distribution in Oregon of *Ixodes pacificus, Dermacentor andersoni*, and *Dermacentor occidentalis* with a note on *Dermacentor variabilis* (Acarina: Ixodidae). J Med Entomol 1977;13:501–6.

46. Furman DP, Loomis EC. The ticks of California (Acari: Ixodida). Bulletin of the California Insect Survey 1984;25:1–239.

47. Blouin EF, Kocan AA, Kocan KM, et al. Evidence of a limited schizogonous cycle for *Cytauxzoon felis* in bobcats following exposure to infected ticks. J Wildl Dis 1987;23:499–501.

48. Keirans JE, Hutcheson HJ, Durden LA, et al. *Ixodes* (Ixodes) *scapularis* (Acari:Ixodidae): redescription of all active stages, distribution, hosts, geographical variation, and medical and veterinary importance. J Med Entomol 1996;33: 297–318.

49. Dennis DT, Nekomoto TS, Victor JC, et al. Reported distribution of *Ixodes scapularis* and *Ixodes pacificus* (Acari: Ixodidae) in the United States. J Med Entomol 1998;35(5):629–38.

50. Ogden NH, St-Onge L, Barker IK, et al. Risk maps for range expansion of the Lyme disease vector, *Ixodes scapularis*, in Canada now and with climate change. Int J Health Geogr 2008;22:7–24.

51. Lane RS, Piesman J, Burgdorfer W. Lyme borreliosis: relation of its causative agent to its vectors and hosts in North America and Europe. Annu Rev Entomol 1991;36:587–609.

52. Rand PW, Lubelczyk C, Holman MS, et al. Abundance of *Ixodes scapularis* (Acari: Ixodidae) after the complete removal of deer from an isolated offshore island, endemic for Lyme Disease. J Med Entomol 2004; 41(4):779–84.

53. Guerra M, Walker E, Jones C, et al. Predicting the risk of Lyme disease: habitat suitability for *Ixodes scapularis* in the north central United States. Emerg Infect Dis 2002;8(3):289–97.

54. Bunnell JE, Price SD, Das A, et al. Geographic information systems and spatial analysis of adult *Ixodes scapularis* (Acari: Ixodidae) in the Middle Atlantic region of the U.S.A. J Med Entomol 2003;40(4):570–6.

55. Fritz CL, Kjemtrup AM. Lyme borreliosis. J Am Vet Med Assoc 2003;223: 1261–70.

56. Wilson ML, Spielman A. Seasonal activity of immature *Ixodes dammini* (Acari: Ixodidae). J Med Entomol 1985;22:408–14.

57. Olsen CA, Cupp EW, Luckhart S, et al. Occurrence of *Ixodes pacificus* (Parasitiformes: Ixodidae) in Arizona. J Med Entomol 1992;29:1060–2.

58. Doggett JS, Kohlhepp S, Gresbrink R, et al. Lyme disease in Oregon. J Clin Microbiol 2008;46(6):2115–8. Epub 2008 Apr 30.

59. Foley JE, Foley P, Brown RN, et al. Ecology of *Anaplasma phagocytophilum* and *Borrelia burgdorferi* in the western United States. J Vector Ecol 2004;29(1): 41–50.

60. Castro MB, Wright SA. Vertebrate hosts of *Ixodes pacificus* (Acari: Ixodidae) in California. J Vector Ecol 2007;32(1):140–9.

61. Dantas-Torres F. The brown dog tick, *Rhipicephalus sanguineus* (Latreille, 1806) (Acari: Ixodidae): from taxonomy to control. Vet Parasitol 2008; 152(3–4):173–85.

62. Little SE, Hostetler J, Kocan KM. Movement of *Rhipicephalus sanguineus* adults between co-housed dogs during active feeding. Vet Parasitol 2007;150(1–2): 139–45.

United States Postal Service

Statement of Ownership, Management, and Circulation
(All Periodicals Publications Except Requestor Publications)

1. Publication Title
Veterinary Clinics of North America: Small Animal Practice

2. Publication Number
0 0 3 - 1 5 0

3. Filing Date
9/15/09

4. Issue Frequency
Jan, Mar, May, Jul, Sep, Nov

5. Number of Issues Published Annually
6

6. Annual Subscription Price
$229.00

7. Complete Mailing Address of Known Office of Publication *(Not printer) (Street, city, county, state, and ZIP+4®)*

Elsevier Inc.
360 Park Avenue South
New York, NY 10010-1710

Contact Person
Stephen Bushing
Telephone *(Include area code)*
215-239-3688

8. Complete Mailing Address of Headquarters or General Business Office of Publisher *(Not printer)*

Elsevier Inc., 360 Park Avenue South, New York, NY 10010-1710

9. Full Names and Complete Mailing Addresses of Publisher, Editor, and Managing Editor *(Do not leave blank)*

Publisher *(Name and complete mailing address)*

John Schrefer, Elsevier, Inc., 1600 John F. Kennedy Blvd. Suite 1800, Philadelphia, PA 19103-2899

Editor *(Name and complete mailing address)*

John Vassallo, Elsevier, Inc., 1600 John F. Kennedy Blvd. Suite 1800, Philadelphia, PA 19103-2899

Managing Editor *(Name and complete mailing address)*

Catherine Bewick, Elsevier, Inc., 1600 John F. Kennedy Blvd. Suite 1800, Philadelphia, PA 19103-2899

10. Owner *(Do not leave blank. If the publication is owned by a corporation, give the name and address of the corporation immediately followed by the names and addresses of all stockholders owning or holding 1 percent or more of the total amount of stock. If not owned by a corporation, give the names and addresses of the individual owners. If owned by a partnership or other unincorporated firm, give its name and address as well as those of each individual owner. If the publication is published by a nonprofit organization, give its name and address.)*

Full Name	Complete Mailing Address
Wholly owned subsidiary of	4520 East-West Highway
Reed/Elsevier, US holdings	Bethesda, MD 20814

11. Known Bondholders, Mortgagees, and Other Security Holders Owning or Holding 1 Percent or More of Total Amount of Bonds, Mortgages, or Other Securities. If none, check box. ☐ None

Full Name	Complete Mailing Address
N/A	

12. Tax Status *(For completion by nonprofit organizations authorized to mail at nonprofit rates) (Check one)*
The purpose, function, and nonprofit status of this organization and the exempt status for federal income tax purposes:
☐ Has Not Changed During Preceding 12 Months
☐ Has Changed During Preceding 12 Months *(Publisher must submit explanation of change with this statement)*

13. Publication Title
Veterinary Clinics of North America: Small Animal Practice

14. Issue Date for Circulation Data Below
September 2009

15. Extent and Nature of Circulation

		Average No. Copies Each Issue During Preceding 12 Months	No. Copies of Single Issue Published Nearest to Filing Date
a. Total Number of Copies *(Net press run)*		3247	3100
b. Paid Circulation (By Mail and Outside the Mail)	(1) Mailed Outside-County Paid Subscriptions Stated on PS Form 3541. *(Include paid distribution above nominal rate, advertiser's proof copies, and exchange copies)*	1866	1805
	(2) Mailed In-County Paid Subscriptions Stated on PS Form 3541 *(Include paid distribution above nominal rate, advertiser's proof copies, and exchange copies)*		
	(3) Paid Distribution Outside the Mails Including Sales Through Dealers and Carriers, Street Vendors, Counter Sales, and Other Paid Distribution Outside USPS®	482	487
	(4) Paid Distribution by Other Classes Mailed Through the USPS (e.g. First-Class Mail®)		
c. Total Paid Distribution *(Sum of 15b (1), (2), (3), and (4))*		2348	2292
d. Free or Nominal Rate Distribution (By Mail and Outside the Mail)	(1) Free or Nominal Rate Outside-County Copies Included on PS Form 3541	133	99
	(2) Free or Nominal Rate In-County Copies Included on PS Form 3541		
	(3) Free or Nominal Rate Copies Mailed at Other Classes Through the USPS (e.g. First-Class Mail)		
	(4) Free or Nominal Rate Distribution Outside the Mail (Carriers or other means)		
e. Total Free or Nominal Rate Distribution *(Sum of 15d (1), (2), (3) and (4))*		133	99
f. Total Distribution *(Sum of 15c and 15e)*		2481	2391
g. Copies not Distributed *(See instructions to publishers #4 (page #3))*		766	709
h. Total *(Sum of 15f and g)*		3247	3100
i. Percent Paid *(15c divided by 15f times 100)*		94.64%	95.86%

16. Publication of Statement of Ownership

☐ If the publication is a general publication, publication of this statement is required. Will be printed in the **November 2009** issue of this publication. ☐ Publication not required

17. Signature and Title of Editor, Publisher, Business Manager, or Owner

Stephen R. Bushing

Stephen R. Bushing – Subscription Services Coordinator

Date: September 15, 2009

I certify that all information furnished on this form is true and complete. I understand that anyone who furnishes false or misleading information on this form or who omits material or information requested on the form may be subject to criminal sanctions (including fines and imprisonment) and/or civil sanctions (including civil penalties).

PS Form 3526, September 2007 (Page 1 of 3 (Instructions Page 3)) PSN 7530-01-000-9931 PRIVACY NOTICE: See our Privacy policy in www.usps.com

PS Form 3526, September 2007 (Page 2 of 3)

Moving?

Make sure your subscription moves with you!

To notify us of your new address, find your **Clinics Account Number** (located on your mailing label above your name), and contact customer service at:

Email: journalscustomerservice-usa@elsevier.com

800-654-2452 (subscribers in the U.S. & Canada)
314-447-8871 (subscribers outside of the U.S. & Canada)

Fax number: 314-447-8029

**Elsevier Health Sciences Division
Subscription Customer Service
3251 Riverport Lane
Maryland Heights, MO 63043**

*To ensure uninterrupted delivery of your subscription, please notify us at least 4 weeks in advance of move.

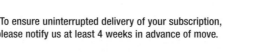
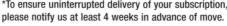